Innovative Teaching Strategies in Nursing and Related Health Professions

Fourth Edition

Martha J. Bradshaw, PhD, RN
Associate Dean and Professor
Louise Herrington School of Nursing
Baylor University
Dallas, Texas

Arlene J. Lowenstein, PhD, RN
Professor Emeritus
MGH Institute of Health Professions
Boston, Massachusetts

JONES AND BARTLETT PUBLISHERS
Sudbury, Massachusetts
BOSTON   TORONTO   LONDON   SINGAPORE

World Headquarters

Jones and Bartlett Publishers
40 Tall Pine Drive
Sudbury, MA 01776
978-443-5000
info@jbpub.com
www.jbpub.com

Jones and Bartlett Publishers
Canada
6339 Ormindale Way
Mississauga, Ontario L5V 1J2
Canada

Jones and Bartlett Publishers
International
Barb House, Barb Mews
London W6 7PA
United Kingdom

Jones and Bartlett's books and products are available through most bookstores and online booksellers. To contact Jones and Bartlett Publishers directly, call 800-832-0034, fax 978-443-8000, or visit our website www.jbpub.com.

Substantial discounts on bulk quantities of Jones and Bartlett's publications are available to corporations, professional associations, and other qualified organizations. For details and specific discount information, contact the special sales department at Jones and Bartlett via the above contact information or send an email to specialsales@jbpub.com.

The authors, editor, and publisher have made every effort to provide accurate information. However, they are not responsible for errors, omissions, or for any outcomes related to the use of the contents of this book and take no responsibility for the use of the products and procedures described. Treatments and side effects described in this book may not be applicable to all people; likewise, some people may require a dose or experience a side effect that is not described herein. Drugs and medical devices are discussed that may have limited availability controlled by the Food and Drug Administration (FDA) for use only in a research study or clinical trial. Research, clinical practice, and government regulations often change the accepted standard in this field. When consideration is being given to use of any drug in the clinical setting, the health care provider or reader is responsible for determining FDA status of the drug, reading the package insert, and reviewing prescribing information for the most up-to-date recommendations on dose, precautions, and contraindications, and determining the appropriate usage for the product. This is especially important in the case of drugs that are new or seldom used.

Production Credits
Executive Editor: Kevin Sullivan
Production Director: Amy Rose
Associate Editor: Amy Sibley
Production Editor: Carolyn F. Rogers
Senior Marketing Manager: Emily Ekle
Marketing Manager: Katrina Gosek
Cover Design: Kate Ternullo
Composition: Auburn Associates, Inc.
Printing and Binding: Malloy, Inc.
Cover Printing: Malloy, Inc.
Cover Image: © Todd Hackelder/Shutter Stock, Inc.

Library of Congress Cataloging-in-Publication Data
Innovative teaching strategies in nursing and related health professions
  / Martha Bradshaw, Arlene J. Lowenstein, editors. — 4th ed.
     p. ; cm.
  Rev. ed. of: Fuszard's innovative teaching strategies in nursing /
edited by Arlene J. Lowenstein, Martha J. Bradshaw. 3rd ed. 2001.
  Includes bibliographical references and index.
  ISBN-13: 978-0-7637-3856-3 (pbk. : alk. paper)
     1. Nursing—Study and teaching.   I. Bradshaw, Martha J.
  II. Lowenstein, Arlene J.   III. Fuszard's innovative teaching strategies
in nursing.
     [DNLM: 1. Education, Nursing. 2. Teaching—methods.   WY 18
  I589 2007]
  RT71.F84 2007
  610.73071—dc22
                                   2006021448

6048

ISBN-13: 978-0-7637-3856-3
ISBN-10: 0-7637-3856-5

Printed in the United States of America
10 09 08 07 06   10 9 8 7 6 5 4 3 2 1

Dedication

This book is dedicated in loving memory and honor of Dr. Barbara Fuszard, a professional educator, leader in nursing, a mentor to both faculty and students, and a caring nurse.

The early editions of this book were prepared by Dr. Fuszard, who was also a leader in nursing education. Upon her retirement, she graciously requested that we continue her work by serving as coeditors on the third edition. This fourth edition of the text will miss her, due to her unfortunate death. However, her presence is with us, and we have endeavored to continue the purposes that Barbara Fuszard envisioned with each edition.

Contents

Section V: Clinical Teaching

Section VI: Evaluation

Preface

In the multifaceted world of health care, nursing no longer stands alone in practice and in education. Interdisciplinary collaboration is critical. To provide more effective care, students from all healthcare professions should learn *about* and learn *from* each other. Each profession brings its own knowledge base and nature of practice to impact patient care outcomes. This edition reaches beyond nursing to capitalize on the contributions of numerous healthcare professionals to the educational process.

Regardless of the health profession to which we belong, those of us involved in student education are teachers first and foremost. Education has a knowledge base that crosses over the disciplinary lines and is one we need to understand in order to be effective in our work. This book incorporates educational principles and techniques suitable for students in all college settings, graduate or undergraduate levels. It is our intent that this book will be a useful resource for educational programs in all health professions.

Every chapter has been reviewed for content and timeliness and revised as needed. Some chapters have been broadened to address related concepts and an interdisciplinary focus. New features in this edition include recognition of student diversity, an expanded section on the use of technology, and additional chapters to reflect current clinical teaching and evaluation of the teaching–learning process.

Rapid changes in technology require that teachers recognize the valuable principles behind the use of specific technologies, rather than focusing on the technology itself. As an example, teachers at one time lectured with the use of overhead projectors and numerous sheets of plastic film. The technique for using the overhead called for clear large type and succinct statements on each slide. The principle involved is that the instructor provided statements that were easy for the reader to see, write down, and remember. These statements were part of a class outline upon which the instructor expanded during teaching and discussion. Presently, instruction is conducted in the same manner, but the overhead has been replaced with the computer and a PowerPoint presentation. The principle remains the same and the presentation, although now enhanced with animation, color, and other features, still requires the instructor to address effective student learning. As technology evolves, teachers can take advantage of new features while adhering to the principles for effective teaching.

Martha J. Bradshaw
Arlene J. Lowenstein

Contributors

Linda C. Andrist, PhD, RNC, WHNP
MGH Institute of Health Professions
Boston, MA

Kristina Gilden Bowen, RN, MSN
Mary Black School of Nursing
University of South Carolina, Upstate
Spartanburg, SC

Kathy P. Bradley, EdD, OTR/L,
    FAOTA
Department of Occupational
    Therapy Research
School of Allied Health Sciences
Medical College of Georgia
Augusta, GA

Martha J. Bradshaw, PhD, RN
Associate Dean and Professor
Louise Herrington School of Nursing
Baylor University
Dallas, TX

Patricia Christensen, PhD, RN

Patricia R. Cook, RN, PhD
Associate Professor
University of South Carolina, Aiken
Aiken, SC

Mariana D'Amico, EdD, OTR/L
Medical College of Georgia
Department of Occupational
    Therapy
Augusta, GA

Kathy Lee Dunham Hakala, MSN
Louise Herrington School of Nursing
Baylor University
Dallas, TX

Brian M. French, RN, MS, BC
Professional Development
    Coordinator
The Knight Nursing Center for
    Clinical and Professional
    Development
Massachusetts General Hospital
Boston, MA

Elizabeth Friedlander, PhD, APRN,
    BC
Clinical Assistant Professor
MGH Institute of Health Professions
Boston, MA

Clive Grainger
Science Education Department
Harvard-Smithsonian Center for
    Astrophysics
Cambridge, MA

Miriam Greenspan, RN, MS
Massachusetts General Hospital
Boston, MA

Alex Griswold, AB
Science Education Department
Harvard-Smithsonian Center for
    Astrophysics
Cambridge, MA

Jill M. Hayes, PhD, RN
Associate Professor & Assistant Dean
University of Texas Health Science
    Center at San Antonio
School of Nursing
San Antonio, TX

Lynn E. Jaffe, ScD, OTR/L
Associate Professor
Medical College of Georgia
Department of Occupational
    Therapy
Augusta, GA

Judy Johnson-Russell, EdD, RN
Texas Woman's University
College of Nursing
Dallas, TX

Charlotte James Koehler, MN,
    IBCLC, RN
Mary Black School of Nursing
University of South Carolina,
    Upstate
Spartanburg, SC

Ellen M. Landis, ADTR, LMFT, PhD
    Candidate in Expressive Arts
    Therapy
Clinical Director of Sharevision, Inc.,
    Family Counseling Center and
    Consulting Group
National Chair of the
    Hadassah–Women's Sports
    Foundation, GoGirlGo! Project
Faculty, Family Institute of
    Cambridge
Adjunct Faculty, Applied Psychology
    Department, Dance Therapy
    Division
Antioch New England Graduate
    School
Amherst, MA

Arlene J. Lowenstein, PhD, RN
Professor Emeritus
MGH Institute of Health Professions
Boston, MA

Alfred E. Lupien, PhD, CRNA
Interim Program Director
Nursing Anesthesia Program
School of Nursing
Medical College of Georgia
Augusta, GA

Jennifer Mackey, MA
Clinical Assistant Professor
Graduate Program in
 Communication Sciences and
 Disorders
MGH Institute of Health Professions
Boston, MA

Hendrika Maltby, PhD, RN, FRCNA
Associate Professor
College of Nursing and Health
 Sciences
University of Vermont
Burlington, VT

Lynn Minnick, RN, BA, MA, FNP,
 MSN
Clinical Assistant Professor
Arnold House
University of Massachusetts,
 Amherst
Amherst, MA

Marjorie Nicholas, PhD
Associate Professor
Graduate Program in
 Communication Sciences and
 Disorders
MGH Institute of Health Professions
Boston, MA

Hollie T. Noveletsky, PhD, RNCS

Jane A. Petrillo, EdD, C&I Health
 Promotion, MS
Associate Professor
Department of Health Physical
 Education and Sports Science
Kennesaw State University
Kennesaw, GA

Carol Picard, PhD, RN
Professor and Graduate Program
 Director
School of Nursing
University of Massachusetts,
 Amherst
Amherst, MA

Judith Schurr Salzer, RN, PhD, MBA,
 CPNP
Interim Associate Dean for Strategic
 Management
Medical College of Georgia
School of Nursing
Augusta, GA

Patricia Solomon, PhD, PT
Professor
McMaster University
Faculty of Health Sciences
School of Rehabilitation Science
Hamilton, Ontario, Canada

Deborah Tapler, PhD, RN
Texas Woman's University
College of Nursing
Dallas, TX

Karen H. Teeley, MS, RN, AHN-C
Clinical Assistant Professor
Simmons College
Boston, MA

Barbara C. Woodring, RN, EdD
Professor and Associate Dean,
 Undergraduate Studies
University of Alabama, Birmingham
Birmingham, AL

Richard C. Woodring, DMin, MDiv,
    BA, AA
Continuing Education Program
    Specialist
Division of Continuing Education
Medical College of Georgia
Augusta, GA

SECTION I

INTRODUCTION

Creating an effective learning environment is not an easy task in today's world, and it is even more complex in education programs for the health professions. Students entering the fields of health care are extremely diverse. Traditional undergraduates, entering college directly from high school, sit side by side with a vast variety of nontraditional students returning to school after experiences in the workplace and/or having completed previous college degrees. There is a wide range of ages and experience within the student body. Educators are challenged to recognize different learning needs and respect and utilize the knowledge and experiences that students bring to the learning settings. The teaching strategies and examples throughout this book may be adapted for use in a variety of situations, at undergraduate and graduate levels, taking into account the diversity of learning needs.

The chapters in Section I provide a foundation for understanding, selecting, and adapting specific teaching strategies to the educator's setting and student body. The contributors provide a theory base for learning and critical thinking and bring in various dimensions of effective learning that include creativity, humor, and exploration of diverse viewpoints and ways of processing information.

CHAPTER 1

Effective Learning: What Teachers Need to Know

Martha J. Bradshaw

"Knowing is a process, not a product."
Jerome Bruner (1966)

What brings about effective learning in nursing students? Is it insight on the part of the student? A powerful clinical experience? Perhaps it is the dynamic, creative manner in which the nurse educator presents information or structures the learning experience. Effective learning likely is the culmination of all of these factors, in addition to others. In this chapter, dimensions of effective learning will be explored as a foundation for use of the innovative teaching strategies presented in subsequent chapters.

THEORIES OF LEARNING

We approach learning individually, based largely on cognitive style (awareness of and taking in of relevant information) and preferred approaches to learning, or learning style. Some students are aware of their style and preference, some gain insight into these patterns as they become more sophisticated learners, and some students have never been guided to determine how they learn best.

Theoretical underpinnings classify learning as *behavioristic* or *cognitive*. Behavioristic learning was the earliest pattern identified through research. Psychologists such as Skinner and Thorndike described learning as a change in behavior and used stimulus response actions as an example. Subsequent theorists have described more complex forms of behaviorist learning. Bandura's (1977) theory of social learning describes human learning to come from others through observation, imitation, and reinforcement. We learn from society, and we learn to be social. This type of learning is evident when we describe the need to "socialize" students to the profession of nursing.

Robert Gagne (1968) formulated suggestions for sequencing of instruction, conditions by which learning takes place, and outcomes of learning, or categories in which human learning occurs. These learning categories are based on a hierarchical arrangement of learning theories, moving from simple to complex learning, and include intellectual and motor skills, verbal information, cognitive strategies, and attitudes. For example, within the category of intellectual skills are the following stages:

- *Discrimination learning*—distinguishing differences, in order to respond appropriately
- *Concept learning*—detecting similarities, in order to understand common characteristics
- *Rule learning*—combination of two or more concepts, as a basis for action in new situations

Gagne's ideas seem to combine behaviorism and cognitive theories. Use of behaviorism in nursing education was especially popular in the 1970s and early 1980s through the use of concrete, measurable, specific behavioral objectives. Even though nursing education has moved away from the concrete methods of learning and evaluation, use of the hierarchical arrangement is seen in curriculum development and learning outcomes.

Cognitive theories address the perceptual aspect of learning. Cognitive learning results in the development of perceptions and insight, also called *gestalt*, that brings about a change in thought patterns (causing one to think, "Aha") and related actions. Jerome Bruner (1966) described cognitive learning as processes of conceptualization and categorization. He contended that intellectual development includes awareness of one's own thinking, the ability to recognize and deal with several alternatives and sequences, and the ability to prioritize. Bruner also saw the benefit of discovery learning to bring about insights. Ausubel's (1968) assimilation theory focuses on meaningful learning, in which the individual develops a more complex cognitive structure by associating new meanings with old ones that already exist within the learner's frame of reference. Ausubel's theory relies heavily on the acquisition of previous knowledge. These principles are useful for introducing the new student to the health care environment by relating information to what the student knows about health and illness. The same principles are fundamental to curriculum development based upon transition from simple to complex situations.

Gardner's theory of multiple intelligences recognizes cognition as more than knowledge acquisition. Based on his definition of intelligence as "the ability to solve problems or fashion products that are valued in more than one setting" (Gardner & Hatch, 1990, p. 5), Gardner has described seven forms of intelligence:

1. *Linguistic*—related to written and spoken words and language, and use and meaning of language(s)

2. *Musical/rhythmic*—based on sensitivity to rhythm and beat, recognition of tonal patterns and pitch, and appreciation of musical expression
3. *Logical/mathematical*—related to inductive and deductive reasoning, abstractions, and discernment of numerical patterns
4. *Visual/spatial*—ability to visualize an object or to create internal (mental) images, thus able to transform or re-create
5. *Bodily kinesthetic*—the taking in and processing of knowledge through use of bodily sensations. Learning is accomplished through physical movement or use of body language
6. *Interpersonal*—emphasizes communication and interpersonal relationships, recognition of mood, temperament, and other behaviors
7. *Intrapersonal*—related to inner thought processes, such as reflection and metacognition, includes spiritual awareness and self-knowledge (Gardner & Hatch, 1990)

Cognitive theories that address learning stages appropriate for college students include Perry's (1970) model of intellectual and ethical development. This model recognizes four nonstatic stages in which students progress: (1) dualism (black vs. white), (2) multiplicity (diversity and tolerance), (3) relativism (decision made by reasoned support), and (4) commitment to relativism (recognition of value set for decision making). Perry's ideas can serve to explain how critical thinking is developed over time.

APPROACHES TO LEARNING

Emerging from learning theories are descriptions of preferred styles or approaches to learning. Categorized as *cognitive styles* and *learning styles*, these approaches to learning are the ways that individuals acquire knowledge, which are concerned more with form or process than content (Miller & Babcock, 1996). Cognitive style deals with information process, the natural, unconscious internal process concerned with thinking and memory. It is the consistent way in which individuals organize and handle information (DeYoung, 2003). The most common example of cognitive style is Witkin and colleagues' field dependent-field independent style (Witkin, Moore, Goodenough, & Cox, 1977). The field dependent-field independent style describes one's field of perception, or how one takes in information or data. Whereas one style generally predominates, people possess the capacity for both styles. Field-dependent individuals are more global, are open to external sources of information, are influenced by their surroundings, and therefore see the situation as a whole, rather than identifying and focusing on the separate aspects of it. Field-dependent people tend to be social, people-oriented, and sensitive to social cues. Learners in which the field-dependent style predominates may be externally motivated and therefore take a more spectator or passive role in the learning process, preferring to be taught rather than to actively participate. Field-independent individuals are less sensitive to the social environment and thus take on a more analytical approach to information. By identifying aspects of the situation separately, they are able to restructure information and to develop their own system of classification. Field-independent learners enjoy concepts, challenges, and hypotheses, and are task oriented (Miller & Babcock, 1996).

An aspect of learning style related to student behavior is *response style*. Kagan (1965) pioneered work, with school-age children, on the concepts of reflection and impulsiveness. These dimensions of cognitive response style describe personal tendencies regarding possibilities to solutions and choice selection. Individuals who have the impulsivity tendency prefer the quick, obvious answer, especially in highly uncertain problems, thus selecting the nearly correct answer as first choice. Reflective individuals identify and carefully consider alternatives before making a decision or choice. The implications for nursing education are apparent and will be discussed further. One problem that emerges with individuals who have a strong tendency in one of these dimensions is that the impulsive individual acts too quickly, based on an instant decision. On the other hand, the reflective individual may be immobilized in decision making, which has outcomes implications.

Reflection, as associated with learning, was described as early as 1916 by John Dewey as being a process of inquiry (Miller & Babcock, 1996). To reflect on a situation, experience, or collection of information is to absorb, consider, weigh, speculate, contemplate, and deliberate. Such reflection serves either as a basis for reasoned action or to gain understanding or attach meaning to an experience. The most notable descriptions of reflection, especially as related to nursing, have been presented by Schon (1983). In his work, Schon related reflection to problem solving. He pointed out that traditional means of teaching and learning result in structured problem solving where the ends are clear and fixed. In the reality of health care, such ends are not always so concrete.

Schon also believes that professionals in practice demonstrate a unique proficiency of thinking, and he has described three aspects of this thinking: (1) knowing-in-action (use of a personally constructed knowledge base), (2) reflection-in-action (conscious thinking about what one is doing, awareness of use of knowledge), and (3) reflection-on-action (a retrospective look at thoughts and actions, to conduct self-evaluation and make decisions for future events). Reflection results in synthesis. This outcome is evident when the individual carries over thoughts, feelings, and conclusions to other situations. Teaching includes reflection-in-action, in which the teacher spontaneously adapts to learner reactions. Thus, reflection is the foundation for growth through experience. Reflection, as a form of thinking and learning, can be cultivated. Educators improve their teaching when they reflect upon episodes of teaching that were successful, as well as those that were failures (Pinsky, Monson, & Irby, 1998).

One of the best known descriptions of learning styles is Kolb's, which emerged from Dewey's seminal theory on experiential learning (Kolb, 1984). Dewey pioneered educational thinking regarding the relationship between learning and experience. The relationship between the learning environment and personal factors such as motivation and goals can lead the learner through a stream of experiences that, once connected, bring about meaningful learning (Kelly and Young, 1996). Using these ideas, Kolb went on to describe learning as occurring in stages: concrete experiences, observation and reflection on the experience, conceptualization and generalization, then theoretical testing in new and more complex situations. Learning is cyclical, with new learning coming from new experiences. Consequently, learning occurs in a comprehensive means, beginning with performance (concrete experience) and ending with educational growth. Kolb further explained that individuals go about this learning along two basic dimensions: grasping experiences (prehension) with abstract-concrete poles and transforming, with action-reflection poles (Kelly & Young, 1996). Applying his experiential learning theory to his dimensions, Kolb identified four basic learning styles:

1. *Convergers*—prefer abstract conceptualization and active experimentation. These individuals are more detached and work better with objects than people. They are problem solvers and apply ideas in a practical manner.
2. *Divergers*—prefer concrete experience and reflective observation. Individuals with this tendency are good at generating ideas and displaying emotionalism and interest in others. Divergers are imaginative and can see the big picture.
3. *Assimilators*—prefer abstract conceptualization and reflective observation. Assimilators easily bring together diverse items into an integrated entity, sometimes overlooking practical aspects or input from others. Theoreticians likely are assimilators.
4. *Accommodators*—prefer concrete experience and active experimentation. These individuals, while intuitive, are risk takers and engage in trial-and-error problem solving. Accommodators are willing to carry out plans, and they like and adapt to new circumstances (Miller & Babcock, 1996).

Svinicki and Dixon (1987) report that average learning style scores for undergraduate nursing majors are predominantly in the converger category, with a tendency toward the accommodator category. Among nursing faculty, however, the average style is that of diverger. Implications for teaching-learning and professional development will be discussed further.

Gregorc's (1979) categorization of learning styles is similar to Kolb's, except that Gregorc believes that an individual's style is static, even in light of the changing educational setting. Thus, even through maturity and further learning, an individual still approaches learning in the same way. Gregorc uses the learning style categories of concrete sequential, concrete random, abstract sequential, and abstract random. In his research, Gregorc determined that individuals have preferences in one or two categories. In studying both first-year and fourth-year baccalaureate nursing students, Wells and Higgs (1990) discovered that these students have preferences in the concrete sequential and abstract random categories (total 81% of first-year students, 74% of fourth-year students).

USE OF LEARNING STYLES AND PREFERENCES: APPLICATION OF RESEARCH

Theoretical foundations regarding learning and descriptive studies of cognitive and learning styles provide insight and understanding of self. It would be difficult to address research on all modes of learning in this one chapter. A summary application of information from the vast field of knowledge about learning theory and cognitive and learning styles has been developed by Svinicki (1994) as six operating principles:

1. If information is to be learned, it must first be recognized.
2. During learning, learners act on information in ways that make it more meaningful.
3. Learners store information in long-term memory in an organized fashion related to their existing understanding of the world.
4. Learners continually check understanding, which results in refinement and revision of what is retained.
5. Transfer to new contexts is not automatic but results from exposure to multiple applications.
6. Learning is facilitated when learners are aware of their learning strategies and monitor their use (Svinicki, 1994, p. 275).

To understand one's own learning styles is to help understand one's own thinking, to be aware of a fit between style and strategies for learning, and thus to select the most effective and efficient means to go about learning. Some students are aware of how they learn best and gravitate toward that strategy. Instructors see this process in students who choose to sit in the front row of the class, take many notes, and feel involved with the topic, or students who choose to not come to class but instead read course material, watch videos, and acquire information as it pertains to a clinical assignment. Some students adhere to tradition-bound forms of learning, such as lecture and reading, yet do not maximize their learning. This result explains why these students benefit more from direct clinical experiences. Many students find learning to be more powerful when they experience something new or significant in a clinical environment, then explore information and reflect on the experience. Learning experiences can be adapted to the environment and are influenced by the environment in which they occur. Awareness and comprehension of one's style of learning enables one to tailor the learning environment for optimal outcomes. A simple test that will guide the student in discovering his or her learning style(s) is presented in the teaching example.

Feedback from an observer, such as the instructor, can heighten awareness of personal styles. The knowledgeable educator also can guide the student in enhancing predominant styles or in beginning to cultivate additional dimensions of thinking and responding. For example, a student who is predominantly impulsive in decision making should be guided to explore outcomes of decisions and encouraged to increase reflection time as appropriate. Conversely, the student who is highly reflective may need to explore reasons that bring about hesitancy or prolonged deliberation and the outcomes of such behaviors.

EFFECTIVE TEACHING FOR EFFECTIVE LEARNING

A knowledgeable and insightful educator is the key to effective learning in many situations. Consequently, the educator should call upon a knowledge base in learning and teaching as well as an extensive repertoire of useful strategies to reach learning goals. Faculty in health profession education are challenged to be directive in their teaching, addressing measurable learning outcomes that are directly linked to professional standards. This is juxtaposed with the importance of freeing the student from linear thinking and encouraging broader approaches to learning that are accomplished through dialogue, expression, and attribution of meaning. Romyn (2001) addresses this dilemma by pointing out the two approaches to teaching: behaviorist and emancipatory. Whereas the behaviorist teacher approaches the world from a measurement perspective and seeks a means to an end, the emancipatory teacher embraces a nonphenomenal view of learning and places greater value on the experience and an understanding of such. Most teachers will have strength in one of these two approaches, but should consider their teaching from the other as well, to enrich learning opportunities.

Regarding the teaching strategies presented in this book, each strategy will have different effects on the attainment of learning outcomes in each student, based on the attributes and use of the strategy, in addition to learning and cognitive styles and learning preferences. Here are some broad suggestions for applying information about learning in teaching situations. The specific strategies addressed in subsequent chapters provide detailed information that enable faculty to use each method in an optimal way.

Underlying assumptions regarding the nature of professional education are derived in part from principles on adult learning, as formulated by Knowles (1978). Key principles include assuming responsibility for one's own learning and recognition of meaning or usefulness of information to be learned. Students in health professions are career oriented and need to see practical value in their educational endeavors. As consumers, adult students need to believe that they are receiving the maximum benefit from learning experiences. Furthermore, taking charge of one's own learning is empowering. Students who gain a sense of self-responsibility can feel empowered in other areas of their lives, such as professional practice. Faculty, in turn, have the responsibility to cultivate empowerment and to affect learning outcomes.

The classroom environment should be fresh and challenging each time the class meets. Faculty should endeavor to provide variety in the manner in which they teach, rather than the same, predictable, albeit comfortable method of telling, rather than teaching. As providers of information, instructors need to remember that learning is best brought about by a combination of motivation and stimulation. The effective instructor should be the facilitator of learning in the students. In professional education, motivation is gained when the relationship to the well-being of the client is pointed out. The value of faculty experience is evident when the nurse-teacher shares from his or her own professional experiences and uses these anecdotes as examples for client outcomes. Nursing students and faculty agree that nontraditional strategies such as collaborative or cooperative learning, active involvement, and participation in the learning experience are desirable for effective learning. Because there is some disagreement regarding how much or often these strategies should be used indicates that both teacher and student are more comfortable with the traditional, teacher-dominated classroom (August, Hurtado, Wimsatt, & Dey, 2002).

Students in professional education programs do respond positively to opportunities to choose or structure some of their learning experiences (Melrose, 2004). This approach should be used frequently by the teacher, to not only promote active learning but to instill in students a sense of empowerment, which is an important attribute for the clinical setting. Technology-based learning activities direct the student to engage in independent learning, research, and use visual cues, such as video, to enhance comprehension.

Students are more likely to remember information with which they can agree or relate, and if they can attach meaning to the item or information (DeYoung, 2003). Disagreement or disharmony should be explored in an objective fashion. Viewpoints can then be strengthened or altered. Questioning and discussion should be based on the diversity that exists among the students. An instructor who is able to establish a sense of trust and confidence with the students can promote the expression of different perspectives likely to be found in the group. Professional educators should support students who are at various levels of cognitive growth, looking upon students from a criterion framework, rather than a normative one. Faculty should show that various viewpoints are welcome, legitimate, and worthy of discussion.

Effective educators guide students to see how their thought processes occur. They ask "what do you know about _____?" "How did you arrive at that answer/conclusion?" Teachers cultivate further development in the individual learners by demonstrating how to critique a theory, develop a rationale, or work through the steps of problem solving. These strategies will facilitate growth in students who are in an early cognitive stage such as dualism, or will challenge more advanced students to a commitment to realism (Perry, 1970).

Delivery of information should be based on instructional theory in addition to content expertise. Using Ausubel's (1968) principles of advanced organizer, the teacher can develop inductive discovery by which students can build on previously acquired, simplistic knowledge to develop new or broader concepts. This strategy operationalizes some of Svinicki and Dixon's (1987) cognitive principles.

Effective learning experiences that emerge from identified styles should be developed and used in both class and clinical settings. Information from Kolb's four dimensions serves as an excellent example. Students who are *convergers* readily become bored with straight lecture, especially with topics that are abstract in nature. These individuals work better by themselves, so they are less likely to participate well in group projects. Learners with the *diverger* style learn from case studies and will actively participate in discussion, but they may have difficulty detaching personal values from the issue. These students often are visionary group leaders. Individuals with the *assimilator* style manipulate ideas well, so they will participate well in discussion or write comprehensive papers; however, these students may be less practical and have difficulty with some of the realism of nursing practice. *Accommodators* usually enjoy case studies, new or unusual teaching strategies, skills lab, and tinkering with new equipment. These learners will be most responsive to a challenging, complex client. With the multitude of learning opportunities available through electronic resources and patient simulation, teachers can readily craft a learning experience that meets most learning styles and preferences. However, one-way learning, such as web-based instruction, will not fully replace competency-based instruction and verification that is needed in the applied disciplines of health care (Knapp, 2004).

In the clinical setting, the instructor may wish to provide introductory motivation through discovery learning. One way to accomplish this goal is to have each student observe or follow an individual in the clinical setting to gain exposure to the myriad tasks and responsibilities of a professional health care provider. Whereas students may have some rudimentary ideas of what health care providers do, they discover the depth and demands required in day-to-day work by observing actual practice. This strategy should broaden their perspectives and set the stage for meaningful learning, which includes increased retention of material and greater inquiry.

As students develop clinical written summaries about their clients, instructors should be flexible with the type of written work submitted. Traditionally, nursing students develop some form of a care plan based on the nursing process. The structured, linear method has taken criticism as the only way to look at clients. As a concrete, methodical strategy, the nursing process care plan is effective for students who are field independent and who can readily discern the data and related information needed for each step.

Additional methods of client summary or analysis should be introduced, and students should be encouraged to try each method. In doing so, students may broaden their ways of seeing clients and nursing problems, thus setting the stage for increased insight, analysis, and confidence. For example, use of the concept map is a way in which a student can envision the client or care situation in a holistic manner. Concept maps provide a fluidity that enhances the ability to determine relationships and make connections. Therefore, this strategy likely will be used positively by students who demonstrate Gardner's categories of visual/spatial or interpersonal intelligence. Learners who are field dependent also should do well with the concept map strategy because of their tendency to see the situation as a whole. Concept mapping should be effective for learners with all of Kolb's styles but for different reasons and with different outcomes.

Guided reflection, especially reflection-on-action, helps the student bring closure to the clinical experience, as well as conduct self-evaluation and gain from the experience. Journal writing is one of the most effective means by which the student can capture thoughts and responses and preserve these ideas in writing for subsequent consideration. This strategy is particularly useful as a means by which students can identify and modify impulsive-reflective tendencies. Journal writing will have the best results with divergers and assimilators, and some students may benefit from open discussion about the experiences entered into their journals. Again, feedback from the faculty is crucial and should be as thoughtful as the entries provided by the student. Faculty reading journals should guide the student in growth of insight and patterns of reflection.

Effective teachers in the health professions are those who possess content expertise, create an active learning environment, and use carefully selected teaching strategies (Wolf, Bender, Beitz, Wieland, & Vito, 2004). One of the greatest challenges for faculty is in developing the blend of strategies to bring about effective learning in all students. Part of the challenge is the fit between the faculty's styles and learning preferences and that of each of the learners. Faculty should become aware of their approaches to learning and how these approaches enhance or hinder the learning of others (Kelly & Young, 1996). Faculty especially should be on guard against favoritism to students who possess the same attributes as the instructor. Conversely, the congruency between styles of the teacher and of the student may enhance a relationship that is especially meaningful and may evolve into professional mentoring.

FUTURE CONSIDERATIONS

From this chapter, many ideas emerge that are worthy of more detailed scrutiny. The majority of research on cognitive styles, learning style, and learning preferences was conducted in the 1970s and 1980s. This was before the widespread accepted use of electronic technology. Use of technology in teaching and learning may be influenced by learning preferences, such as in visual and kinesthetic learners. Have some students learned to modify their preferences in order to become more comfortable with technology? Online education is widely accepted, but has not been embraced by all learners. The extent to which learners continue to value the presence of the instructor for spontaneous teaching is worthy of investigation. Currently, there is a shift in education toward student-centered, active learning for the development of critical thinking, coupled with emerging generations of students who are used to immediate feedback and a variety of stimulation. Educators must determine if selected strategies are useful for genuine learning, or if not used properly, merely providing entertainment.

CONCLUSION

Effective learning is more than merely the results of good teaching. It is enhanced by a learning environment that includes active interactions among faculty, students, and student peers. Effective learning is achieved through the use of creative strategies designed not to entertain but to inform and stimulate. The best ways faculty can bring about effective learning are by recognizing students as individuals, with unique, personal ways of knowing and learning, by creating learning situations that recognize diversity, and by providing empowering experiences in which students are challenged to think.

TEACHING EXAMPLE

How Do I Learn Best?

This instrument typically takes 4–6 minutes to complete and can be self-scored. The style categories are visual, aural, read/write, and kinesthetic, which correspond with categories found in Gardner's multiple forms of intelligence. Students are directed to answer the brief questions, then are shown the learning modalities that best fit predominant styles.

HOW DO I LEARN BEST?

This test is to find out something about your preferred learning method. Research on left brain/right brain differences and on learning and personality differences suggests that each person has preferred ways to receive and communicate information.

Choose the answer that best explains your preference and put the key letter in the box. If a single answer does not match your perception, please enter two or more choices in the box. Leave blank any question that does not apply. Once you have completed the test, find the totals for each of the letters (V, A, R, K) that correspond with a learning preference. Then look at the Table of Learning Modalities (Table 1-1) to see what strategies best support your learning preference.

1. You are about to give directions to a person. She is staying in a hotel in town and wants to visit your house. She has a rental car. Would you:
   V) draw a map on paper?
   R) write down the directions (without a map)?
   A) tell her the directions by phone?
   K) collect her from the hotel in your car?

2. You are staying in a hotel and have a rental car. You would like to visit a friend whose address/location you do not know. Would you like him to:
   V) draw you a map on paper?
   R) write down the directions (without a map)?
   A) tell you the directions by phone?
   K) collect you from the hotel in his car?

3. You have just received a copy of your itinerary for a world trip. This is of interest to a friend. Would you:
   A) call her immediately and tell her about it?
   R) send her a copy of the printed itinerary?
   V) show her the itinerary on a map of the world?

4. You are going to cook a dessert as a special treat for your family. Do you:
   K) cook something familiar without need for instructions?
   V) thumb through the cookbook looking for ideas from the pictures?
   R) refer to a specific cookbook where there is a good recipe?
   A) ask for advice from others?

5. A group of tourists has been assigned to you to find out about national parks. Would you:
   K) drive them to a national park?
   R) give them a book on national parks?
   V) show them slides and photographs?
   A) give them a talk on national parks?

6. You are about to purchase a new stereo. Other than price, what would most influence your decision?
   A) A friend talking about it.
   K) Listening to it.
   R) Reading the details about it.
   V) Its distinctive, upscale appearance.

7. Recall a time in your life when you learned how to do something like playing a new board game. Try to avoid choosing a very physical skill, e.g., riding a bike. How did you learn best? By:
   V) visual clues—pictures, diagrams, charts?
   A) listening to somebody explaining it?
   R) written instructions?
   K) doing it?

8. Which of these games do you prefer?
   V) Pictionary
   R) Scrabble
   K) Charades

9. You are about to learn to use a new program on a computer. Would you:
   K) ask a friend to show you?
   R) read the manual that comes with the program?
   A) telephone a friend and ask questions about it?

10. You are not sure whether a word should be spelled *dependent* or *dependant*. Do you:
    R) look it up in the dictionary?
    V) see the word in your mind and choose the best way it looks?
    A) sound it out in your mind?
    K) write both versions down?

11. Apart from price, what would most influence your decision to buy a particular textbook?
    K) Using a friend's copy.
    R) Skimming parts of it.
    A) A friend talking about it.
    V) It looks OK.

12. A new movie has arrived in town. What would most influence your decision to go or not go?
    A) Friends talked about it.
    R) You read a review about it.
    V) You saw a preview of it.

13. Do you prefer a lecturer/teacher who likes to use:
    R) handouts and/or a textbook?
    V) flow diagrams, charts, slides?
    K) field trips, labs, practical sessions?
    A) discussion, guest speakers?

Source: Gardner & Hatch, 1990.

Table 1-1 Learning Modality

	In class	When studying	For exams
Visual	Underline Use different colors Use symbols, charts, arrangements on a page	Recall visual aspects of presentation Reconstruct images in different ways Redraw pages from memory Replace words with symbols and initials	Recall the pictures on the pages Draw, use diagrams where appropriate Practice turning visuals back into words
Aural	Attend lectures and listen Discuss topics with students Use a tape recorder Discuss overheads, pictures, and other visual aids Leave space in notes for later recall	May take poor notes because of preference for voices Expand your notes by talking out ideas Explain new ideas to another student Read assignments out loud	Speak your answers/tutorials Practice writing answers to an old exam Read questions to self or have someone read them to you
Reading/ writing	Use lists, headings Write out lists and definitions Use handouts and textbooks	Write out the words Reread notes silently Rewrite ideas in other words Use lecture notes/read	Practice with multiple-choice questions Write paragraphs, beginnings, endings Organize diagrams into statements
Kinesthetic: use all your senses	May take notes poorly because topics do not seem relevant Go to lab, take field trips Use trial-and-error method Listen to real-life examples	Put examples in note summaries Talk about notes, especially with another kinesthetic person Use pictures and photos to illustrate	Write practice answers Role-play the exam situation in your head

REFERENCES

August, A. L., Hurtado, S., Wimsatt, L. A., & Dey, E. L. (2002). *Learning styles: Student preferences vs. faculty perceptions.* Paper presented at the annual forum for the Association for Institutional Research, Toronto, Ontario.

Ausubel, D. P. (1968). *Educational psychology: A cognitive view.* New York: Holt, Rinehart and Winston.

Bandura, A. (1977). *Social learning theory.* Morristown, NJ: General Learning Press.

Bruner, J. (1966). *Toward a theory of instruction.* New York: W. W. Norton & Co.

DeYoung, S. (2003). *Teaching strategies for nurse educators.* Upper Saddle River, NJ: Prentice-Hall.

Gagne, R. M. (1968). Learning hierarchies. *Educational Psychologist, 6,* 1–9.

Gardner, H., & Hatch, T. (1990). *Multiple intelligences go to school: Educational implications of the theory of multiple intelligences* (Technical Report No. 4). New York: Center for Technology in Education.

Gregorc, A. F. (1979). Learning/teaching styles: Their nature and effects. In *Student learning styles* (pp. 19–26). Reston, VA: National Association of Secondary Principals.

Kagan, J. (1965). Reflection-impulsivity and reading ability in primary grade children. *Child Development, 36,* 609–628.

Kelly, E., & Young, A. (1996). Models of nursing education for the 21st century, pp. 1–39. In K. Stevens (ed.), *Review of Research in Nursing Education. Vol. vii.* New York: National League for Nursing.

Knapp, B. (2004). Competency: An essential component of caring in nursing. *Nursing Administration Quarterly, 28,* 285–287.

Knowles, M. A. (1978). *The adult learner: A neglected species* (2nd ed.). Houston, TX: Gulf Publishing.

Kolb, D. A. (1984). *Experiential learning theory.* Englewood Cliffs, NJ: Prentice-Hall.

LeFrancois, G. (1988). *Psychology for teaching* (6th ed.). Belmont, CA: Wadsworth Publishing.

Melrose, S. (2004). What works? A personal account of clinical teaching strategies in nursing. *Education for Health, 17,* 236–239.

Miller, M.A., & Babcock, D. E. (1996). *Critical thinking applied to nursing.* St. Louis, MO: Mosby.

Perry, W. G. (1970). *Forms of intellectual and ethical development in the college years: A scheme.* New York: Holt, Rinehart and Winston.

Pinsky, L. E., Monson, D., & Irby, D. M. (1998). How excellent teachers are made: Reflecting on success to improve teaching. *Advances in Health Sciences Education, 3,* 207–215.

Romyn, D. M. (2001). Disavowal of the behaviorist paradigm in nursing education: What makes it so difficult to unseat? *Advances in Nursing Science, 23*(3), 1–10.

Schon, D. A. (1983). *The reflective practitioner: How professionals think in action.* New York: Basic Books.

Svinicki, M. D. (1994). Practical implications of cognitive theories. In K. A. Feldman & M. B. Paulsen, (Eds.), *Teaching and Learning in the College Classroom* (pp. 274–281). Needham Heights, MA: Ginn Press.

Svinicki, M. D., & Dixon, N. M. (1987). The Kolb model modified for classroom activities. *College Teaching, 35,* 141–146.

Wells, D., & Higgs, Z. R. (1990). Learning and learning preferences of first and fourth semester baccalaureate degree nursing students. *Journal of Nursing Education, 29,* 385–390.

Witkin, H. A., Moore, C. A., Goodenough, D. R., & Cox, P. W. (1977). Field-dependent and field-independent cognitive styles and their implications. *Review of Educational Research, 47,* 1–64.

Wolf, Z. R., Bender, P. J., Beitz, J. M., Wieland, D. M., & Vito, K. O. (2004). Strengths and weaknesses of faculty teaching performance reported by undergraduate and graduate nursing students: A descriptive study. *Journal of Professional Nursing, 20,* 118–128.

CHAPTER 2

Diversity in the Classroom

Arlene J. Lowenstein

Today's classrooms are very different from those in the past. Immigration, both forced and voluntary, has shaped the face of this country. Each new wave of immigrants adds to the mosaic that is the United States. A mosaic is made up of many pieces, each different in size and shape; some may be brightly colored, others pale, transparent, or with no color added. Each piece does not mean much by itself, but when put together, the pieces change, forming new designs and an overall effect very different from the component pieces. The strength of that mosaic is the ability to capitalize on new and different ideas. Its weakness is the clash between cultures that feeds prejudice and discriminatory behaviors. Health professions educators and leaders have recognized this change, and cultural competence of practitioners is now being stressed in both education and service. By using the strengths and originality of diverse students, the final classroom product can be much stronger than the product of an assimilated, cookie cutter one.

A new emphasis on civil rights, feminism, sexuality, and morality issues in the late 1960s and 1970s brought about drastic change in what had been considered accepted societal behavior. Those changes shaped the move toward increased diversity of both patients and student body in our world today, and provided new and different opportunities and challenges from those of the past. Change continues, and classrooms in the future may look very different. Educators need to be flexible, aware of trends and patterns, and able to respond to continuing challenges. This chapter presents a brief glimpse at some of the diversity issues in the past and present day, and it discusses some of the issues and strategies involved in working with a diverse classroom population.

THE PAST

In the 1950s, health care professional education was almost nonexistent for African Americans (Blacks), other minorities, and persons with disabilities. Men went into medicine, while women became nurses. Other health professions may have had some of each gender, but women were often in the majority (Moffat, 2003). Educational facilities were often segregated culturally and religiously, not only in the South, which had a history of legal segregation at that time, but in the North as well (Carnegie, 1991; Carnegie, 2005). Catholic and Jewish hospitals often had their own schools of nursing, and there were religious and ethnic student quotas in many colleges and universities. This meant that most classes were homogenized, with a large majority of Caucasian (White) and Protestant students in all but the religious sponsored or minority established programs, and those were few and far between. Very few Hispanic, Asian, Islamic, or Muslim students were admitted to the schools. For minorities who were admitted, retention rates were often low (Carnegie, 1991).

Nursing education was founded in hospital diploma programs using the apprentice system of education. From the early days in the late 1800s through the 1950s, there were very few graduate nurses in hospitals. Most graduate nurses moved into private duty after graduation, with some going into public health and a few staying on primarily in managerial or teaching positions. Student nurses were the major providers of care for hospital patients. Very ill patients on the hospital wards were most often assigned a private duty nurse to care for them, usually paid for by the patients and their families, although hospitals absorbed the cost in some instances.

In 1946, shortly after World War II, the Hill-Burton Act was passed in Congress and signed into law. It provided funds to hospitals for renovation, expansion, capital projects, and new hospital buildings. As hospitals expanded, more nurses and other health care professionals were needed. Another trend of the time was the development of intensive care units in the mid-1950s, and skilled nurses were needed for those areas as well. The nursing labor pool during those years was still primarily Caucasian and Protestant with few minorities.

During that time, although it seems hard to believe in today's world, very few nursing schools admitted married students. Female students were dismissed from the program if they chose to get married, especially if the secret marriages that occurred were found out by school authorities, and even if they were almost ready to graduate. In the few schools where married students were permitted, pregnant women were excluded, and pregnancy out of wedlock was an unforgivable sin for health professions education.

Nursing was viewed as a woman's profession, and few men were permitted in, and those who were had severe restrictions in clinical experiences such as obstetrics and gynecology, but could be welcomed in psychiatric facilities because it was thought that they were stronger and could work better with distraught and violent patients. It was generally considered that students with disabilities would not be able to participate in providing all aspects of care, and therefore were not admitted to programs. There were no allowances made.

In Augusta, Georgia, from the early 1900s through the early 1960s, University Hospital had two schools of nursing, the Lamar school for Blacks, and the Barrett school for Whites (Lowenstein, 1994). The two schools joined together in 1965, after the passage of civil rights legislation. The Barrett school accepted more nursing students and had a higher graduation rate than the Lamar school. One year, three Asian students applied and were admitted to the Barrett school, but only one graduated. In Augusta, as in most of the South, and often in the North (although no one talked about that), Black students were assigned to the units with Black patients, and White students with Whites. Supervisors, administrators, and teachers were almost always White.

The late 1960s and early 1970s brought a revolutionary change, which has continued expanding since that time. The civil rights movement sparked a feminist movement, and those movements opened previously closed doors in education. Women had more opportunities to be admitted to health care professions that were previously male dominated. A few men were admitted into programs that had only women students, although the numbers were still small, and discrimination prevalent, especially the belief that male nurses were homosexual. The sexual revolution of those years also brought a change in thinking about sexual orientation, although many attitudes of the past still exist today, and discrimination still occurs. In nursing, the rules against marriage were dropped, and women could attend school while pregnant. Although the changes have been gradual, the face of the classroom is continuing its transformation.

During this period of time the community college movement began. It provided more access to minorities, to those who could not afford private college tuition, and to students who needed educational facilities closer to their homes. This was a boon to older women, including minority women, and those with families, who could then attend less expensive schools that were closer to home. Part-time attendance was possible in some programs, and nursing students no longer needed to live at the hospitals. Graduates of associate degree programs in nursing were eligible for licensure as registered nurses and took less time to graduate than the typical three-year diploma program students. Many hospital diploma schools began to close, although that was a prolonged fight. During those years, nursing leaders recognized the discrimination against women in college and university admissions. They were pleased that nursing education had moved out of the hospital program, but were not satisfied. In an effort to raise the status of women in the profession, they began a move toward baccalaureate collegiate education for all nurses by 1984, which also contributed to the demise of hospital programs. However, for many reasons, the baccalaureate goal was not achieved.

The physical therapy profession and its professional organization, the American Physical Therapy Association (APTA), were begun by women, but men were recognized in the profession by the 1920s. However, even with the feminist movements of the 1960s and 1970s, it took until the early 1990s for the APTA to feel it important enough to address women's issues and the inequities in the profession as it pertained to the disparities in the professional and economic status of women. The board of directors appointed the first committee on women in physical therapy, and in 1994 an office of women's issues was created at APTA headquarters in Alexandria, Virginia. The office of minority affairs also became an integral part of the APTA headquarters at that time, as the profession tried to recruit more minorities (Moffat, 2003).

Those years also saw the beginning of affirmative action, and an increased number of minorities began to be admitted to colleges, although the numbers were still small. The end of the Vietnam War began an Asian migration to the United States, and we have seen other migrations since that time, creating increased Latino/Hispanic, Muslim, Indian, and Russian-Jewish populations, among others. Those migrations have meant more diverse students accepted into health professions programs.

In 1990, the Americans with Disabilities Act (ADA) was passed by Congress and signed into law. This required educators to think differently about what could be done to provide access and retention for disabled persons who would be able to work in some, if not all, aspects of their chosen health profession, and thereby provide a valuable service for the profession and its patients.

THE PRESENT

So what has this history led us to in the classroom in today's world? The health professions classroom is more diverse than ever before. However, diversity no longer means ethnic background alone. The age range may be wide and gender ratios may have changed, although nursing still has a minority of male students. In medicine, it worked the other way around, and more women have gone into that field than ever before. There is diversity in sexual orientation, which can result in discrimination.

There are diverse social and family issues in the classroom. Many divorced and single parents have gone back to school, but they often have great responsibility in raising their children alone, and that may interfere with the amount of time that can be allotted to school work (Grosz, 2005; Ogunsiji & Wilkes, 2005). In some places, disadvantaged students have come into the health professions classrooms as new economic relief programs are put into place (Wessling, 2000). Students, especially older ones, may have caretaker responsibilities for their parents or other relatives, including children with disabilities. Those in the "sandwich generation" may have caretaker responsibilities for both their parents and their children.

We also have wealthy students, for whom textbook purchases and other expenses are not a problem, and need-based scholarship students and other students who may have real concerns about the financial issues that can impact on their doing well and completing their program. Tuition increases and the spectre of repayment of student loans may create additional stress. Financially secure students do not always have it easy just because they have the financial means, but they may have other family and social problems that affect them and their classroom abilities.

The number of disabled students, with both physical and/or learning disabilities, has increased. Due to technological advances and better awareness, educational institutions are now able to provide more accommodations for students with disabilities. This may include policy modifications, equipment, and physical changes to increase handicap access. Students with disabilities often have concerns about how they are being perceived by others and worry that other students and faculty are expecting them to fail. Research has shown that creative problem solving and faculty support can be developed for students with disabilities, and health professions education programs can be enriched by their presence (Carroll, 2004).

Colleges and universities are being encouraged to promote diversity in both hiring faculty and in student recruitment and admissions, although success rates are still low (Silver, 2002; Barbee & Gibson, 2001). Even though affirmative action has been under fire, it is recognized that there is still a need to make higher education more accessible for both minorities and students with disabilities. Although diversity in admissions and hiring may be strongly encouraged, retaining diverse students and faculty is often difficult. However, Splenser (2003) and his colleagues, in a study of physical therapy educational programs, found that when schools provided special retention efforts, they were effective in increasing the numbers of graduating minority students. They also found a positive correlation between increased minority applications and the presence of minority faculty in a program.

Other researchers have found that many minority students experience significant culture shock when entering the collegiate world, which may be very different from their previous life experiences. In schools or programs with low numbers of diverse students and faculty, the recruited minority students often had feelings of isolation, loneliness, and anxiety. These feelings could be compounded by impersonal, and sometimes hostile, treatment from faculty, who were still predominately White. Minority faculty also face these feelings, and, in turn, this often leads to students dropping out of school and faculty leaving educational positions (Evans, 2004; Kosowski, Grams, Taylor, & Wilson, 2001; Vasquez, 1990).

Kirkland (1998) found a difference in psychological stress between Black and White nursing students. Blacks often felt more stress and perceived their environments differently. Because of the history of discrimination and their previous experiences with discrimination, Blacks may perceive discrimination, even though White students, employers, or other employees in a health care setting do not feel that discrimination exists (Lowenstein & Glanville, 1995). Kosowski and others (2001) noted that the failure rate for Black students can be higher than for their White counterparts.

There are many causes for the lack of success. Because Blacks are frequently in the minority in such a classroom, feelings of isolation, alienation and loneliness, as well as perceived racism can cause academic difficulties. Inadequate academic preparation for the rigors of college, family conflicts, and lack of financial resources can contribute to that failure. In many cases support services are offered by institutions, but may not be used (Kosowski et al., 2001). Bain (2004) reported that negative stereotypes are often internalized by minority students. That can apply to disabled persons as well. Think about the term *minority*. What does that label mean to students? The connotation is that they are out of the mainstream, not as good as the majority students, and are often expected to fail. Bain noted that even students who had a strong self-image could fall into the trap of feeling that they needed to prove themselves, leading to increased anxiety, stress, and eventually failure. Teachers who have been successful with this population have set up situations where positive expectations are verbalized and integrated into the classroom. Letting minority students know that there is respect for their abilities has been shown to lead to improvement in pass rates (Bain, 2004).

These issues are not limited to Blacks, but often affect other minorities, as well as White students from poorer economic strata. Evans (2004) found Hispanic/Latino and Native American nursing students struggled with similar feelings. Those in the study described the impact of perceived lack of options for minorities. Even before they entered the program, it was difficult for them to imagine themselves successful in a health care profession. Language issues can be difficult to overcome. Lack of family support due to financial or cultural expectations and ignorance of academic demands was also identified as a barrier to success for some students, especially those who were the first in their families to attend college. Students who successfully confronted those barriers were helped by faculty who recognized these stressors, worked to respect students' intense obligation to family and community, and provided long-term, personal encouragement to continue in the program (Evans, 2004).

WORKING WITH A DIVERSE STUDENT BODY

Diversity can have a positive impact on teaching and learning. When encouraged by faculty, recognition and understanding of differences and an introduction to other cultures can broaden viewpoints and stimulate discussion and ideas (Villaruel, Canales, & Torres, 2001). However, it is important to point out that although this chapter discusses some cultural traits, there is a wide range in cultural responses and traits within a single culture. Members of a racial or cultural group may or may not adhere to some of the traditions of their background culture and ethnic group, and may not even identify as a member of that group. Faculty members must remember that people are individuals who react differently and must be treated individually. Students who are members of a cultural group cannot be expected to be a spokesperson for their group. There are too many variations within the groups themselves, and what is appropriate for one sect within a group may not be acceptable to another sect in that group.

Discrimination is always a difficult issue, and faculty, staff, administrators, and patients are not immune. We all have our likes, dislikes, and moral beliefs. Because of their previous experiences, many minorities will see discrimination where others do not. That needs to be respected and cannot be brushed off, but sometimes it also needs to be faced, corrected, or worked with. The major thrust here needs to be concentration on providing appropriate learning opportunities and meeting learning objectives. Seeking ways to help students learn about each other can be a positive force in changing discriminatory attitudes. Many myths of prejudice and discrimination can be dismantled and dismissed when students who have led sheltered backgrounds begin to know those who are different from them and understand that although there are cultural differences, there are also many similarities.

However, conflict between cultural groups does occur in the classroom. There can be other sources for conflict that have nothing to do with ethnicity, as well as conflicts that are ethnicity and values led. In some instances mediation may be helpful to define limits and focus the groups back onto the learning tasks at hand. Separation may work for other groups, but that is usually a temporary situation until the strong feelings calm down. Encouraging groups to learn about each other is a strategy that can be used to defuse potential conflict, but this strategy needs to be carefully managed and the instructor needs to observe group dynamics and be on the alert for peer-influenced negative ideas and peer pressure to adopt those ideas.

Developing a welcoming and supportive environment is essential, not only for ethnic minority students, but also for the other groups mentioned as part of the diverse classroom, including single parents, disabled students, and age and gender disparities. Faculty availability and interest are critical elements in developing a positive environment. Instructors need to be aware of potential issues, know their students, and demonstrate interest in them and their success in the program. The importance of cultural and linguistic role models (e.g., community health professionals of color and/or those from minority-based professional organizations, including those who speak a similar language) cannot be overemphasized because it has a universal effect on overcoming obstacles and achieving academic success for students of color and English-as-a-second-language (ESL) students (Heller & Lichtenberg, 2003; Yoder, 1996). Mentoring has shown success, whether it comes from outside the school or from an advanced student of one's own ethnic or cultural origin, especially when there are no faculty members of color. Those same principles apply to gender-based minorities who may also feel isolated or unwelcome in the profession.

When learning difficulties appear in any group of students, it is important to look for behavioral patterns that may be impacting on their success or other stresses or anxieties that seem present. Some students may need to be encouraged to be tested for learning disabilities. A diagnosis of a learning disorder, confirmed by testing, allows the student access to the resources required under ADA regulations. Faculty need to learn about student support services in their college. They need to know to whom and how to make referrals for students in areas such as financial aid, study skills, test-taking skills and tutorial assistance, mental and physical health services, and social services. It is extremely important that students are supported and encouraged to take advantage of those services.

Age Range

Older students will have a sense of history during their lifetime that is very different from the 18-year-olds', and they have learned how to deal with many situations that 18-year-olds haven't yet faced, which can be valuable when there are opportunities for sharing. However, depending on their success or frustration levels in working with those situations, older students can also hold a cynical or ingrained view that comes through and needs to be worked with and mediated at times. Older students may not value the young lifestyle and find younger students immature. Building on some of the strengths of the younger groups growing up in the technology age can be helpful to older students who are not comfortable with the technology.

Young students can be bored by the older student experiences, tired of listening to them, unable or unwilling to relate those experiences to their own, or they can be interested and learn from them. Younger students may relate to older students as parental figures, which can be good or bad, viewing them as caring or the other extreme of dictatorial or authoritarian, which is often based in their experiences with older adults. The most important task is getting students in different age groups to respect and learn from each other. Small group work can create diverse working groups. Monitoring group work is important to identify conflict areas. However, when students in different age levels get to know each other better and have success in working together towards a common goal of meeting learning objectives, negative perceptions can change, and they can be a positive support for each other.

Communication

Communication can be problematic between cultural and ethnic groups and the majority group. The learning goals and objectives need to be clearly understood by both students and teacher in a diverse classroom. Communication is often an issue and at the same time is the key to understanding and acceptance of those goals. Diverse students may have their own individual goals and objectives based on their interest and learning experiences, and they may or may not be willing to share them with the instructor. An instructor needs to be open to listen to and encourage ideas that can be different than the ones he/she planned for the class and allow for appropriate analytic, creative, and practical knowledge to be utilized. It may be easier for ESL students to read English than it is to understand English conversation, so written instructions or handouts may be helpful and allow students more time to clarify concepts. Instructors need to speak slowly and clearly in classroom presentations, and conversational pauses may need to be longer so that students can be encouraged to speak up, but also allow them to catch up with what is being said and with note taking.

Some minority students come from cultures where eye contact and/or active participation are not normal experiences and may be uncomfortable for them (Suinn, 2006). This can include minimal participation in class discussion, and they may sit back and not offer comments in class, even when they have a good understanding of the material and would have information that would be helpful to the class, or when they need clarification and additional help with a concept. Many of these students may do better in small discussion groups. Some cultures feel strongly about and use collaboration as a norm, and participants may not want to stand out from the group, while the American culture tends to be more individualistic and often competitive, with class discussion more acceptable because it is what they are used to, and it offers an opportunity to show off their knowledge base. Of course, students raised in the American culture can also be shy or nonparticipating, especially in large classes, and small-group discussions can be helpful for them as well.

Students and faculty may have a difference in perception, especially if English is not the primary language. Ideas may not translate well. American ideals and values may be different from what they are used to. One of the most important aspects in working with all students, but especially with minorities and ESL students, is what I call "know your PVCs." This is not the cardiac term most of us are familiar with, but instead stands for *perception, validation,* and *clarification.* Each person perceives an event differently. An inquiry to see if there are any questions or areas they do not understand needs to have more depth than just asking if the students understand and expecting and getting a yes answer. Students need to be encouraged to articulate what they think was said, and that's where the differences show up. Formal classroom assessment techniques can also be helpful in identifying problem areas (Angelo & Cross, 1994).

When an instructor feels a student lacks understanding of the materials, it is important to question that *perception* with the student, *validate* that what was meant to be communicated is in reality what the student understood to be communicated, and, when there is a difference, *clarification* is in order. Students who are not proficient in English may smile and seem to understand, but often do not, and they may not want to ask in front of the whole class for clarification or statements to be repeated. It is important for faculty to be aware of this possibility, and follow-through outside of the classroom environment may be necessary.

Accommodation

The passage of the Americans with Disabilities Act in 1990 has made a major difference in today's classroom. Instructors need to adjust to accommodations that may be necessary. Think about the following: if a health professional is injured or comes down with a debilitating illness or is wheelchair bound, can accommodations be made so they can continue working? In most cases, employees can and will be accommodated in various jobs within the profession, even those employees who become deaf or legally blind. These jobs may not be the usual clinical care, but they are still jobs that need a health professional to perform and are essential for quality care. Think about jobs that a disabled person could perform in your specialty—those that may be possible, despite the fact that some individuals will be limited or unable to perform certain job functions. Assistive devices can often be used to allow the employee to perform safely and appropriately in limited activities if they have the appropriate clinical knowledge required for the specific position. If that is true, why does the door to the profession need to be closed and applicants with disabilities be turned away? Think about ways in which a disabled student could be prepared to work in those jobs within the profession, and the types of clinical experiences that a disabled student can carry out that will provide appropriate experiences for a future job. The technology field is rapidly expanding, and assistive devices are improving and becoming more cost-effective and more available.

Faculty must become well aware of the disability regulations and student support services that colleges have set up because of those regulations. Faculties need to develop awareness of the barriers and regulations that are present for disabled students and which need to be addressed, and where resources can be found to help both faculty members and students. One question that needs to be addressed in a positive manner is "are these accommodations fair to the nondisabled students?" What does *fair* mean? A disability may not be visible to others, in particular, learning disabilities or certain physical disabilities such as back problems. Rules of privacy may not allow a faculty member to discuss a disabled student's condition, but they can encourage the student to discuss this with others and provide support as necessary.

For many years, teachers were authoritarians in the classrooms, with rigid standards and rules and regulations. Things are different today. Student demonstrations in the late 1960s and early 1970s began a students' rights movement that altered college cultures. But some questions need to be asked. How much can be compromised, and how do we work within regulated issues? A very positive part of students' rights has been that faculties have had to look at what they were doing and assessing whether they were working by ritual or providing real learning opportunities. Those faculties have learned to work successfully with students who, in the past, would not have had the opportunities available to them today.

Making accommodations is also an important concept to those with heavy personal responsibilities. Older students may be faced with family issues, such as caring for children and/or elderly parents. They and single parents may have responsibilities that interfere with their ability to meet deadlines or come to class. Rigid attendance policies are often more ritualistic than real. The focus needs to be on what is necessary for the learning experience. Sitting in a class does not guarantee that a student is attentive and learning. Teachers are well aware that students daydream, have conversations with their classmates, and even fall asleep, and that they will forget a good portion of what was presented, even though we as teachers believe that every word we give them is valuable. It may be more important for a student to attend a small seminar-type class because the learning is dependent on participation in discussion more than it is for sitting in a large lecture session. The important determining issue is what are the goals and objectives for the course, and are there other ways to meet them without perfect attendance? That may sound heretical, but there are other ways for conscientious and motivated students to meet learning objectives and set priorities. The use of the Internet, library services, and out-of-class assignments can afford some flexibility if needed. Attendance in clinical experiences may be more problematic because of the need for scheduling and faculty availability, but there are ways to design a program with a student that may afford some flexibility for specific instances. Again, it is important to keep the learning goal of the experience or class in mind and consider creative and flexible ways to work with students to plan for what they feel they can accomplish.

Financially challenged students may not be able to participate in some activities because they may need to work in addition to their school responsibilities. They may have difficulty in buying books and special or technological equipment or participating in outside learning opportunities, such as conferences or lectures that have a fee attached. These students may not be able to spend hours in the library because of their work and family schedules, and finding study time may be difficult. Anxiety and worry over finances can impact their learning experience.

There is no easy answer to these issues, but again, student services can often be an ally. Student lives outside the classroom need to be respected, but the responsibility for learning is theirs, not yours. Students and faculty can work together to assess what is needed to achieve the objectives of the learning experiences, and to facilitate their learning. Are there alternative ways of achieving those objectives that don't meet up with the "is it fair to others" question? It is important for instructors to meet with student services to find out just what they do, and how they do it. Student services can help students set up workable schedules, tutorial services, and study and testing guidance. They can also counsel students on student life issues and refer students to outside resources when needed. Faculty should also be familiar with financial aid issues and regulations, which can be quite complicated because of differences in governmental and private sources, and with outside services for referrals when appropriate.

Academic Issues

Students with academic problems need to be identified early and encouraged to discuss the issue with faculty without the spectre of punishment or embarrassment. It is important to discover patterns of negative behavior, discuss them directly with the student involved, and develop a plan on which the student and faculty agree and believe can be implemented and carried out. Unfortunately, not all students can be helped, and some will drop out or fail out, but others will be successful and benefit from the encouragement.

Students with learning disabilities and ESL students may have problems with timed tests. ESL students may need more time to read and digest test questions, because they may be translating the questions back into their primary language, and some words and phrases do not translate well. The learning disability students are supported in the need for additional time by the ADA regulations, but that is not true for ESL students. In order to evaluate and accurately grade the level of knowledge, faculty can provide opportunities for various types of testing other than timed tests—take home tests being one example. There may be a limit to this, however, when students need to improve in timed testing because they will be subjected to that in the licensure testing. Again, learning disability students can have additional time because the regulations support them, but ESL can be a cause for failure in timed tests, and those students may need practice and/or tutorial assistance to become more proficient in testing in order to pass a licensing exam and enter the profession.

CONCLUSION

Although working with diverse students can be challenging, it can also be stimulating and exciting. As health care professionals, we and our students are in a clinical environment, and learning about new cultures and disabilities can hopefully be translated into increased cultural competence when working with patients. Remember that the responsibility for learning lies with the learner, but feelings of anxiety and isolation can cause stress that impacts the learning process, and it may affect graduation rates and successful entrance into the profession. Family responsibilities can also interfere with a student's ability to carry out the required work. Faculty members need to learn to develop sensitivity and awareness of issues that impact the learning process and work with students to meet the learning goals. They need to develop their knowledge of services and resources that can be utilized by students. Flexibility, patience, and creativity are needed to develop a supportive environment that enhances learning. A major role of faculty is offering support, guidance, and referrals as appropriate and developing a community of students who view diversity as a strength that provides an opportunity to learn from each other as well as from their teachers. It is painful but necessary to understand that this will not work for all students, but it will be appreciated by and benefit many students. Our reward for efforts expended is that we can rightly celebrate and be proud of the successful students that we have helped enter the profession and who are now providing a valuable service to their patients, communities, and profession.

Although the teaching example for this chapter has been used to provide understanding of gender issues, the techniques can be adapted to increase understanding of cultural and social issues among students.

TEACHING EXAMPLE

Effective Communication Related to Human Sexuality Issues

Dr. Jane A. Petrillo

Associate Professor, Department of Health, Physical Education and Sport Science, Kennesaw University, Kennesaw, Georgia

One of the most important topics and tasks in teaching human sexuality is examining communication and gender-related issues. The development of effective communication skills among and between the genders has been an ever-present challenge. Honest, open, and often unsolicited communication about personal and often complex subject matter related to sexual issues is highly difficult and can contribute to further misunderstanding and problems in a relationship. Thus, this classroom strategy has been designed to teach, develop, and further nurture open and effective communication among undergraduate and/or graduate students in a human sexuality class with particular emphasis on relationship and gender issues and effective communication between and among males and females. This instructional strategy is intended to be utilized directly following lecture and discussion in the classroom setting on text and course content specific to the principles and skills of effective communication and gender and relationship issues.

The strategy is most appropriate in a human sexuality course at the undergraduate and/or graduate level following instruction on the core content areas in sexuality including but not limited to: the sociological, cultural, psychological, and physiological concepts of human sexuality; historical and cross-cultural issues; research methods and current findings in sexuality; male and female sexual anatomy and reproduction; phases of human sexual response; methods of contraception; sexuality across the life span; and gender development, gender related issues, and relationship issues. During the instruction on gender development, gender issues, and relationships, it is suggested that a multitude of information sources, resources, and strategies that reinforce and further expand on text information and serve to stimulate student learning, dialogue, and critical thinking be employed. Suggested resources and strategies include a review of the current literature on gender and relationship issues and the use of content-related video clips from popular television shows and movies, television commercials, popular magazine advertisements, and music videos. The content on gender should address gender role development and issues, gender behaviors and expectations, social and cultural norms, media and popular culture influences, and sexual activity and preferences. The employment of the above mentioned strategies and resources also provide multiple opportunities for students to become more engaged in the learning process.

Content on effective communication principles and skills should then be introduced. Though the content on effective communication may vary depending upon text content and course objectives, critical foundation content on communication should include types and contexts of communication (verbal and nonverbal communication, social and cultural contexts); influences on communication (age, gender, social, and work status, type of relationship, length of relationship, trust in a relationship); barriers to effective communication (lack of trust, relationship inequity); and steps to effective communication (speaking with clarity, using *I* statements, matching nonverbal with verbal communication, maintaining direct eye contact, engaging in active listening, repeating what was heard from the speaker, asking for clarification if and when necessary, and listening and responding with empathy). It must be emphasized to the students that the utilization of effective communication skills is critical in all interactions, both personal and professional in nature.

The class period prior to implementing this strategy, students are instructed to compose and type three questions related to human sexuality with particular emphasis on gender and relationship issues. On the top of the question page, the females type the phrase, "Questions to Ask the Males," and the males will title theirs, "Questions to Ask the Females." All questions are collected and carefully reviewed by the course instructor and those that are redundant or inappropriate may be eliminated at the instructor's discretion. This all must be conducted prior to beginning the activity. Students will include their name in pencil on the question page and each student will earn a total of 30 points (10 points per question) for the three clearly stated and typed questions. After the instructor records the 30 points for each student in the course grade book, student names are erased as a means of maintaining student anonymity.

When beginning the instructional strategy, females and males arrange their desks to directly face one another. The instructor has the question sheets arranged in two stacks. Stack one is labeled "Questions to Ask the Males" and stack two is labeled "Questions to Ask the Females." The instructor, as activity facilitator, will alternate reading a question to be addressed by the males and then a question to be addressed by the females, drawing from each stack of questions. The instructor encourages the students to continue dialogue on each question and related issue until clarity and understanding of each student's perspective is attained.

The instructor monitors, corrects, and reinforces the utilization of effective communication skills, as does each student, throughout the activity. A common occurrence in this strategy is that of an unequal ratio of males versus females in the class. This will result in the underrepresented gender having a greater number of written questions to address from the opposite and overrepresented gender. Should this be the case, the instructor can supplement questions to add to the underrepresented group's stack. The instructor can use questions that have been accumulated from formerly conducted activities on this exercise. The supplementing of questions can also be done when there are a limited number of questions due to small class size.

In addition, the principles and skills of effective communication are posted on the chalkboard, whiteboard, or poster board, and the instructor and students review and clarify each principle and skill thoroughly prior to beginning the activity. The success of this activity is dependent upon the consistent use of effective communication skills among all students. In addition, honesty, clarity, and mutual respect are critical to the effectiveness of the activity. Throughout the strategy, effective communication principles and skills are practiced and reviewed if necessary. This strategy is best suited for a class period of at least sixty minutes and should be consistently monitored and facilitated by the course instructor. If additional time is necessary to address all critical questions and concerns among the students, the activity can continue at the onset of the following class meeting. A conclusion and summary is facilitated by the course instructor and consists of a review of the major issues and concerns related to human sexuality, communication, and gender and relationship topics which were discussed during the activity.

Several events and related consequences may occur prior to, during, and/or upon completion of this instructional strategy. First, most students look forward to this activity and come to class prepared and eager to participate in open discussion and dialogue on critical gender, sexual, and relationship issues relative to their daily lives. Yet, some students may feel anxious or hesitant to discuss personal sexual issues and concerns in such an open format and may decide not to come to class on the day the strategy is being conducted. The earning of 30 points for each student's questions and attending and fully participating in class on the day of the activity serves as an incentive for all students. The instructor also clarifies to all students that the activity and related discussions will be conducted in an informal yet caring manner and the application of effective communication principles and skills will continually be reinforced. Also, some students may have a concern of being judged or of disclosing highly personal or intimate information relative to the sexual topics being discussed. An effective way of addressing this issue at the onset of the activity is to clearly indicate to the class that students' responses may not necessarily be based on direct or first-hand experience and that judgment of any individual based on his or her response will undermine the integrity of the activity and be counter to the intention and outcome of the activity. On occasion, a student, depending on age and maturity level, may use a term or phrase that is slang or inappropriate in a classroom setting. In that case, the instructor must briefly stop the activity and clarify to the students that correct and appropriate terminology in reference to sexual behaviors and issues must be consistently used during this and all class discussions. The use of appropriate terminology can also serve to diffuse much of the laughter and embarrassment that can occur during class discussions.

Another occurrence during this strategy is that of only a few uninhibited and outgoing students monopolizing the activity. An effective approach to addressing this situation is to have alternating students ask the questions and alternating students answer the questions, at least in the initial phase of query and response. Often though, various students will ask another question which builds upon the preceding question, and numerous students will respond to the questions being asked as a means of further clarifying and addressing each question thoroughly. Therefore, the instructor must be careful not to stifle or limit open and thorough discussion of a critical issue by placing overly stringent rules on the activity. Once a question has been thoroughly addressed as determined by the instructor and students, then the next student is directed to ask another question. The overall outcome of the strategy is highly positive on many levels. As evidenced in an instructor-led review of the issues and discussions at the completion of the strategy, students will typically indicate that an increased understanding of the opposite genders' perspective specific to sexual and relationship issues is achieved. During the review, students also indicate that the activity helped to reinforce the development of effective communication skills, particularly in the areas of asking for clarification and engaging in active listening. **Table 2-1** provides samples of discussion questions chosen by the students and summaries of student responses.

The evaluation of learner attainment is both formal and informal. Formal evaluation methods include the three clearly stated and typed questions submitted by each student prior to the beginning of the strategy. Another formal method of evaluating student learning is via the inclusion of content specific to the principles and effective methods of communication on a course examination. An informal method of learner attainment is conducted by the instructor as well as the students via the practice and reinforcement of effective communication skills by each student throughout the activity in accordance with those identified on the board and specific to the course text. Another means of informally assessing student learning is through the review, clarification, and summary of critical information that was discussed during the activity.

The resources needed for this activity include class time of approximately one hour; classroom desks and chairs that can be moved in a pattern conducive to open classroom dialogue and discussion among all students; pencil or pen; paper; bulletin board, whiteboard, or chalkboard; and textbook and/or supplemental materials identifying effective principles and practices of effective communication. Current undergraduate and/or graduate level textbooks in human sexuality for course and instructional strategy content include:

Blonna, R., & Levitan, J. (2005). *Healthy sexuality*. Belmont, CA: Thomson-Wadsworth Publishing.

Kelly, G. F. (2006). *Sexuality today: The human perspective* (8th ed.). New York, NY: McGraw-Hill Companies.

McAnulty, R. D., & Burnette, M. M. (2004). *Exploring health sexuality: Making health decisions* (2nd ed.). Boston, MA: Pearson Education, Inc.

Westheimer, R. K., & Lopater, S. (2005). *Human sexuality: A psychological perspective* (2nd ed.). Baltimore, MD: Lippincott, Williams and Wilkins.

Table 2-1   Sample Questions and Summary of Student Responses and Discussions

Questions to ask the females:	Summary of responses/discussions:
1. Why does a woman want a man to dig so deep into his feelings?	1. Females explained that it is very important to them to know what a man is feeling is very important and necessary in formulating and maintaining intimacy and connection in the relationship. Expressing feelings helps the females understand what matters to men, what is important, and also how the men feel about the females. It eliminates second-guessing for the females, makes them feel more secure, and builds trust in the relationship. It also makes it easier for the females to share their feelings when men can be open about their own feelings.

Table 2-1   Sample Questions and Summary of Student Responses and Discussions (*continued*)

Questions to ask the females:	Summary of responses/discussions:
2. What are the three most important characteristics a woman wants a man to have?	2. A multitude of characteristics were identified including being physically fit, having kind eyes, having broad shoulders, and other physical characteristics. Nonphysical characteristics were caring, being self-assured but not cocky, being a good listener, being thoughtful, being honest, being goal oriented, liking children, having integrity, and loving his family. Many women said that it depended on what type of relationship was being sought (sexual, short-term, long-term, etc.).
3. How does it feel to have multiple orgasms?	3. Some women indicated that they have not experienced multiple orgasms. Others said they are still working on it. Those who have been multiorgasmic responded immediately, saying that it was wonderful, fantastic, and incredible. Women also indicated that they aren't consistently multiorgasmic. Others indicated that it takes a lot of concentration, comfort, trust, and communication between partners and that the partners needed to know one another well.
4. Why do so many girls lie about masturbating?	4. Many females said that they do not lie about self-pleasure and masturbation. Others indicated that they are not comfortable with the idea of masturbation, and some females indicated that they are embarrassed about admitting to masturbating. Several women said that for either religious, cultural, or inhibition-related reasons, they do not masturbate.
5. How frequently do women think about sex?	5. The majority of women indicated that they don't think that females think about sex as much as men do. Many also said that they think about sex more when they are having sex more

	frequently, especially with a new part-ner. Several women indicated that they think about sex in terms of how to get out of having it.
6. How soon is too soon to have sexual intercourse when beginning a new relationship?	6. Women's responses varied. Some women thought it depended on the age of the persons involved. Others indicated that it depended on how well and/or how long they have known the man. Religion, number of dates, level of connection, and amount of trust were also included as factors that are considered. Others indicated that they will not have sexual intercourse until they are married and on their honeymoon. Several women wanted to know how the men felt about this issue. Again, the responses varied and depended upon most of the same factors listed above.
Questions to ask the males:	**Summary of responses/discussions:**
1. Why are males so interested in pornography?	1. Males responded with many answers such as it turns them on, it is what men do, it is fun to watch (especially two women together), they like watching pornography with their partner, they do so for entertainment, it's addictive, and it is readily available (magazines, videos, Internet). Other men indicated that they did not enjoy watching pornography and others said it only turned them on initially, and then they tend to get bored with it. The discussion led to the conclusion that a large number of women indicated that they are turned off by pornography and found it demeaning to women. Some women said watching pornography made them feel dirty. Other women indicated that they would only watch pornography with a partner they really were comfortable with and a small number of women said that watching pornography with their partner did work effectively in getting them in the mood for sex.

Table 2-1   Sample Questions and Summary of Student Responses and Discussions (*continued*)

Questions to ask the males:	Summary of responses/discussions:
2. Why do guys hate to talk about relationships?	2. The men's responses were varied and included the idea that women want to talk about and dissect every aspect of a relationship, leaving the men to feel there is nothing left to talk about. Also, men said that they want relationships to evolve and develop but women have to continually push for talking about relationship issues. The men felt that women always look for issues and problems in a relationship. Several men continued to project their reasons back on women. The women responded that they felt the need and pressure to talk about relationships because they never know where they stand with the men or what the men are feeling.
3. Is it true that when heterosexual males engage in sexual activity, they often fantasize about other women? If so, why?	3. Many men said yes and even shared the identities of some of their female fantasies (usually a high profile celebrity or female athlete or model such as Angelina Jolie). The reasons provided for fantasizing included fixation on certain females' body parts (Pam Anderson's breasts, for example), and desires for particular sexual activities (fellatio or anal sex, for example). Some women admitted to sexual fantasizing during lovemaking about either a person (such as Brad Pitt) and/or also a certain sexual act that they wanted to have performed on them.
4. Why are men so turned on by two women making love together?	4. The majority of men admitted to being turned on by the mere thought of two women making love and the reasons included were that it makes them feel like a voyeur and that the women are

	doing it because they know they are being watched and that in itself turns the men on. Other reasons included that just seeing women please each other and perform sexual acts and enjoy it is a tremendous turn on. Several men said it turns them on because they fantasize that the women are getting ready for the man to join them.
5. Why do men have such a problem with commitment?	5. The men said that women push for commitment too soon in a relationship and that makes the men more commitment phobic. Other men indicated that they just have not found the right woman to whom they wish to commit.
6. Does a girl's sexual history matter to you?	6. Men had a number of responses to this question. Some men felt that what women did in the past and with whom is not an issue, even when selecting a long-term partner. Others indicated that it was important to them that females they are interested in dating not have an excessive number of partners in their past. Many men said that it depended on the female's age (older women may accumulate a higher number of sexual partners over the years). The men often then asked the women the same question. The women believed that society puts less emphasis on men's sexual history than on females'.

REFERENCES

Angelo, T. A., & Cross, K. P. (1994). *Classroom assessment techniques: A handbook for college teachers* (2nd ed.). San Francisco: Jossey-Bass.

Bain, K. (2004). *What the best college teachers do.* Cambridge, MA: Harvard University Press.

Barbee, E., & Gibson, S. (2001). Our dismal progress: The recruitment of non-whites into nursing. *Journal of Nursing Education, 40*(6), 243–244.

Carnegie, M. E. (1991). *The path we tread: Blacks in nursing 1834–1990.* New York: National League for Nursing.

Carnegie, M. E. (2005). Educational preparation of Black nurses: A historical perspective. *ABNF Journal, 16*(1), 6–7.

Carroll, S. M. (2004). Inclusion of people with physical disabilities in nursing education. *Journal of Nursing Education, 43*(5), 207–212.

Evans, B. C. (2004). Application of the caring curriculum to education of Hispanic/Latino and American Indian nursing students. *Journal of Nursing Education, 43*(5), 219–228.

Grosz, R. (2005). The forgotten (?) minority. *The Internet Journal of Allied Health Sciences and Practice, 3*(3). Retrieved May 10, 2006, from http://www.nova.edu/cwis/centers/hpd/allied-health/journal/articles/vol3num3/grosz_commentary.htm

Heller, B. R., & Lichtenberg, L. P. (2003). Addressing the shortage: Strategies for building the nursing workforce. *Nursing Leadership Forum, 8*(1), 34–39.

Kirkland, M. L. S. (1998). Stressors and coping strategies among successful female African American baccalaureate nursing students. *Journal of Nursing Education, 37*(1), 5–13.

Kosowski, M. M., Grams, K. M., Taylor, G. J., & Wilson, C. B. (2001). They took the time . . . they started to care: Stories of African-American nursing students in intercultural caring groups. *Advances in Nursing Science, 23*(3), 11–27.

Lowenstein, A. (1994, September). *Racial segregation and nursing education in Georgia: The Lamar experience.* Paper presented at the annual convention of the Transcultural Nursing Society. Atlanta, GA.

Lowenstein, A. J., & Glanville, C. (1995). Cultural diversity and conflict in the health care workplace. *Nursing Economics, 13*(4), 203–209, 247.

Moffat, M. (2003). The history of physical therapy practice in the United States. *Journal of Physical Therapy Education, 17*(3), 15–25.

Ogunsiji, O., & Wilkes, L. (2005). Managing family life while studying: Single mothers' lived experience of being students in a nursing program. *Contemporary Nurse, 18*(1–2), 108–123.

Silver, J. H., Sr. (2002). Diversity issues. In R. Diamond (Ed.), *Field guide to academic leadership* (pp. 357–372). San Francisco: Jossey-Bass.

Splenser, P. E., Canlas, H. L., Sanders, B., & Melzer, B. (2003). Minority recruitment and retention strategies in physical therapist education programs. *Journal of Physical Therapy Education, 17*(1), 18–26.

Suinn, R. M. (2006). Teaching culturally diverse students. In W. J. McKeachie & M. Svinicki (Eds.), *McKeachie's teaching tips* (12th ed., pp. 152–171). Boston: Houghton Mifflin.

Vasquez, J. (1990). Instructional responsibilities of college faculty to minority students. *Journal of Negro Education, 59,* 599–610.

Villaruel, A. M., Canales, M., & Torres, S. (2001). Educational mobility of Hispanic nurses. *Journal of Nursing Education, 40*(6), 245–251.

Wessling, S. (2000, Fall). Coming home: Two unique programs are giving homeless and disadvantaged persons an opportunity to start again as nursing professionals. *Minority Nurse,* 32–35.

Yoder, M. (1996). Instructional responses to ethnically diverse nursing students. *Journal of Nursing Education, 35,* 315–321.

RECOMMENDED READING

Barbee, E., & Gibson, S. (2001). Our dismal progress: The recruitment of non-Whites into nursing. *Journal of Nursing Education, 40*(6), 243–244.

Byrne, M. (2001). Uncovering racial bias in nursing fundamentals textbooks. *Nursing and Health Care Perspectives, 22,* 299–303.

Dickerson, S., & Neary, M. (1999). Faculty experiences teaching Native Americans in a university setting. *Journal of Transcultural Nursing, 10*(1), 56–64.

Edward, J. (2000). Teaching strategies for foreign nurses. *Journal for Nurses in Staff Development, 16*(4), 171–173.

Evans, B. C. (2004). Application of the caring curriculum to education of Hispanic/Latino and American Indian nursing students. *Journal of Nursing Education, 43*(5), 219–228.

Griffiths, M., & Tagliareni, E. (1999). Challenging traditional assumptions about minority students in nursing education. *Nursing & Health Care Perspectives, 20*, 290–295.

Grosz, R. (2005, July). The forgotten (?) minority [Commentary]. *The Internet Journal of Allied Health Sciences and Practice, 3*(3). Retrieved May 10, 2006 from http://www.nova.edu/cwis/centers/hpd/allied-health/journal/articles/vol3num3/grosz_commentary.htm

Kosowski, M. M., Grams, K. M., Taylor, G. J., & Wilson, C. B. (2001). They took the time . . . they started to care: Stories of African-American nursing students in intercultural caring groups. *Advances in Nursing Science, 23*(3), 11–27.

Maruyama, G., Moreno, J. F., Gudeman, R. H., & Marin, P. (2000). *Does diversity make a difference? Three research studies on diversity in college classrooms.* Washington, DC: American Association of University Professors. (ERIC Document No. ED444409)

Maville, J., & Huerta, C. (1997). Stress and social support among Hispanic student nurses: Implications for academic achievement. *Journal of Cultural Diversity, 4*(1), 18–25.

Miller, J. E., & Hollenshead, C. (2005). Gender, family, and flexibility—why they're important in the academic workplace. *Change, 37*(6), 58–62.

Splenser, P. E., Canlas, H. L., Sanders, B., & Melzer, B. (2003). Minority recruitment and retention strategies in physical therapist education programs. *Journal of Physical Therapy Education, 17*(1), 18–26.

Taylor, V., & Rust, G. (1999). The needs of students from diverse cultures. *Academic Medicine, 74*, 302–304.

Vasquez, J. (1990). Instructional responsibilities of college faculty to minority students. *Journal of Negro Education, 59*, 599–610.

Weaver, H. (2001). Indigenous nurses and professional education: Friends or foe? *Journal of Nursing Education, 40*, 252–258.

Yoder, M. (1996). Instructional responses to ethnically diverse nursing students. *Journal of Nursing Education, 35*, 315–321.

Yurkovich, E. (2001). Working with American Indians toward educational success. *Journal of Nursing Education, 40*, 259–269.

ELECTRONIC RESOURCES

Center for Teaching and Learning—University of North Carolina at Chapel Hill (1997). *Diversity in the college classroom.* Retrieved May 10, 2006, from http://ctl.unc.edu/tfitoc.html

Gurin, P., Dey, E. L., Hurtado, S., & Gurin, G. (2002). Diversity and higher education: Theory and impact on educational outcomes. *Harvard Educational Review, 72*(3). Retrieved May 10, 2006, from http://gseweb.harvard.edu/~hepg/gurin.html

U.S. Department of Justice. *ADA regulations and technical assistance materials.* Retrieved May 10, 2006, from http://www.usdoj.gov/crt/ada/publicat.htm

CHAPTER 3

Strategies for Innovation

Arlene J. Lowenstein

The scope of change in health care has been enormous, and the rate at which change occurs continues to accelerate. Today's technology and therapeutics were inconceivable even a few decades ago. Over time, the growth of the health professions has been influenced by those new technologies and therapeutics, but there are many other influencing factors and forces, including, but not limited to:

- The appearance of new diseases, such as HIV/AIDS, Lyme disease, and bird flu.
- War and its consequences, which brought new techniques to care for burns and radiation, growth of the use of penicillin and other antibiotics, treatments for posttraumatic stress syndrome, growth of nursing and rehabilitation services in the military, and veterans' systems.
- Sociocultural issues, including the civil rights movement, the feminist movement, the consumer revolution of the late 1960s and 1970s, and changing immigration and demographic patterns, which brought dramatic changes in maternity care from shortened length of stay to sibling visitation, increased focus on care of the elderly, and end of life care. Diversity has increased in health care education and practice, and more emphasis has been placed on culturally competent care.
- Religious issues brought in ethical components of care and the development of parish nursing.
- Changing economics and political/legal issues, which brought us Medicare, Medicaid, managed care, and legalized abortion.
- Changes in education that brought nursing into academic settings and gave rise to nursing science and nursing research, thereby changing practice and creating new roles, such as advanced practice nursing. Physical therapy has embraced the doctor of physical therapy (DPT) as an entry-level degree, and other health professions have developed and evolved.

These forces are not isolated, but are part of the total environment in which we live and work. They are ever-changing and interacting, challenging health professions educators to keep on top of the trends, technologies, and resources, while enabling self-directed student learning. Graduates who are self-directed learners understand and are responsive to health care system changes when they are in practice and out of the school setting, where there are no faculty members with whom to consult.

Health care educators straddle the fields of health care practice and education. They need to be knowledgeable about changes in practice and technology in both fields. What health care practitioners learn, as well as how they are taught, must keep pace with the changing milieu. The field of education has also changed over the years through many of the same forces that affected health care. Technology and therapeutics in health care can be compared to a new understanding of learning theories and teaching methods in education. The student entering a health care profession from high school today is most likely much more comfortable with the use of computers than the RN returning to school or an older student who has chosen a health profession as a second career. Online courses are now in the mainstream.

Health professions classrooms are also more culturally diverse than ever before. More men are entering the nursing profession and more women are going to medical schools. Younger students may have had very different cultural experiences in the secondary schools than did older students. Older students may be dealing with the added stress of parenthood and job responsibilities. Different cultures and experiences may produce different expectations of teaching and learning. Respecting learning-need differences and establishing an innovative climate in the classroom can help to prepare students for the changes they will face in practice. An educational climate that values different viewpoints and experiences among students encourages those students to create their own innovations. Those innovations will serve them in good stead by enhancing positive interactions with the wide variety of persons for whom they will be caring and with whom they will be working.

Sources of information have multiplied. The Internet has laid at our doors the possibility of learning over long distances. The barrier of geography has been breached. Even nurses in rural communities have access to continued learning by highly qualified nurse educators. Innovative computer-based materials can provide technical training within the classroom—audio and video combining to offer a breadth of exposure previously only available through many hours at the bedside. The use of simulators has increased. This capability is becoming much more important as productivity pressures make clinical sites for student experience harder and harder to find.

How do we teach more and more information to our students without overwhelming them? And how do we maintain the underlying paradigm of care and compassion? How do we maintain the threads of patient-centered, holistic, and compassionate care within the complex scientific information our students must master? In this textbook, we hope to provide health professions educators with ideas and examples that have been used to allow students to master the facts and theory as well as the perspective of a caring professional. Implementing and adapting these methods will lead to further discovery of successful teaching strategies to keep pace with changes in the profession.

EXAMPLES OF INNOVATION

Innovative teaching strategies can range from simple to complex. Innovations can be developed for an exercise within a course to the method by which the entire course is taught. Teaching innovations can be developed for whole programs or even whole schools. They can be developed by one faculty member or by groups of faculty members. The prime objective is that the teaching strategies selected must address what needs to be learned in relation to the learning needs of students.

Think back to a favorite teacher or any strongly remembered event. Why does it stand out? What makes it unique among similar events? A major factor can be the realization that one object was completely different or out of its usually defined place, whereas the surrounding objects appeared normal. The teachers we remember often stood apart from our perception of others by only one or two details, but these details were out of the normal range. We remember the different much more than the normal, yet we can grasp only a small amount of the different and a large amount of the usual. The occasional, nondigestible, completely different piece in the sea of the expected forces our energies on analyzing not just the different piece, but also the other 99% rote material normally not given much attention and easily forgotten. Kirp, a professor of public policy, asked a former student who had become a college professor what she remembered about his teaching. He was astonished to hear that she remembered his baseball stories. She elaborated that the baseball anecdotes prodded her into thinking of him as more approachable and more human. Once she felt that way, she began to pay attention (Kirp, 1997).

Exhibit 3-1 is an example of using something different in a lesson: an analogy of pain management to the sinking of the *Titanic*. The objective is to allow students to discover how what they know applies to other situations. Students will remember more if they can make the discovery.

Art, literature, story telling, humor, and technology-assisted learning can all be used in innovative ways. Whitman and Rose (2003) had students choose their media to express their nursing philosophy. This technique required students to think differently about what they were doing and what they believed. One student

EXHIBIT 3-1

Analogy: Pain Management and the Sinking of the *Titanic*

The aftermath of bone surgery, such as ankle fusion, is a very painful procedure for patients. To create a more dynamic understanding of a patient's experience with pain and the need for appropriate pain relief measures, an analogy was used to discuss the issues involved. The choice of the *Titanic* disaster as an analogy actually came from a patient's description of the pain he felt in the postoperative period and his feeling that the nursing staff needed to pay more attention to pain relief. He felt there were times when he was totally immersed with the pain, and relief could have been started sooner and on a more even keel.

The *Titanic* was constructed with six watertight compartments that were expected to withstand a breach and keep the ship afloat. The compartments had very high walls but, unfortunately, no top. The design was appropriate for most possibilities, but not for the accident that actually happened. Students were told to think of the walls as the job of the pain medication and water as the pain. The wall of the pain medication isolates the water from the ship and the passengers' realization that they are surrounded by water. The pain is hidden. The danger lies in what happens if the water in the first compartment overflows its limit and then starts filling the second compartment. If up to three of these compartments fill with water (pain), it may not interfere with the ship's normal function; however, as the effect cascades into more of the compartments, the ship sinks by the bow until it's "all hands lost."

Patients initially don't understand that a sea of pain surrounds them. As the pain relief diminishes and they suddenly (perhaps by waking from sleep) find themselves immersed, a fear of this unexpected and uncomfortable situation is formed. This fear becomes a constant presence even after pain relief is restored, leading to anxiety and apprehension over the possibility of a repeat experience. In very painful procedures, this fear can result in clock watching over the medication schedule, as well as a compulsion to do anything to stay ahead of the pain curve. Appropriate pain relief measures, timing of administration, and other nursing measures can be discussed, continuing use of the analogy (e.g., use of lifeboats in the pain relief cycle). Students can also be taught to develop and share their own analogies to improve learning retention.

used a guitar and song to express his philosophy of healing. Another painted a brain within a heart, which symbolized her need to incorporate compassion as well as intellect into patient care. A third wrote a poem to express her feelings and beliefs. This technique used sight, touch, and movement in addition to listening, which encouraged retention postclass for both the creator of the piece and the viewer.

DEVELOPING INNOVATIVE STRATEGIES

Innovation can occur at all levels of an educational organization. Support for innovation in education may begin at the top of the organization or be developed and implemented at program or individual class levels. Success is enhanced when administrators and faculty members work side by side to plan strategically and implement changes to improve the educational milieu (Woods, 1998).

Innovation at the school level was demonstrated by a group of business school educators. These schools chose to focus more on entrepreneurship and to move away from the traditional management that prepared students to work in large organizations. This strategic innovation recognized the realities of the marketplace in a changing world. These schools set the pace for others to follow (They Create Winners, 1994). Nursing education has grown through innovation. Mildred Montag's introduction of the associate degree program in nursing, developed through research to meet an assessed need, changed the landscape of nursing education. The introduction of nurse practitioner programs also created a revolution in the profession. The physical therapy profession has endorsed the doctor of physical therapy (DPT) as the entry-level degree and strongly encouraged schools to provide transition programs for physical therapists currently in practice. The introduction of distance learning in all the health professions is the latest revolution and is growing rapidly, offering students different choices that are unfettered by the barrier of geography.

Successful innovation does not come easily and requires creativity, planning, and evaluation. **Exhibit 3-2** describes a process for educators to work through to develop innovative teaching strategies. Just as health professions call for patient assessments, the educational process calls for learning and program assessments. *Assessment* of a course, which is the first step of the process, requires a look at both strengths and problems. How can the strengths be enhanced? What needs to be changed? Educators must focus on what the expected learning outcome should be with awareness of learning theory and student learning styles and needs. Specific content requirements change often in health care, as new techniques, technologies, and research bring new knowledge needs. With the overwhelming amount of information available in today's health care world, it will not be possible to include everything students need. They will need to have appropriate resources to supplement classroom or clinical learning. The instructor must decide what and how much content will be needed, a decision that is often difficult. While addressing the content to be learned, it is also important to consider student learning needs. An understanding of the diversity in learning needs provides a foundation for the development of effective strategies.

To *define options* (the second step), the literature should be searched for research, suggestions, or techniques that could address the identified needs.

EXHIBIT 3-2

The Process of Innovation

Assessment

What is the content to be learned? What are the student learning needs? How are those needs being met? What is working and what is not?

Defining Options

How else can I look at this? Does the literature provide suggestions that would address the identified needs? Do students or other faculty members have suggestions that I could utilize?

Planning

1. Does this change require working with curriculum committees, collaborating with other faculty members, or individual instructor planning? How should this change be approached?
2. Will there be a need to work with technical specialists in the use of computer technology? Do I need additional technological knowledge to carry out this change?
3. How can I best use change theory in this planning? Who are the stakeholders who need to be considered? How and where will I meet resistance? How will I develop support?
4. How will I plan to evaluate the effectiveness of this innovation?

Gaining Support for Innovation

What resources will be needed? How will they be acquired and funded? What is the level of administrative support required and available? What strategies will I use to gain additional support if needed?

Preparing Students for the Innovation

Do I need written student instructions? If so, are they clear? Have I provided a mechanism for troubleshooting problems, and do students know how to address problems?

Preparing Faculty Members for the Innovation

If other faculty members are involved, do they need additional education? How will that be carried out? Is everyone in agreement as to how the strategy will be run? Is rehearsal time needed?

Implementing the Innovation

How much flexibility is available if the intervention is not going well? Will follow-up be needed?

Evaluating the Outcome

How will I measure the learning outcome? How have students reacted to the strategy, and can they provide input for change or improvement? If other faculty members are involved, can a consensus be reached about the direction for needed change and/or support for continuation?

Asking students or other faculty members for suggestions can also be helpful. This is the place where creativity reigns. It is important to look at many different ways to address the learning objective before selecting one. Asking the question, "Is there another way to look at this?" can be fun and lead to additional options.

Once a strategy has been selected, the third step, ***planning***, is all important. Understanding who the stakeholders are and what their investment is in the status quo or in change can be helpful in planning strategies to bring them on board. Many stakeholders, including students, do not like change and will resist new approaches. Using change theory can assist in demonstrating need and provide information that can make resisters more amenable to change. Some strategies will require curricular change, which is a complicated process and one that needs to be started early to avoid implementation delays. It is important to take time to develop support for the strategy. If this is a simple change within a course, then the instructor will need the support of students to participate effectively and not sabotage the effort. In more complex strategies, it may be important to bring in other faculty members or administrators.

Some strategies will require getting help from technical specialists, who may be able to offer support and/or instruction for using the required equipment. Time must be allotted for adequate instruction to enable faculty members and students to reach a comfort level. Most important, the technical staff must be available to help solve problems, which are bound to occur. Planning strategies for troubleshooting and providing access for problem solving for both faculty members and students need to be thought out in advance of implementation.

A part of the planning step is planning for the evaluation of the strategy. This is the time to decide what needs to be evaluated and how it should be done. This can range from how the strategy will be used in student grading to evaluating learning outcomes for the class as a whole and needs to be developed to allow student and faculty input for future development. This can also be the time to develop an educational research project, if appropriate. Educational research and publication of results are needed and can assist all of us in understanding and applying an effective educational process.

Gaining support for the innovation is the next step. Some strategies require little or no resources to implement, whereas others require significant physical and/or financial resources. If resources are needed, then gaining support for acquisition of those resources is essential. Looking at alternative sources of funding is helpful. Grants can provide a good funding source but require time and effort to secure and may be for a limited time. Administrative support may be required, but administrators may also be an excellent resource to tap to discuss potential funding or acquisition of physical resources. Once the project has been developed, it is important to validate the support of stakeholders.

Class preparation is a given in education. ***Preparing students for the innovation*** is an important step. Student instructions need to be clear and specific.

This is the time for motivating students to want to try this process and for gaining their support. Students need to know how to address problems, especially when technology is involved. There may be a learning curve required with some strategies. Students need to feel comfortable that they will not be punished for mistakes, but rather will benefit from those mistakes as part of the learning process. Evaluation methods or grading must be made clear.

Faculty members may also need preparation for the innovation. For some strategies, rehearsal time may be needed, or additional education may be required. Planning sufficient time for those activities will increase everyone's comfort level with the process. This is the time to be sure that everyone agrees about how the strategy will be run. Use of *perception, validation,* and *clarification* (I like to use the mnemonic *PVCs* when I teach students about this. Health professionals are familiar with cardiac premature ventricular contractions as PVCs, but using this term in a different context can help students relate to the term and remember it better) can be valuable here. Too often, people interpret statements differently. Checking that everyone has the same perceptions (validating) and clarifying differences can provide unity in approach to students and reduce problems of students playing one instructor against another. The guideline, "Remember your PVCs," reminds us to think about this issue.

The best part of the process is *implementing the innovation.* It is hoped that things will go well, but flexibility may be required if problems arise. Sometimes, unintended consequences, such as surfacing of emotional issues, can occur. Instructors should be alert to the need for follow-up or referral if problems arise.

Evaluating the outcome is the final step in the process. Remember that learning can continue to occur long after implementation of the strategy. It may be possible to measure short-term attainment of learning outcomes, but it may or may not be possible to explore long-term effects. For certain strategies that were developed to provide a foundation for other learning experiences, it may be possible to remeasure students at the end of their program. Students and faculty members should be able to provide input for future development and use of the strategy. A strong evaluation process provides an opportunity to participate in educational research. Even if a strategy is not suitable for research, it still may be appropriate for publication. Sharing teaching strategies presents the opportunity to improve the educational process. A catchphrase in health care today is *evidence-based practice.* We also need evidence-based practice in education.

CONCLUSION

Innovative teaching strategies must be based on both learning objectives and student learning needs. The wide diversity of student learning needs means that educators must recognize that, although most students will benefit from the new approaches, some will not. This perspective can be disappointing, but it is realistic, and educators must take pride in what they have accomplished. Problems that you could not foresee despite any amount of planning will occur. These problems, although disturbing at the time, often become humorous memories and can be addressed to improve future offerings. Developing effective teaching strategies is challenging and requires effort and persistence but can also be exceedingly rewarding and fun. Sharing those strategies with others will benefit students and faculty alike. We hope you will take advantage of the strategies presented in this book and go on to develop, implement, and share your own innovative strategies.

TEACHING EXAMPLE
Interdisciplinary Case Study Analysis

An example of an innovative strategy at the school level was the introduction of interdisciplinary case studies to health profession students. Health care providers interact daily with members of other disciplines. The mission statement of the health professions school, with programs in nursing, physical therapy, and communications sciences disorders included the following:

> While health professionals must be prepared to provide expert care within their respective disciplines, they contribute to evaluating and improving health care delivery by working in close cooperation with professionals from other disciplines. Students educated in an interdisciplinary setting, one that integrates academic and clinical pursuits, will be well-equipped to function as members of the health care team. The involvement of active practitioners from different fields in program planning, student supervision, and teaching supports such an integrated program (MGH Institute of Health Professions, 2000, p. 13).

Faculty members and administrators felt the need to strengthen the manner in which that portion of the mission statement was being addressed. Although students were exposed to a few multidisciplinary courses such as research and ethics, there was overall agreement that they needed more useful exposure to other disciplines within a clinical context. An interdisciplinary faculty task force was developed to explore possibilities. The academic dean staffed the task force and provided administrative support. After much discussion, the task force settled on a series of four required interdisciplinary clinical seminars as the preferred method.

The mechanics of developing and implementing the program were daunting, but the group was committed to the project. They enlisted other members of their departments to develop four case studies—one for each seminar. The subject of the case study would require care from each of the three disciplines, nursing, physical therapy, and speech pathology. Thought was given to the need for students to be involved with different age groups and various clinical settings. Teams of faculty members with expertise in each area developed the following cases:

- **Seminar Case 1.** Pediatric patient with cerebral palsy who is starting school.
- **Seminar Case 2.** Elderly patient with cerebral vascular accident and dysphagia in an acute care setting.

- **Seminar Case 3.** Middle-aged adult with HIV and family issues in the community (end stages of illness).
- **Seminar Case 4.** Young teen with traumatic brain injury in a rehabilitation center.

The intensive involvement of many faculty members in the development of the cases had some very beneficial effects. Interdisciplinary cooperation was necessary as the cases were developed. Faculty members were able to learn from each other and appreciate the role of the other disciplines. The faculty members who developed the cases were then invested in the project and were able to support and commend it to other faculty members and to students in their classes, which reduced some resistance.

Each program was responsible for determining which students would be required to attend the seminars. The nursing program selected students who were in the spring semester of the second year of an entry-level master's program and were enrolled in the Primary Care I course. Nursing students in this program held a baccalaureate in any field prior to entry into the program. They had completed the first year and second fall semester in the generalist level of the nursing program. They were in the process of taking the RN licensing exam during the semester (they all passed). They were in advanced-level coursework that would lead to a master's of science in nursing degree and eligibility to sit for certification as a nurse practitioner. Interdisciplinary seminar attendance was mandatory and counted as part of the clinical component in the Primary Care I course so that students would not be required to add hours to the course. Compromise and negotiation were needed on the part of the course faculty to recognize and accept that the interdisciplinary seminar was a legitimate learning experience appropriate to the course.

Scheduling the seminars was a major problem. Coordinating three programs with students in different classes and in clinical sites was very difficult. The seminars were held in the late afternoon, and students in clinical placements were asked to leave their clinical site early enough to return to the school. There is no easy answer to this problem. Each student was sent a letter outlining the purpose of the seminars and given the dates and times. The letter explained that attendance was mandatory and that the seminar would count as class hours.

Approximately 60 students were expected to attend the seminars. Four faculty members from each department were recruited to facilitate each seminar. In smaller departments, this meant that department faculty members participated in more than one seminar. The case discussions were designed so that students had an opportunity to participate in multidisciplinary groups, meet with students in their own specialty, and meet as a total group. The sessions were planned to last two hours each.

The role of the faculty members was to facilitate but not to lead the discussion among students. Faculty members were available to correct wrong information, but the focus was to have students take responsibility for explaining their discipline's role in working with the patient. Faculty members were not expected to be experts in the area under discussion or to introduce new material. The faculty role was explained to the students at the beginning of the session.

Prepreared case materials presented assessment tools used by each discipline and questions to be addressed. The goals of the seminar were presented and clarified to all of the students before breaking the large group into smaller groups. Students presented their assessments and plans for working with the patients, defining priorities of care. Faculty facilitators encouraged participation by all. Each small group took notes to be presented to the entire group for general discussion.

Evaluations of the seminars from both faculty members and students were excellent. As discussed earlier, the time selected for the seminars was problematic for many participants and seemed to be the major concern of students. Some students had various excuses for not being able to attend. Snow forced the cancellation of one session. All students attended a minimum of one seminar, but most attended the sessions as scheduled. Students remarked that the discussions were excellent and that they had gained new knowledge from each other as the different disciplinary approaches were presented. Faculty members also benefited from the discussions, and interdepartmental communications were enhanced. Some faculty members were uncomfortable at first with the expectation of their role and were concerned that they did not know enough about specific cases; however, most soon realized that the objectives of the session were valid for the level of their expertise and the expectation of facilitation, not instruction. Overall, the project was deemed a strong success and was presented again, with minor changes.

The program has now evolved toward a grand rounds format, but the commitment to interdisciplinary education remains and has expanded. Students will have at least one interdisciplinary learning experience in each year. Each department is responsible for developing the experience for their students and schoolwide presentations will be carried out each semester. A full evaluation will be completed at the end of the spring semester.

REFERENCE

MGH Institute of Health Professions. (2000). Mission statement. *MGH Institute of Health Professions Self-Study.*

REFERENCES

Kirp, D. L. (1997). Those who can't: 27 ways of looking at a classroom. *Change, 29*(3), 10–19.

They create winners. (1994). *Success, 41*(7), 43–46.

Whitman, B. L., & Rose, W. J. (2003). Using art to express a personal philosophy of nursing. *Nurse Educator, 28*(4), 166–169.

Woods, D. R. (1998). Getting support for your new approaches. *Journal of College Science Teaching, 27*(4), 285–286.

RECOMMENDED READING

Butell, S. S., O'Donovan, P., & Taylor, J. D. (2004). Educational innovations: Instilling the value of reading literature through student-led book discussion groups. *Journal of Nursing Education, 43*(1), 40–44.

Abstract: With the desire to instill the value of lifelong reading, nursing faculty and a librarian developed a student-led book discussion group as an innovative teaching strategy for a senior seminar course. Inclusion of the librarian was unique and influenced the shape and rigor of the assignment. In this assignment, students chose one of the faculty-selected books, researched its author(s), read relevant professional book reviews, and developed questions for their peer discussion groups. Student and faculty responses were positive and clearly demonstrated the benefits of this assignment for students' personal development and professional growth.

Jesse, D. E., & Blue, C. (2004). Mary Breckinridge meets Healthy People 2010: A teaching strategy for visioning and building healthy communities. *Journal of Midwifery & Women's Health, 49*(2), 126–131.

Abstract: In both midwifery and nursing education, it is essential to include innovative teaching strategies that address the health of communities. This article presents a creative learning activity for midwifery and/or nursing education that integrates Mary Breckinridge's historical example with today's national goals for building communities. The establishment of the Frontier Nursing Service in 1925 is an excellent example of the mobilize, assess, plan, implement, and track (MAP-IT) framework for building health communities. Advanced practice nursing and midwifery students can use this historical template to implement their ideas for building healthy communities today.

Kirp, D. L. (1997). Those who can't: 27 ways of looking at a classroom. *Change, 29*(3), 10–19.

Nof, L., & Hill, C. (2005). On the cutting edge—a successful distance PhD degree program: A case study [Electronic version]. *The Internet Journal of Allied Health Sciences and Practice, 3*(2). Retrieved May 10, 2006, from http://www.nova.edu/cwis/centers/hpd/allied-health/journal/articles/vol3num2/nof.htm

Travis, L., & Brennan, P. F. (1998). Information science for the future: An innovative nursing informatics curriculum. *Journal of Nursing Education, 37*(4), 162–168.

Woods, D. R. (1998). Getting support for your new approaches. *Journal of College Science Teaching, 27*(4), 285–286.

CHAPTER 4

Critical Thinking in Nursing Education

Patricia R. Cook

INTRODUCTION

Let's set the stage: The patient is a 62-year-old female admitted with anemia. Twenty-four hours prior to admission the patient fainted in the grocery store. Because of the patient's history of uterine cancer 6 years ago and the possibility of metastasis, she is admitted for a comprehensive evaluation. As a registered nurse, you admit the patient to the unit and conduct your initial interview. The patient informs you that her stools have been very dark and that she has been taking an anti-inflammatory drug for her swollen knee. Is this information related to her admitting diagnosis? What components of the patient's history should the nurse consider as relative to the current situation?

Each day health care providers are faced with situations such as this example. Nurses are required to think critically in order to deliver safe and competent nursing care. The challenge facing health care education today is to develop a curriculum that contains effective teaching/learning strategies for students to develop skills in critical thinking. Utilization of critical thinking provides a care provider with the advantage of looking at things from a point of view that is grounded in purposeful and methodical thinking. This challenge seems at face value to be fairly simple, but this task is difficult and complex for those responsible for educating tomorrow's health care professionals.

DEFINITION OF CRITICAL THINKING

Scholars from various disciplines have examined the concept of critical thinking to gain a better understanding of this process. Dewey, in an early (1933) discussion, used the phrase *reflective thinking* to describe this process. Following Dewey's contributions to understanding critical thinking, Watson and Glaser (1980) looked at critical thinking and identified three elements that make up this thinking process, namely attitude, knowledge, and skill. First, the critical thinker must have the attitude or desire to approach the problem and to accept that the problem needs to be solved. Next, the critical thinker must have knowledge of the problem's subject matter. The critical thinker then must have the necessary skills to use and manipulate this knowledge in the problem-solving process.

Ennis (1985) studied critical thinking and defined it as "reflective and reasonable thinking that is focused on deciding what to believe or do" (p. 45). He added that critical thinking is a practical activity that requires creativity in identifying hypotheses, questions, options, and ways of experimentation. Based on a philosophy background and an in-depth study of critical thinking, Paul (1993) identified critical thinking as thought that is "disciplined, comprehensive, based on intellectual standards, and as a result, well-reasoned" (p. 20). Paul related seven characteristics of the critical thinker:

1. It is thinking which is responsive to and guided by intellectual standards such as relevance, accuracy, precision, clarity, depth, and breadth.
2. It is thinking that deliberately supports the development of intellectual traits in the thinker, such as intellectual humility, intellectual integrity, intellectual perseverance, intellectual empathy, and intellectual self-discipline, among others.
3. It is thinking in which the thinker can identify the elements of thought that are present in all thinking about any problem, such that the thinker makes the logical connection between the elements and the problem at hand.
4. It is thinking that is routinely self-assessing, self-examining, and self-improving.
5. It is thinking in which there is integrity to the whole system.
6. It is thinking that yields a predictable, well-reasoned answer because of the comprehensive and demanding process that the thinker pursues.
7. It is thinking that is responsive to the social and moral imperative to not only enthusiastically argue from alternate and opposing points of view, but also to seek and identify weaknesses and limitations in one's own position. (pp. 20–23)

Probably the most substantial definition of critical thinking was developed in the late 1980s by a group of theoreticians and published by the American Philosophical Association (APA) in 1990. This group identified the critical thinker as one who is:

Habitually inquisitive, well-informed, trustful of reason, open-minded, flexible, fair-minded in evaluation, honest in facing personal biases, prudent in making judgments, willing to reconsider, clear about issues, orderly in complex matters, diligent in seeking relevant information, reasonable in the selection of criteria, focused in inquiry, and persistent in seeking results which are as precise as the subject and the circumstances of inquiry permit. (p. 3)

Nursing has used these critical thinking definitions from education and philosophy to formulate its own view of this important concept. Facione and Facione (1996) described critical thinking as purposeful, self-regulatory judgment that gives reasoned consideration to evidence, content, conceptualization, methods, and criteria. Using the APA's definition of critical thinking, Facione and Facione identified the role of one's disposition in this thinking process. Within one's disposition there are seven elements: truth-seeking, open-mindedness, analyticity, systematicity, self-confidence, inquisitiveness, and maturity. Using these seven elements, Facione and Facione (1994) developed *The California Critical Thinking Disposition Inventory (CCTDI) Test Administration Manual*. This inventory was specifically put together to assess "one's opinions, beliefs, and attitudes" (p. 3).

Bandman and Bandman (1995) discussed the issue of critical thinking and the role of reasoning in this thinking process. If individuals are critically thinking, then they will "examine assumptions, beliefs, propositions, and the meaning and uses of words, statements, and arguments" (p. 4). They continued by identifying four types of reasoning that constitute critical thinking, namely deductive, inductive, informal, and practical reasoning.

Alfaro-LeFevre (2004) discussed critical thinking and noted that critical thinking is a synonym for "reasoning . . . that involves distinct ideas, emotions, and perceptions . . ." (p. 4). She delineated a description of critical thinking and noted that critical thinking in nursing:

1. Entails purposeful, outcome-directed (results-oriented) thinking that requires careful identification of key problems, issues, and risks involved.
2. Is driven by patient, family, and community needs.
3. Is based on principles of nursing process and scientific method (for example, making judgments based on evidence rather than guesswork).
4. Uses both logic and intuition, based on knowledge, skills, and experience.
5. Is guided by professional standards and ethics codes.
6. Requires strategies that make the most of human potential (for example, using individual strengths) and compensate for problems created by human nature (for example, over-coming the powerful influence of personal views).
7. Is constantly reevaluating, self-correcting, and striving to improve. (p. 5)

IMPORTANCE IN NURSING

Enter any health care setting today, and the need for critical thinking is clearly evident. Situations in typical health care settings present a level of complexity that requires nurses to make rational and responsible decisions. Specific reasons critical thinking is needed in health care today include:

1. Situations require the nurse to process and utilize a great deal of information.
2. Information related to health care continues to expand on a daily basis.
3. Trends in health care have forced sick patients home prematurely, requiring extensive and complex home health care.

4. Changing staffing patterns in acute care facilities challenge nurses to care for high acuity patients.
5. Changes in health care—many of which we cannot begin to imagine—will continue to occur.
6. Trends in technology show continued advances in diagnostics and treatment modalities.
7. Society continues to grow in complexity, with many diverse cultures represented in American society—a trend that is expected to continue.

Today's nurse and the nurse of the future must have the ability to use valuable time to think in an effective, organized, goal-directed, and open-minded manner. Nurses must solve problems using a variety of mental processes, such as reasoning, reflection, judgment, and creativity. Nursing education has the responsibility to produce graduates who possess and utilize critical thinking. The future of the graduate depends on nursing programs that continuously evaluate their programs and implement needed changes to ensure graduates' success on the National Council Licensure Examination for Registered Nurses (NCLEX-RN) and success as a member of the nursing workforce. Therefore, teaching/learning strategies that promote the development of critical thinking need to be identified.

THE ROLE OF NURSING EDUCATION

In nursing education, the challenge of producing students who think critically needs to be met by first examining all components of the teaching/learning process—curriculum, teaching/learning strategies, and evaluation measures. If nursing education implements an effective and comprehensive curriculum, identifies useful teaching/learning strategies to teach critical thinking, and applies appropriate evaluation measures, then students will be assured that they are leaving nursing programs with skills in critical thinking. Teaching/learning strategies can be identified based on key elements of critical thinking identified by Watson and Glaser (1980), namely attitude, knowledge, and skill.

Attitude

Given any situation in nursing, students must first recognize that a problem exists and is worthy of solving. Faculty must utilize teaching/learning strategies that instill an attitude of curiosity and caring. From the first day of class until graduation, nursing faculty present common health care problems and relate them to needed nursing interventions. Clinical experiences provide students with opportunities to apply the concepts of nursing care in real-life situations. This introduction to real-life situations promotes the interest of students and develops beginning awareness of the many problems to be solved. Instructors play an important part in developing an attitude of inquiry by guiding students to ask questions, examine or challenge current practices, look for answers, and evaluate various factors in the delivery of nursing care.

Knowledge

The issue of what to include in a nursing curriculum continues to frustrate nursing faculty. Today's knowledge of disease and illness has never been greater. Therefore, nursing faculty must evaluate the content of their curricula and include concepts that focus on developing a knowledge base that is applicable to multiple situations. Curriculum forms the structure for presenting concepts that provide the foundation for the development of critical thinking in nursing.

With a sound curriculum in place, nursing education is faced with identifying teaching/learning strategies that promote learning and the development of critical thinking. Unfortunately, there is no simple answer to developing the skill called "critical thinking." In her discussion of teaching methods, Klaassens (1988) identified four principles for teaching critical thinking: First, the teaching method should move systematically through the stages of readiness, introduction, reinforcement, and extension. Second, it should be focused, moving from introduction of task and explanation of steps to presentation, supervised practice, and return demonstration by the student. Third, this method should blend with the typical topics, and fourth, it should guide students through the steps of knowledge acquisition—ending in formal thinking.

The traditional strategy for imparting knowledge in a nursing classroom has been lecture. Although students often prefer this teaching strategy, it does little to stimulate critical thinking. Today, nursing education has many teaching/learning strategies that promote the development of critical thinking. Using a variety of tools assists students with various learning styles to be effective learners. Selection and utilization of a variety of teaching/learning strategies requires the commitment of instructors to seek teaching/learning strategies that match students' cognitive level as well as the content being presented.

In 1979, Steinaker and Bell identified an experiential taxonomy for use in planning and evaluating educational programs. Using a taxonomy reinforces that teaching/learning strategies should be evaluated and implemented based on the strategy's ability to reinforce learning where the student is at the time of the expected learning. The taxonomy developed by Steinaker and Bell has five categories, with varying levels within each category. These categories include exposure, participation, identification, internalization, and dissemination. The categories of exposure, participation, and identification are used to discuss the framework for appropriate teaching/learning strategies. The categories of internalization and dissemination are not being used because they require more experience within the practice of nursing following graduation from nursing programs.

Exposure

The category of exposure is used at the introduction level, at which the student is aware of the experience, begins to form mental reactions to the stimuli, and becomes prepared for more experience. At this level, the instructor is setting the stage for learning—in other words, presenting basic concepts. The goal is to develop skill in applying knowledge in the delivery of nursing care, but students must acquire knowledge prior to application. At this stage in learning, lecture is an effective strategy for the introduction of the content; however, students need additional teaching/learning strategies that offer them the opportunity to manipulate and process basic content.

The following strategies are effective tools in applying basic concepts:

1. ***Study Guides:*** In this strategy, students seek out basic information related to the subject topic. The guide directs students to answer questions about the subject. Instructors can be creative in developing study guides and can use patient scenarios to promote beginning application thinking. Use of study guides encourages students to independently seek out information, which was supported by Rubenfeld and Scheffer (2006) in their comment that educators must "move toward learning partnerships focused on students discovering things for themselves" (p. 85). For many students, this beginning level of empowerment encourages them to be more responsible for their learning—a basic need for the critical thinker. As students study new material, ample opportunity that encourages students to ask why or how must be provided because this increases the value of one's learning new information (Nugent and Vitale, 2004).

2. ***Case Studies:*** Using case studies to apply concepts is nothing new to nursing education. Using examples of how concepts are applied in a clinical setting encourages students to think about how concepts relate to real-life situations. Case studies can be developed with varying levels of difficulty—ranging from the simple application of principles of hot and cold to the application of multiple concepts in the care of the burn patient.

When using case studies at the exposure level, simple situations, focusing on specific focus concepts, should be included. Although case studies are often used as independent work for the student, they also are useful in the classroom. Case studies can be used as a class activity to teach students to think on their feet and to reinforce the need to understand concepts in real-life situations. In other words, case studies take facts and use them in practical ways. This type of application shows students how selected interventions focus on outcomes for the patient (Youngblood & Beitz, 2001).

3. ***Group Discussions:*** With the participation of students in classroom discussions, students learn from other students while developing their personal thinking skills. In this setting, students challenge each other's ideas and opinions, which is an important component to critical thinking (Linderman & McAthie, 1999). When using an in-class activity such as group discussions, faculty need to continuously monitor the use of thinking and thoughtfulness and intervene as appropriate to redirect the group—if necessary.

4. ***Writing:*** Students at all levels of a nursing curriculum can benefit from writing. At the basic level, students use concepts and build them into current knowledge as well as previous experiences. Development of papers requires the application of various tools of critical thinking, such as blending of concepts, determining priorities, and formulating conclusions (Nugent & Vitale, 2004). Using writing assignments provides the faculty with an opportunity to assess what students are learning and how well they process the new concepts.

Participation

At the second level of the taxonomy, students have purposeful interaction with the experience. Many of the exposure strategies also are suitable for the participation level, namely writing, case studies, and computer-based interactive programs. Teaching/learning strategies at the participation level require recurrent thinking, however, because previously learned foundational concepts need to be used as students build on and learn beyond the basics. Writing, for example, requires students to move beyond the basic concepts and to use or apply them to a situation.

Writing at the participation level promotes student recognition that patient situations are not textbook and that they require the selection of interventions appropriate to that specific patient. In her discussion of a writing project conducted in California, Olson (1992) identified four levels or domains of writing—sensory/descriptive, imaginative/narrative, practical/informative, and analytical/expository. The domain of sensory/descriptive is writing built on concrete concepts or points. The goal at this level is to center and focus on basic information. At the next level, students construct a story by means of identifying, sequencing, and capturing significant details. At the practical/informative level, students "learn accuracy, clarity, attention to facts, appropriateness to tone, and conventional forms" (p. 23). At the last level of the domain, students are expected to use the tasks of analysis, interpretation, and persuasion. Olson noted that these domains are not completely separate, and interdependency does exist among the levels.

Case studies used at the participation level should involve more creativity and reasoning than those used at the exposure level. With more knowledge, students can be challenged to bring together concepts that have an increasing number of variables. For example, at the exposure level, students learn to identify the role of vital signs in the assessment of their patients. At the participation level, students should begin identifying the alterations in vital signs that occur when diseases affect the body and should identify needed interventions.

Other teaching/learning strategies appropriate for the participation level include:

1. ***Problem-Solving Team:*** Using groups to work as a team provides an opportunity for the students to share ideas and knowledge while working on a common goal or outcome. For this strategy to be effective, the instructor must provide clear objectives with specific instructions. Brookfield (1987) identified themes characterizing critical thinking. One of those themes related to critical thinkers is the use of imagination and exploration of alternatives. Teamwork provides ample opportunity to spark imagination and creativity for the situation presented. Typically, group discussion leads to the identification of many alternatives; the group then evaluates and selects the needed interventions. This type of teaching/learning strategy promotes a second theme identified by Brookfield, namely, the importance of context in critical thinking. No nursing or patient care situation is identical to another. Students must be able to assess each situation and to implement the required interventions. According to Linderman and McAthie (1999), when knowledge guides practice, it takes into consideration all other information gained through complementary means.

2. ***Computer-Assisted Instruction (CAI):*** CAI programs are effective tools to reinforce concepts. At the participation level, students using CAI programs are called on to problem solve using a variety of components of crit-

ical thinking. Today, a variety of computer-based interactive programs are available for students. Many continue to use a linear format, taking students through a series of screens with little to no variation. Other, more creative software programs use a branching format that allows more student control. According to Nugent and Vitale (2004), as CAI meets student needs, learning is more efficient, study time is managed better, and students are more motivated. It is important that nursing faculty select CAI programs that are appropriate for the students' knowledge and problem-solving level.

3. ***Reflective Journals:*** Students' use of journals is an important tool to encourage reflection on an experience and to evaluate one's performance and/or responses to the experience. Reflection provides an opportunity to weigh, consider, and choose (Adams & Hamm, 1994). Use of a reflective journal encourages students to think about their experiences and to examine the components as well as the overall experience. To be effective, instructors need to give specific guidelines on what information to include in the journal. For example, the student first describes the patient care situation. Next, students provide an analysis of significant events in the delivery of patient care and an exploration of feelings, reactions, and responses. Critical thinking is developed further when students are asked to identify decisions made or priorities set during the clinical experience. In the last phase of journal writing, students "examine the outcomes of the reflective process" (Bratt, 1998, p. 1). After this examination, students often identify changes to be made in future experiences.

4. ***Problem-Based Learning:*** This teaching/learning strategy focuses primarily on process. A small student group works on a case study with the assistance of a faculty facilitator. This strategy links theory with clinical situations and encourages reasoning in a realistic situation using collaboration and negotiation within the group. See Chapter 9 for more information on this strategy.

5. ***Mind (Concept) Mapping:*** This simple, but effective teaching/learning strategy requires students to develop word pictures for a specific patient problem. There are a variety of ways these maps can be constructed, but they all focus on helping students to reason, prioritize, and link the various components to a patient problem with nursing actions. Students conclude this activity with a holistic view of the situation at hand (Schuster, 2002). See Chapter 26 for more information on this strategy.

6. ***Questioning:*** Using questioning to reinforce learning is an excellent tool in the development of critical thinking. The use of questioning as a teaching tool can be traced back to Socrates in ancient Greece. Socratic questioning examines basic concepts or points, explores deeper into these

concepts, and attends to problem areas of one's thinking (Paul, 1993). One effective way to use questioning is in a game format. It is easy to adapt popular games to the content being discussed. Gaming can be very effective because it infuses fun into learning.

Identification

At the identification level, students become more active learning partners. Students identify with the experience at an emotional and personal level. As the experience becomes a part of the students, they desire to share the experience with others. As previously noted, teaching/learning strategies such as writing, case studies, and CAI continue to be important learning tools in the category of identification. With each of these strategies, there needs to be increasing complexity with more variables.

Additional teaching/learning strategies at the identification level should focus on organizing and applying concepts. Instructors play an important role at this level because they must rely on teaching/learning strategies that engage students to think in more complex situations with more variables. Other teaching/learning strategies for the identification category include:

1. ***Defensive Testing:*** Students at this level need to be challenged more on why they select one option over another. They need to recognize that nursing care is based on principles and knowing which principle matches a specific situation, in other words, matching knowledge to the appropriate context. This strategy also provides students the opportunity to reflect on their understanding of the material being tested. Additionally, they are providing rationalization to their answers.
2. ***Debates and Critiques:*** Having students critique an article or other type of work provides a means of reinforcing the six critical thinking abilities identified by Linderman and McAthie (1999). These abilities include identifying possibilities/innovations, formulating and analyzing arguments, constructing meaning, using knowledge as context, negotiating, and critically reflecting on one's thoughts and actions. Seeking information and analyzing its meaning move students beyond basic concepts and challenge traditional use of these concepts. The strategy of debating is effective to developing critical thinking because it prepares students "to doubt, to challenge what is held to be true" (Smith, 1990, p. 104). If a student is required to debate the issue of abortion, he or she will formulate in-depth critical thinking about the purpose of abortion, its impact on a woman, and how society views access to this intervention. See Chapter 11 for information on the use of debate.

3. ***Problem-Based Learning:*** With this teaching/learning strategy, students actively participate in problem solving. Discussion focuses on the problems presented in the case study and the identification of knowledge from previous experience with the identified problem(s).

Skill

Once students have developed an attitude of inquiry and the knowledge base needed, they need an opportunity to develop and apply knowledge in real-life situations. In nursing, these real-life situations are found in clinical settings. According to Adams and Hamm (1994), knowledge is beneficial only to the degree that it can be used to produce new knowledge.

The learning lab typically is located at the school of nursing and provides a tremendous opportunity for simulated learning. Although the learning lab traditionally has been used for learning of psychomotor skills, it offers students a safe, controlled environment to develop critical thinking. As students' nursing knowledge increases over the span of the curriculum, instructors can use a high-fidelity patient simulator to create situations in the learning lab that promote student exploration into the various options available for nursing care (without injury to the patient). In this nonthreatening environment, students are provided the opportunity to question, explore, and experiment using a simulated patient scenario. Students can apply reasoning skills without the constraints of limited time and reflect upon decisions made during the course of the experience. See Chapter 15 for more discussion of the use of high-fidelity simulators to promote student learning.

The clinical setting is identified as any setting where students provide nursing care to real patients. Today, clinical settings range from in-hospital units to homeless clinics in the community. In these clinical settings, learning opportunities to develop critical thinking abound. The challenge of all clinical instructors is to construct clinical experiences that maximize student learning. The clinical setting requires students to be familiar with their patients' health problems, medications, procedures, and lab data. Using their knowledge of the textbook patient, students are challenged to develop skills in critical thinking in their efforts to implement appropriate care for an actual patient.

Care of patients in real-life situations reinforces that critical thinking is contextual. Although the textbook lists specific interventions for patients with pneumonia, students must recognize the care needed for a *specific* patient at a *specific* time. Using a variety of mental processes, such as reasoning, prioritizing, judging, and inferring, students are able to select needed interventions. As knowledge and clinical skills develop, students' skills in critical thinking increase.

There is no best style for instruction in the clinical setting; however, several points should be considered to increase the effectiveness of the clinical experience.

1. Questioning by the instructor is an important part of the clinical experience. This process encourages students to think about the options available and to select an intervention appropriate to a *specific* patient. A good technique to use when questioning students is asking the student to talk aloud while answering the instructor's questions (Corcoran, Narayan, & Moreland, 1988). Using this technique assists instructors in evaluating students' processing skills. Did they use appropriate reasoning skills? Was there a logical correlation between data and problem identification? Was the nursing process used appropriately, with logical sequencing of data, problem, goals, strategies or interventions, evaluation, and follow-up with changes? Was there effective prioritization for the patient?

2. Students should be encouraged to test their thinking. Many health care alternatives are available today, and students need to explore what is best for their patients. The clinical setting provides the instructor with the opportunity to teach students on a one-on-one basis. Instructors need to seek every occasion when students perform correctly to verbally praise the student. Although clinical training is stressful and challenging, students need and deserve positive reinforcement of effective problem solving using critical thinking.

3. Instructors need to empower students to think critically. Students who feel a sense of empowerment take responsibility for the process of problem solving.

4. Instructors must see the importance and impact of role modeling. Using the teaching/learning strategy of modeling includes "leading the student through thoughts and experiences to one's own conclusions" (Reilly & Oermann, 1992, p. 331).

5. Written work related to clinical experiences is an important component in developing critical thinking. Students have the opportunity to take textbook patients and to select suitable interventions for their patients. The exercise of individualizing nursing care reinforces the conceptuality of critical thinking and the need to explore all available options for patient care.

Kurfiss (1988) discussed the elements of what she called *cognitive apprenticeship*, which include modeling or demonstration, coaching or assisting, guiding with gradual removal of the guidance, articulating or reasoning, reflecting or comparing, and exploring goals and options. All of these elements can be accomplished with clinical experiences. Clinical experiences expose students to the dynamic world of health care and practice with multiple concepts. Whether collecting data and relating their role to the patient's condition or developing an argument on why one intervention is better than another, students are developing skills in critical thinking. See Chapters 21 and 27 for more discussion of clinical instruction.

EVALUATION OF CRITICAL THINKING

In 1991, the National League for Nursing revised its criteria for accreditation and incorporated the need for evaluation of critical thinking in undergraduate nursing programs. The National League for Nursing Accrediting Commission (2005) recently reiterated its support of the need for critical thinking as noted in its core competencies for nursing educational programs. The American Association of Colleges of Nursing also emphasized critical thinking, as noted in its *Essentials of Baccalaureate Education for Professional Nursing Practice* (1998). Since this notable recognition of critical thinking and its role as a competency for nursing, educators have explored, pondered, and discussed how critical thinking should be evaluated. While there is agreement on the need for critical thinking for all nurses, a consensus is absent on how critical thinking is defined and how it can be measured (Ali, Bantz, & Siktberg, 2005); however, evaluation of critical thinking is an important component of nursing education. Work within nursing education over the last few years has seen the identification of alternative options to evaluating critical thinking skills, such as concept maps and context-dependent testing (Daley, Shaw, Balistrieri, Glasenapp, & Piacentine, 1999; Oermann, Truesdell, & Ziolkowski, 2000).

Teaching and evaluation clearly go hand in hand. Nursing education is challenged to identify and/or develop tools for evaluating critical thinking that reflect the individual program's definition and philosophy. With the use of multiple means of evaluation, nursing education gains a better understanding of teaching critical thinking and the impact of this instruction on student learning. Students should see evaluation as a learning tool; it is a positive means for determining the need for additional learning, further clarification, and/or added directions by instructors.

CONCLUSION

Nursing education's challenge to produce a nurse who can think critically has never been greater. Changing health care, increased acuity of patients, and a dynamic culture offer a tremendous challenge for nurses. Nursing education must attune itself to the task of reexamining the concept of critical thinking.

This reexamination includes evaluation of all components of the teaching/learning process—curriculum, teaching/learning strategies, and evaluation measures. With the development of an effective curriculum, nursing education must create an attitude of inquiry in its students, develop the knowledge base needed, and provide ample opportunities for students to use their knowledge. Using a taxonomy such as the Steinaker and Bell (1979) model provides an excellent framework to approach the development of critical thinking skills. In selecting approaches to develop critical thinking skills, nursing faculty can assure their students that as health care workers of tomorrow they will possess the necessary skills needed to deliver safe and competent nursing care.

REFERENCES

Adams, D. M., & Hamm, M. E. (1994). *Cooperative learning: Critical thinking and collaboration across the curriculum.* Springfield, IL: Charles C Thomas Publisher.

Alfaro-LeFevre, R. (2004). *Critical thinking and clinical judgment: A practical approach.* Philadelphia: W. B. Saunders.

Ali, N. S., Bantz, D., & Siktberg, L. (2005). Validation of critical thinking skills in online responses. *Journal of Nursing Education, 44*(2), 90–96.

American Association of Colleges of Nursing. (1998). *The essentials of baccalaureate education for professional nursing practice.* Washington, DC: Author.

American Philosophical Association. (1990). *Critical thinking: A statement of expert consensus for purposes of educational assessment and instruction. The Delphi report: Committee on pre-college philosophy* (ERIC Document Reproduction Service No. ED 315-423).

Bandman, E. L., & Bandman, D. (1995). *Critical thinking in nursing.* Norwalk, CT: Appleton & Lange.

Bratt, M. M. (1998). Reflective journaling: Fostering learning in clinical experiences. *Dean's Notes, 20*(1), 1–3.

Brookfield, S. (1987). *Developing critical thinkers: Challenging adults to explore alternative ways of thinking and acting.* San Francisco: Jossey-Bass.

Corcoran, S., Narayan, S., & Moreland, H. (1988). Thinking aloud as a strategy to improve clinical decision making. *Heart & Lung, The Journal of Critical Care, 17*(5), 463–468.

Daley, B. J., Shaw, C. R., Balistrieri, T., Glasenapp, K., & Piacentine, L. (1999). Concept maps: A strategy to teach and evaluate critical thinking. *Journal of Nursing Education, 38*(1), 42–47.

Dewey, J. (1933). *How we think: A restatement of the relation of reflective thinking to the educative process.* Chicago: Regnery.

Ennis, R. N. (1985). A logical basis for measuring critical thinking skills. *Educational Leadership, 43*(2), 44–48.

Facione, N., & Facione, P. A. (1994). *The California Critical Thinking Disposition Inventory (CCTDI) test administration manual.* Millbrae, CA: The California Academic Press.

Facione, N., & Facione, P. A. (1996). Externalizing the critical thinking in knowledge development and clinical judgment. *Nursing Outlook, 44*(3), 129–136.

Klaassens, E. L. (1988). Improving teaching for thinking. *Nurse Educator, 13*(6), 15–19.

Kurfiss, J. G. (1988). *Critical thinking: Theory, research, practice, and possibilities.* College Station, TX: Association for the Study of Higher Education.

Linderman, C., & McAthie, M. (1999). *Fundamentals of contemporary nursing practice.* Philadelphia: W. B. Saunders.

National League for Nursing. (1991). *Criteria and guidelines for evaluation of baccalaureate nursing programs.* New York: Author.

National League for Nursing Accrediting Commission. (2005). *Accreditation manual with interpretive guidelines.* New York: Author.

Nugent, P. M., & Vitale, B. A. (2004). *Test success: Test-taking techniques for beginning nursing students.* Philadelphia: F. A. Davis Company.

Oermann, M., Truesdell, S., & Ziolkowski, L. (2000). Strategy to assess, develop, and evaluate critical thinking. *The Journal of Continuing Education in Nursing, 31*(4), 155–160.

Olson, C. B. (1992). *Thinking/writing: Fostering critical thinking through writing.* New York: HarperCollins.

Paul, R. W. (1993). *Critical thinking: What every person needs to know to survive in a rapidly changing world.* Pohnert Park, CA: Center for Critical Thinking.

Reilly, D. E., & Oermann, M. H. (1992). *Clinical teaching in nursing education.* New York: National League for Nursing.

Rubenfeld, M. G., & Scheffer, B. K. (2006). *Critical thinking TACTICS for nurses: Tracking, assessing, and cultivating thinking to improve competency-based strategies.* Sudbury, MA: Jones and Bartlett Publishers.

Schuster, P. M. (2002). *Concept mapping: A critical-thinking approach to care planning.* Philadelphia: F. A. Davis Company.

Smith, R. (1990). *To think.* New York: Teachers College Press.

Steinaker, N. W., & Bell, M. R. (1979). *The experiential taxonomy: A new approach to teaching and learning.* New York: Academic Press.

Watson, F., & Glaser, E. M. (1980). *Watson-Glaser critical thinking appraisal.* Dallas: Psychological Corporation.

Youngblood, N., & Beitz, J. M. (2001). Developing critical thinking with active learning strategies. *Nurse Educator, 26*(1), 39–42.

CHAPTER 5

Creativity: A Collaborative Process

Carol Picard, Ellen M. Landis, and Lynn Minnick

According to Bohm (1998), the Nobel prize-winning physicist, creativity is an elemental process and the natural order of the universe. We are inherently and constantly in a creative process responding to our context in a biological effort of survival. For human beings, creativity is the ability to perceive patterns of relationship and intentionally construct patterns in relatively novel ways. Creativity engages one's imagination. It takes shape through reflection on one's experience in the world. Philosopher and paleontologist Teilhard de Chardin (1959) identified the human capacity for reflection and creative expression as its contribution to evolution—the noosphere, or thinking layer of the world.

Though the health care professions acknowledge the importance of creativity to practice, Fasnacht (2003) suggests that the refinement of the concept of creativity still needs clarification. For example, despite Corita Kent's statement, "To create is to relate" (1992, p. 5), creativity is still too often regarded as an individual process rather than a collaborative one. Some educators, however, are beginning to emphasize collaborative generativity. Kent would have applauded this approach, because she believed that learning exercises that encourage the ability to connect and see new relationships foster a creative response to living. To be in a creative state of mind, one must have an attitude of interest that is wholehearted and total. Energy is not expended on protecting the self, but instead, energy is released and free from the creative imaginative process.

Bohm described the need for openness, acknowledging barriers to the creative process in human beings. Cultural blocks or conditions may prevent creativity from being expressed. Society, as well as educational institutions, tends to "conformist, imitative and mechanical states of mind" that do not disturb the established order (Bohm, 1998, p. 16). Faculty face these barriers as they work to prepare professionals who are competent and creative as beginning practitioners. An additional barrier particular to educating health care practitioners is the amount of content required to be competent, which can sometimes overshadow the process of reflection and creativity. Watson (1999) cautions that current health care practitioner education often values the powerful prevailing medical discourse, where data and content are emphasized over experience and reflection. Charon (2001) agrees, stating, "a scientifically competent medicine alone cannot help a patient grapple with the loss of health or find meaning in suffering" (p. 1897). Watson faults the technical and instrumental focus in the current health care environment as contributing to the lack of time devoted to the ontology of competence in clinical education and practice.

Watson, as well as Benner et al. (1996) critique teaching strategies in health care practitioners' education that value critical thinking devoid of emotion. Also, Rees (2004) points out that the ritual of routine and the speed at which health care practitioners must often respond to patients are disincentives to creativity. The challenge is to foster creative responses to professional situations that are grounded in clinical knowledge. On this basis, Charon (2001) has advocated for the cultivation of narrative competence in medical education. Narrative competence is defined as "the ability to acknowledge, absorb, interpret, and act on the stories and plights of others" (p. 1897). Cultivating openness and self-awareness can support this goal. It is an openness of mind that Belenky and colleagues (1986) say is responsible for conception of ideas necessary for accepting health conditions and options. A creative exploration of boundaries in academic and clinical sites is an essential practice throughout career development. Though some educators may not be comfortable with an attitude of openness when curricula is content driven, reflection remains an important element in cultivating critical thinking. Bateson (1994) explains that emphasis on a single activity teaches us to devalue multisensory awareness. She further recognizes the learning potential in attending to relational as well as technical information. Today, such multimodal learning is thought of in terms of interdisciplinary reflexive learning and expanded systemic thinking (Landis, Baldwin, & Thompson, 2004).

The innovative methods included in this text are examples of collaborative creativity in health care professionals' education. Fostering creativity enhances the potential for knowledge development in all disciplines because no two students are alike, and their ways of exploring phenomena of concern to their profession will also be unique.

THEORETICAL RATIONALE

The goal of creative strategies in clinical education is to foster openness and a creative attitude in students. Creative strategies present opportunities for students to increase their awareness, which is a process of self-discovery. Watson recommended that health care practitioners develop an awareness of self-in-relation, which is an essential component of transpersonal caring-healing, and the essence of postmodernism. Watson encourages practitioners to reflect on energy, consciousness, and caring as the basis for practice. Newman's (1994) theory of health as expanding consciousness describes the uniqueness of each person's pattern. Philosopher Bachelard (1994) illustrates the role of imagination in creativity as the link between what is and what is not, our subjective world and the experience of others, putting imagination at the very center of what it is to be human. Shotter (1993) affirms the creative process as primary to avoid becoming entrapped within the confines of narratives, metaphors, and theories about life. The extent to which someone is enmeshed in and estranged from a system is related to one's ability to affect and be affective in that system (Pearce & Cronen, 1980). Skills for imaginative inquiry support opening new avenues of communication to explore existing knowledge.

Expanding cognition is supported by creative activities. By collaboratively reflecting on one's own patterns of response and engagement with others and the environment, consciousness expands. Newman (1994) encourages practitioners to embody theory, melding theory and practice in a praxis approach to caring in the human health experience. Her theory is not something so much to apply as it is to become. The teacher establishes a mindful presence to foster openness in students as a mirror or model for what students can later do with patients and families. Vacarr (2001) approaches her role as an educator with a strategy that includes public expressions of vulnerability. By normalizing unexpected and unpredictable action, teachers and students become aware of transformational opportunities. Baldwin (2005) recognizes:

> Collaborative creativity as one of the most powerful resources we have for transforming difficult situations into opportunities for growth. Yet, when we are overwhelmed by situations we feel we cannot resolve, we tend to lose this capacity, reacting, instead of responding reflectively, narrowing our range of behavior, often isolating ourselves from others. (p. 1)

A creative approach is one requiring alertness and sensitivity. Although establishing a knowledge base can sometimes require habitual processes of thinking such as rote learning and memorization of facts, such activity can become a barrier to mindfulness. Calling students' attention to their capacity for expanding awareness can support energy availability for creative responses to situations. Using resources and methods that are not typical for the health professions, students can enhance the creative process because these methods are antidotes to ordinary habits of mind. Techniques involving several senses, or the use of poetry or film as artistic expressions of concepts and situations in the classroom example can enliven focus on the subject at hand. Developing a practice that prioritizes practitioners' own creativity also helps prevent burnout (Albarran, 2004).

CONDITIONS

Two important conditions support creative strategies. The first is safety. Because creative strategies foster openness, students may feel vulnerable as a result. Students must have confidence that the teacher is going to create a safe place for any risk taking of sharing ideas or feelings. As part of this creation of safe space, students must feel free to pass on any part of an activity. This freedom allows students their sense of empowerment and encourages their ability to make important choices. Secondly, the teacher sets the tone of respect for the contributions of all participants. Because some activities, such as those described in the teaching example, might cause a student to feel uncomfortable, the tone of respect is also the expectation of the teacher for the attitude of the whole group.

Creative activities can be part of a wide variety of teaching situations. The teacher is limited only by his or her own imagination and of course codes of ethical conduct. The goal is to cultivate an open, wholehearted spirit of inquiry. This creative act is teaching at its best. In preparing a lecture, ask yourself: How will students understand this new knowledge? How does it come alive? This is part of the teacher's creative process. In planning a lecture, sift through multiple sources on the topic, both from within and without the discipline. Let students know that it is assumed they have read from some sources and will come together in dialogue. The goal is to make the material come alive so the students can engage with it.

TYPES OF LEARNERS

These strategies can be used with both graduate and undergraduate students and have been used in professional development programs by the authors.

USING THE METHOD

In preparing for a lecture/discussion on caring for patients with mood disorders, the knowledge needed to care for a depressed person includes not only diagnostic criteria, etiological theories, and standard professional care interventions, but also an appreciation of the cultural experience of depression. To invite the students to reflect on this state, Carol Picard starts the class with a poem by Sharon Olds entitled, "Summer Solstice, New York City" (1987). The poem depicts a suicidal person on a rooftop and those who rescue him. Other poetry on illness and disability by health care professionals is available in anthologies (Belli & Coulehan, 1998; Davis & Schaefer, 1995). Weaving the poetic knowledge with the clinical descriptions and personal stories of patients, as well as inviting students to share their own knowledge of how depression is experienced, begins to color the class.

Frequently, students have cared for a person with depression in their clinical setting that week and can illustrate with their new experiences. Others draw on experiences with close friends, relatives, or sometimes personal experiences. Former patients and expert practitioners are invited to the classroom to share their experiences. For example, when discussing the value of electroconvulsive therapy (ECT), we use a patient-education videotape on the topic, which brings the students to the bedside while the treatment is occurring. Because the treatment is still perceived by much of the lay public as something to be feared, Picard also shows them why older people may have a great deal of anxiety. Many younger students have never seen the film *One Flew Over the Cuckoo's Nest*. Using excerpts from the film helps students to appreciate an American iconic image of ECT, which their patients may remember. Class is over when students collaboratively examine the learning and consider what all of this means to their practice.

Creative Identification

Creativity may also be seen as the stretch of ourselves beyond what we perceive as pedestrian and inattentive behavior and reaching in to an exaggerated multisensory experience. Creativity looks different in different people. However, there are similar components to how people describe the experience for themselves. Thinking about one's own creativity, relating to it, acknowledging it as an important part of life makes it easier to bring creativity to the everyday experiences of problem solving in training experiences as well as to professional collaboration with clients and colleagues.

Visualization

1. Visualize yourself being creative, whether that be dancing, playing basketball, playing music, designing an outfit, cooking a meal or developing a creative program for your family, or professionally. Then, write, draw, sculpt, or move about the experience of being creative; your impressions, thoughts, feelings, even body memories are useful information to reflect on. You can break it down into stages of creativity.

Dialogue and Action

2. The class breaks into small groups of two or three people. Divide up the remaining time for this activity so each person has the same amount of

time to talk. One person at a time talks about his or her creativity. The listeners are invited to share ideas based on how they are impacted by witnessing how the presenter expresses an understanding of his or her creativity. Then the next person shares what she or he chooses to about creativity and the listeners are again invited to give feedback (Baldwin, 2005).

3. Include time for the facilitator to wrap up with the learning opportunity, applying themes from the exercise that represent the learning goals of the course.

TEACHING EXAMPLE

Developing Collaborative Creativity Skills

This activity by Ellen Landis was first used in a play therapy course for master's candidates in a variety of health care professions at Lesley University in Cambridge, Massachusetts. Most of these students had worked professionally in the health care field prior to returning to school or had experiences in the field through internships. The theme for the day was self-care for the professional. The class began with a lecture on burnout prevention, introduced the frequency and risk of secondary trauma for professionals as well as thoughts and behaviors to watch out for. An experience on self-care followed, addressing the sociocultural elements of creating an environment that meets the needs of a diverse workforce.

Landis brought out just one box full of inexpensive supplies such as balloons, ribbon, colored markers, paper, and scissors. The class divided into small groups of four people. They were all instructed to collaboratively create a safe place for them as students and professionals to decompress from the stress of their job. They needed to make decisions about their priorities and find a way to express their ideas using the simple supplies. They were asked to create a performance piece that could include the development of creating a safe place. Each group took supplies, discussed their concerns and came up with a performance piece. The activity was followed up with a group discussion. Themes that emerged include: bringing a spirit of fun to difficult work, bringing a sense of calm to the job, being a good listener, bringing ideas to the table, as well as bringing conflict resolution skills to the job.

Since people often seek health care when there is an acute situation, a crisis, or an emergency, students recognize the inherent stress related to their work. This trilogy of evidence-based, theory-driven, reflective practice brought students together in affirmation of their goal to be part of a work environment that brings out the best in people, whether that is the patient or the professional.

REFERENCES

Albarran, J. W. (2004). Creativity: An essential element of critical care nursing practice. *Nursing in Critical Care, 9*(2), 47–49.

Bachelard, G. (1994). *The poetics of space.* Boston: Beacon.

Baldwin, R. (2005). *Sharevision.* Amherst, MA: Sharevision, Inc.

Bateson, M. C. (1994). *Peripheral visions: Learning along the way.* New York: HarperCollins Publisher.

Belenky, M., Clinchy, B. M., Goldberger, N. R., & Tarule, J. M. (1986). *Women's ways of knowing: The development of self, voice, and mind.* New York: Basic Books.

Belli, A., & Coulehan, J. (Eds.). (1998). *Blood & bone.* Iowa City: University of Iowa Press.

Benner, P., Tanner, C., & Chesla, C. (1996). *Expertise in nursing practice.* New York: Springer.

Bohm, D. (1998). *On creativity.* New York: Routledge.

Charon, R. (2001). Narrative medicine: A model for empathy, reflection, profession, and trust. *Journal of the American Medical Association, 286*(15), 1897–1902.

Davis, C., & Schaefer, J. (Eds.). (1995). *Between the heartbeats.* Iowa City: University of Iowa Press.

Fasnacht, P. H. (2003). Creativity: A refinement of the concept for nursing practice. *Journal of Advanced Nursing, 41*(2), 195–202.

Kent, C. (1992). *Learning by heart: Teaching to free the creative spirit.* New York: Bantam.

Landis, E., Baldwin, R., & Thompson, L. (2004). Expressive arts therapy: A voice from the USA. In *Context.* London: The Invicta Press.

Newman, M. (1994). *Health as expanding consciousness.* Sudbury, MA: Jones & Bartlett.

Olds, S. (1987). *The gold cell.* New York: Alfred Knopf.

Pearce, W. B., & Cronen, V. (1980). *Communication, action, and meaning: The creation of social rules.* New York: Praeger.

Rees, C. (2004). Celebrate creativity. *Nursing Standard, 19*, 14–16, 20–21.

Shotter, J. (1993). *Conversational realities: Constructing life through language.* London: Sage Publications.

Teilhard de Chardin, P. (1959). *The phenomenon of man.* New York: Harper & Row.

Vacarr, B. (2001). Moving beyond political correctness: Practicing mindfulness in the diverse classroom. *Harvard Educational Review, 71*(2), 285–295.

Watson, J. (1999). *Postmodern nursing and beyond.* New York: Churchill Livingstone.

RECOMMENDED READING/VIEWING

Brookfield, S. (1995). *Becoming a critically reflective teacher.* San Francisco: Jossey-Bass.

Bryner, A., & Markova, D. (1996). *An unused intelligence.* Berkeley, CA: Conari Press.

Diaz, A. (1992). *Freeing the creative spirit.* San Francisco: Harper.

Forman, M. (1975). *One flew over the cuckoo's nest.* Los Angeles: Warner Home Video.

Gadamer, H. G. (1993). *Truth and method* (2nd ed.). New York: Continuum Publishing Company.

Gardner, H. (1983). *Frames of mind.* New York: Basic Books.

Gardner, H. (1993). *Multiple intelligences: The theory in practice.* New York: Basic Books.

Gelb, M. (1998). *How to think like Leonardo daVinci.* New York: Delacorte.

Hervey, L. W. (2000). *Artistic inquiry in dance/movement therapy: Creative alternatives for research.* Springfield, IL: Charles C Thomas, Publisher.

Kent, C. (1992). *Learning by heart: Teaching to free the creative spirit.* New York: Bantam.

Richards, M. C. (1989). *Centering.* Middletown, CT: Wesleyan.

Root-Bernstein, R., & Root-Bernstein, M. (1999). *Sparks of genius.* Boston: Houghton Mifflin.

Thiboutot, C., Martinez, A., & Jager, D. (1999). Gaston Bachelard and phenomenology: Outline of a theory of the imagination. *Journal of Phenomenological Psychology, 30*(1), 1–17.

CHAPTER 6

Lighten Up Your Classroom

Mariana D'Amico and Lynn Jaffe

"Humor is also a way of saying something serious."
T. S. Eliot

"At its best, humor simultaneously hurts and heals, makes one larger from a willingness to make oneself less. It has essentially much more breadth than wit, from being much more universal in appeal and human in effect. If harder to translate or explain, it often need not be explained or translated at all, revealing itself in a sudden gesture, a happy juxtaposition."
Louis Kronenberger

Most educators take learning very seriously, especially those in health care. They overlook the fact that humor is a lifeline to sanity and reality. Humor is not a primary teaching strategy—it is quite difficult to measure the educational effect of humor in isolation from other teaching methods—yet, the judicious use of humor can influence the cognitive and behavioral aspects of learning by engaging at least six of Gardner's seven forms of intelligence (as identified in Chapter 1, Effective Learning: What Teachers Need to Know). Research on humor has been a multidisciplinary endeavor, including a focus on its use in classrooms and health care (Wrench & McCroskey, 2001; Ziegler, 1998). Well-placed humor can make the classroom environment a safe, comfortable, and effective arena for cognitive and professional growth. Educators have used humor to alleviate classroom stress and facilitate knowledge acquisition and application for decades. Humor contributes to a positive affect and, to that end, humor has been used as a teaching tool for generations. Effectively using humor in the classroom requires knowledge, art, and skill, all of which can be learned (Hillman, 2001; Ziegler). This chapter will highlight humor as an educator's tool and describe specific strategies for humor use in the classroom.

DEFINITION AND PURPOSE

Humor is a communication that induces amusement. Thus, it must be shared. It makes the learning environment a shared, pleasurable experience. In education, the most positive forms of humor are funny stories or comments, jokes, and professional humor. Sarcasm has been recorded as common in the classroom, but tends to be a negative form of humor. Mirth is the emotional reaction to humor, joy, and pleasure. Wit is the cognitive process that elicits humor. Laughter or smiling is a physical expression of humor. With all these elements, the formal study of humor in the classroom has been a challenge. One reviewer declared that the literature on the use of humor in health care education was predominantly opinion pieces or reviews as opposed to actual evidence (Ziegler, 1998). However, that reviewer went on to cite at least a dozen studies of humor in educational settings. Whether the evidence is as sound as it should be remains equivocal, but the majority of authors praise its contributions to the educational experience (Hillman, 2001; James, 2004; Southam & Schwartz, 2004; Torok, McMorris, & Lin, 2004).

Humor has been studied and discussed from a variety of approaches—the physiological, psychological, emotional, and cognitive. Recent reviews have summarized these studies (Southam & Schwartz, 2004; Torok et al., 2004; Ziegler, 1998), confirming the bottom line that humor can promote health as well as learning through the physical benefits of reduced stress, increased productivity, and enhanced creativity. Humor has been deemed a primary vehicle for enhancing the learning environment through enlivening potentially dreary topics, keeping lectures engaging and enjoyable, and humanizing faculty in students' perceptions. The cultivation of the abilities to laugh at oneself and with others bridges many gaps between people and broadens the pathway from student to professional (Flowers, 2001).

The use of humor in the classroom can be productive, promoting comfortable, safe interactions between faculty and students. It has been shown to increase teacher credibility (Torok et al., 2004). The effective use of humor promotes creativity, learning, retention, and enculturation of professionals (Boerman-Cornell, 2000; Flournoy, Turner, & Combs, 2001; Girdlefanny, 2004; Southam & Schwartz, 2004; Thorne, 1999). Counterproductive humor can cause fear and hostility, decrease self-esteem and motivation, and disrupt the community within the classroom (Boerman-Cornell; Girdlefanny; Weber, 2000).

White (2001) and Torok and colleagues (2004) studied whether perceptions regarding the use of humor were correlated between professors and students, whether students thought more favorably of professors who used humor, and what types of humor were preferred. Their findings had strong correlations between perceptions in the use of funny stories, funny comments, jokes, and professional humor. Students were not supportive of humor in testing, nor of the use of sarcasm. Shibles' (n.d.) analysis of humor declares ridicule and sarcasm are used as a superiority differentiation or as a defense mechanism and therefore does not qualify as a type of humor. Educators need to be cognizant of this because such a misuse of humor will be counterproductive in the classroom. Students tended to find humor facilitated attention, morale, and comprehension.

Gender differences in students' perceptions of humor use, with female faculty's use of humor less likely to be recognized, has also been noted (White, 2001). White's study identified agreement between professors and students regarding humor as a tool to relieve stress, create a healthy learning environment, gain attention, and motivate students. An item of greatest variation between faculty and student perceptions was in the use of humor to handle unpleasant situations—students believed it could be used, but faculty did not.

THEORETICAL FOUNDATIONS

Humor is a complex phenomenon with a long and rich history. While no one has been able to establish when the first joke actually occurred, we know the Greek theatre B.C. used both comedy and drama to entertain and enlighten. Many authors, such as Dickens and Swift, used satire to comment on society. Theoretical foundations of humor are multiple (see inexhaustible description in Shibles, n.d.). They have been categorized by discipline (biological, cognitive, physiological, linguistic, etc.) and construct (incongruity, superiority, etc.) (Ziegler, 1998). Effective use of humor may be a component of all learning theories. Humor and laughter contribute to all necessary principles of learning: enjoyment; creativity; interest; motivation; a relaxed, open, warm environment; a positive student-teacher relationship; and decreased tension and anxiety. To be authentic is one of the most important qualities of an educator. Having a sense of humor is an aspect of authenticity. Humor used constructively builds a positive self-image (Hillman, 2001).

Cognitive and affective theories appear the most important for education, because they account for linguistic, intellectual, and emotional aspects of learning. Some humor theories state that laughter or amusement occurs as an intellectual reaction to something unexpected, illogical, or inappropriate in some way (Morreall, 1983, as cited in Hillman, 2001, and Shibles, n.d.). Research indicates that the recognition of incongruity begins in infancy (Hillman). Cognitive theory focuses on an understanding of language, knowledge, situation, and reasoning that addresses recognition of mistakes, incongruity, and wordplays. Puns, irony, and satire require analysis and synthesis of words, knowledge, and context. Without such understanding, students do not perceive the humor and may take affront or feel put down by the instructor. When students understand a concept well they can make jokes or funny remarks about it, indicating their synthesis of the material. Cognition is shaped by culture, and humor has been defined as culturally appropriate incongruity (Wrench & McCroskey, 2001).

According to Kathwohl, Bloom, and Masia (1964), affect is an important domain of learning. Those theorists who subscribe to affective theory stress emotional components of humor. However, it seems inadequate to treat affect as separate from cognition, because emotion is largely constituted by thought (Shibles, n.d.). There has been extensive discussion regarding the emotional and physiological benefits of releasing psychic energy through laughter. Because of this, humor is an invaluable contribution to the educational process. Research supports its use to reduce anxiety and stress, build confidence, improve productivity, reduce boredom, heighten interest, and encourage divergent thinking and the creation of new ideas (Hillman, 2001; Weber, 2000; Ziegler, 1998).

The affective component of humor engages the limbic system, thereby enhancing short- and long-term memory and increasing the willingness of the learner to apply knowledge and skills (Flournoy et al., 2001; Hillman, 2001; Southam & Schwartz, 2004). The expression of feelings, such as empathy and anger, can be more constructive when approached in a witty manner (Hillman). Both sides of the brain are actively engaged during laughter and the perception of humor (Southam & Schwartz). The right side of the brain involves reading and interpreting the visual, nonverbal information of humor while the left side of the brain interprets the language nuances of humor. Novelty, imagination, and visualization help move information into long-term memory through the engagement of multiple brain cells firing simultaneously (Wrench & McCroskey, 2001; Southam & Schwartz; Van Oech, 1990 as cited by Weber, 2000).

The use of humor can be learned and has a growing evidence base, yet it remains highly individualized. Gender, culture, ethnicity, and context impact the acceptance or rejection of this teaching strategy (Ziegler, 1998). Wanzer & Frymier (1999) found that witty, rather than funny, professors were considered interesting, entertaining, and motivating by adult learners. Robinson is often cited (Hillman, 2001; Southam & Schwartz, 2004) as proposing four interrelated aspects to be considered in the area of education and humor: (1) enhancing the learning process itself through humor; (2) using humor to facilitate the process of socialization; (3) teaching the concept of humor as a communication and intervention tool; and (4) modeling the use of humor as a vehicle for facilitating the other three. Using humor in the classroom is not attempting to become a comedian. It is assuming an attitude of authenticity and comfort within the classroom. The ability to learn to use humor has been questioned by a few authors (Wrench & McCroskey, 2001). These authors distinguish sense of humor, a culturally taught trait, from the act of being humorous, which may be a genetic trait. However, most authors promote the idea that the use of humor not only can be learned, but ought to be learned by educators to enhance the teaching-learning process (Flowers, 2001; Girdlefanny, 2004; Yura-Petro, 1991). Employing humorous methods is within every educator's reach and will enhance the educational experience for students.

TYPES OF LEARNERS

Humor is a type of playfulness that spans multiple ages and venues. Developmentally and intellectually appropriate humor can be employed with all levels of learners. Classroom humor relevant to course content is more appreciated by the adult learner than random humor. Studies have provided mixed reviews about students' acceptance and appreciation of humor used by the teacher. Some studies have shown that gender impacts the acceptance and use of humor, as does the match between the educator's and students' sense of humor (Martin, Puhlik-Doris, Larsen, Gray, & Weir, 2003). The associations found between intellectual ability and sense of humor suggest that educators need a firm check on the cognitive status of their students when employing wit or they risk offending rather than amusing them.

Gorham and Christophel (1990, as cited by Southam & Schwartz, 2004) found that learning outcomes of female students were not as influenced by teacher humor as were those of male students, and that females preferred personal stories that illustrated pertinent points related to course content. Student reaction to humor has been differentially related to the gender of the educator as well, with female educators eliciting less overall appreciation of their efforts to be humorous (White, 2001). Acceptance of humor in the classroom has been shown to be positively associated with a student's psychological health (Dziegielewski, Jacinto, Laudadio, & Legg-Rodriguez, 2003; Kuiper, Grimshaw, Leite, & Kirsh, 2004).

CONDITIONS FOR LEARNING

Humor can be used judiciously throughout a class session or course and in all types of classroom situations: lecture, lab, fieldwork, and various course assignments. Positive and constructive humor can be used to put the learner and the teacher at ease with the subject matter. Humorous activities or icebreakers might begin a class. They can also be inserted at intervals to reaffirm the open, relaxed atmosphere that is most conducive to learning. Tension relievers before exams are usually helpful. As long as the humor remains embedded in the content, learners will internalize the new knowledge, otherwise the flow of the lesson can be lost or misdirected (Weaver & Cotrell, 2001). Humor can be used to facilitate creativity and retention of material at any point in a lesson—from initial setup, through final review.

Relationship between class size and classroom size may impact the effective use of humor as Berk (2002 as cited by Torok et al., 2004) noted that laughter is likely to be greater in larger, more crowded classes, than in smaller classes in larger rooms. Laughter, like yawning, is contagious; so once a large group gets going it may take time to bring them back to focus. Dziegielewski et al. (2003) encourage the group leader—the educator in this case—not to stop the laughter but to let it stop on its own accord. They perceive that this laughter helps reduce anger and tension and may build cohesion and well-being, both of which are essential to productivity and learning.

Humor is a part of communication and not dependent upon the natural comedic ability of an instructor. It is an attitude and permission for enjoyment of the educational process (Weaver & Cotrell, 2001). It can be spontaneous or planned. Weaver and Cottrell recommend inserting humorous breaks every fifteen minutes. Essential to creating open communication and allowing humor within the classroom is the teacher's nonverbal communication and voice tone as these can convey openness or constrict enjoyment of learning. If the humor style of the teacher and that of the class do not mesh, then the use of humor in the learning process will not be effective. It is important to understand your audience, which, in this case is the class, to know one's own sense of humor, and be willing to experiment with others (Girdlefanny, 2004; Hillman, 2001).

McMorris, Boothroyd, and Pietrangelo (1997) summarized studies that used humor in testing situations with mixed results. Positive results depended on the type of humor used. Some studies found humor to reduce tension, but this was not a universal finding. Humor was often found to be distracting in a testing situation. Humor with a strong linguistic base may also disadvantage international students. Likewise, as mentioned previously, any use of sarcasm was seen to be detrimental to learning (Torok et al., 2004).

Humor can be very useful in the enculturation of novices into one's profession, especially when dealing with elements of embarrassing intimacy and reality shocks that may occur in health care provision (Southam & Schwartz, 2004). According to Sultanoff (1995), a lack of sense of humor is related to lower self-esteem. On the other hand, a healthy sense of humor is related to being able to laugh at oneself and one's life without degrading oneself. Those who enter the health professions must be able to cope with adversity and be able to help others cope as well. The development of a healthy sense of humor, beginning in preservice classes and continuing through professional in-service meetings benefits everyone.

RESOURCES

As with any teaching strategy, the effective use of humor needs to be learned and refined. Before using humor in teaching situations, educators may want to assess their own sense of humor using a humor profile such as the one developed by Richmond, Wrench, and Gorham (2001) (see Appendix A). The score obtained on the humor profile reflects one's use of humor during communications. Completion of a humor profile is a preliminary step to learning one's current facility with humorous content.

Some ways to increase one's use of humor is by exposing oneself to humorous experiences, such as comics, sitcoms, joke books, and comedy clubs, collecting print and electronic humor samples, and even looking for the humor around oneself. This may include viewing the world through exaggeration or broad, silly perspectives. Using exaggeration is a method to clarify concepts—the contrast assists understanding. Incongruity is another technique for promoting humor in the classroom. One such example is comparing a stripper and a corporate CEO regaining work skills (see applied example). Using props in the classroom for role playing may also enhance the humor of a lesson (Sultanoff, 1995). The cinema is a treasure trove of humorous situations waiting to be tapped by the health care professional looking for examples of exaggeration, incongruity, or basic fun.

Articles about infusing humor into online courses have suggested a number of techniques to promote a positive learning environment in the virtual classroom that mirror applications of humor in the regular classroom. Primary among these techniques is the use of humor to project an authentic representation of the educator. The humor used, by necessity, is primarily linguistic, although cartoons are readily available (James, 2004). Being humorous online requires extensive commitment, time, and effort as it needs to be planned, personalized to the students, and monitored for receptivity (Boynton, as cited by James).

Web Resources

Humor Matters bibliography and resources can be accessed at: http://www. humormatters.com/bibtherapy.htm

A listing of potentially relevant films (primarily on mental illness) can be accessed at: http://www.disabilityfilms.co.uk/mental1/men1dex.htm

or

http://faculty.dwc.edu/nicosia/moviesandmentalillnessfilmography.htm

Sources for Cartoon Humor

CartoonBank.com cartoons from the *New Yorker* magazine can be accessed through: http://www.cartoonbank.com/search_results_category.asp?mscssid= Q5UWM7B2HQ169GHHAE3PF21GRV2J41M4&sitetype=1&keyword= family&section=prints&title=Family&whichpage=4&sortBy=popular

Single cartoons by Randy Glasbergen, often about business or family, can be accessed at: http://www.glasbergen.com

A variety of popular newspaper cartoon serials is accessible at: http://www. mycomicspage.com/free/offers.html

Print Resources

Print versions of cartoons (Far Side; For Better or Worse; Calvin and Hobbes; etc.), local newspapers, the humor section of bookstores

Tibballs, G. (Ed.) (2000). *The mammoth book of humor*. New York: Carroll & Graf.

USING THE METHOD

Using humor in the learning process can take several forms (see **Figure 6-1** for a brief summary). It is easy for most faculty to use spontaneous storytelling by relating their own experiences to enhance the learning process. Other faculty may need to collect jokes, cartoons, movie excerpts, and humorous exercises to insert into their regular teaching activities to enhance the learner's receptivity to information and participation during content presentations. As has been mentioned, faculty must realize that what works for some people does not necessarily work for others (Hillman, 2001).

Some specific techniques for including humor in a class situation include posting humorous situations on a bulletin board to teach interactive concepts (see Flournoy et al., 2001 for complete description). Using irony to contrast expected outcomes and actual occurrence enhances remembrance because of incongruity (Thorne, 1999). Case studies with funny names related to topical

---

Figure 6-1   Tips for using humor in the classroom.

1. Create a casual (and safe) atmosphere.
2. Smile; adopt a laugh-ready attitude.
3. Relax, use open, nonverbal posture; increase interpersonal contact through eye-to-eye and face-to-face contact.
4. Remove social inhibitions; establish nonjudgmental forum for discussion.
5. Begin class with a humorous example, cartoon, anecdote, or thought for the day.
6. Use personal stories, anecdotes, current events related to class content.
7. Plan frequent breaks in content for application, humorous commercials, or exaggerated examples; provide humorous materials.
8. Encourage give and take with students; laugh at yourself occasionally.

Adapted from Weaver & Cotrell, 2001; Provine, 2000.

Figure 6-2   An example of a joke that may be appropriate for a class on clinical reasoning.

Sherlock Holmes and Dr. Watson went camping. After a good meal and an excellent bottle of wine, they lay down and went to sleep. A couple of hours later, Holmes woke up and nudged his faithful friend.

"Watson, Watson," he said. "Look up at the sky and tell me what you see?"

"I see millions and millions of stars," replied Watson.

"And what does that tell you?" inquired the master detective.

Watson thought for a moment. "Well, Holmes, astronomically, it tells me that there are millions of galaxies and potentially billions of planets. Astrologically, I observe that Saturn is in Leo. Horologically, I deduce that the time is approximately two twenty-five. Theologically, I can see that God is all powerful and that we are small and insignificant. Meteorologically, I believe we will have a glorious day tomorrow. What does it tell you, Holmes?"

"Watson, you imbecile! Some thief has stolen our tent!"

Joke 2470 from *The Mammoth Book of Jokes*, edited by Geoff Tibballs (2000). Reprinted by kind permission of Constable & Robinson Ltd (London).

content also enhance memory of the examples. (For example: Petunia Potter liked working in her garden. She needed some ergonomic changes to facilitate her participation in this avocation; how would you adapt this occupation for her?) Use of exaggerations and unusual professions increases awareness of people's needs in the health care arena. Personal stories about real life experiences, challenges in one's role as a new professional, or unexpected circumstances (or embarrassing moments) can have teaching value. Sometimes when students are called upon to do group presentations on a given topic they will use humor (often in the form of mimicry or parody of the instructors) to engage their classmates, and possibly, to alleviate their own stress. Humor usage will be as variable as those using it, which can be quite diverse. See **Figure 6-2**.

POTENTIAL PROBLEMS

Not everyone gets a joke. Some people are too serious. Some do not value humor in the educational process. Some find it too distracting to their learning. Using sarcasm, ridicule, and put-down humor can be counterproductive. Humor has the potential to be offensive, especially with ethnic or gender issues.

Incongruence between innate or cultural humor perceptions can be disruptive to the coordination of the learning environment. Besides potentially offending some members of a class, the use of deprecatory humor may affect students' perceptions of the faculty and undermine their effectiveness. Class clowns, who use humor for personal gain, also abuse the strategy and detract from the learning environment (Martin et al., 2003).

CONCLUSION

It has been said that Plato believed one could discover more about a person in an hour of play than in a year of conversation. The same could be said about the culture of a classroom, cohort, or department. Teaching-learning communities are built upon engagement and communication among students and faculty. The development of respect and desire to learn can be facilitated with the thoughtful use of humor. All involved will find their creativity, enjoyment, and problem-solving boosted by this cognitively stimulating and emotionally safe learning environment.

APPLIED EXAMPLES

At the beginning of a class, in this case a pediatrics class on toddler development, cartoons that related to the lecture topic were used as a starting point for discussion. The cartoons had been selected from the daily newspaper over a span of years, and so there were many examples of toddler behaviors from which to choose. Students who had their own children or younger siblings were able to immediately relate to the cartoon situations and discuss the behaviors depicted as well as other toddler behaviors and observations they had seen. Students without children and siblings participated in the discussion by asking questions of those with more experience. A lively discussion ensued. When presented with the accompanying reading material or tested on the material at a later date, students exhibited better retention and recall of the information and the discussion that occurred around the visual cue of the cartoon.

Another example of a humor-enhanced class discussion revolved around activities of daily living related to client-centered evaluation by using exaggerated comparison and contrast of a stripper and a CEO's daily activity routines, expectations, and needs. Students started discussing their perceived stereotypes of these exaggerated individuals, and as new elements of typical daily living were tossed out to the students to analyze for these individuals, another lively discussion occurred. When assessed for their understanding of activities of daily living evaluations, analyses, and syntheses for treatment plans, students exhibited a greater understanding of these processes related to individualized care with attention to details.

REFERENCES

Boerman-Cornell, W. (2000). Humor your students. *English Journal, 88*, 66–69.

Dziegielewski, S. F., Jacinto, G. A., Laudadio, A., & Legg-Rodriguez, L. (2003). Humor: An essential communication tool in therapy. *International Journal of Mental Health, 32*(3), 74–90.

Eliot, T. S. As quoted on The Quotations page. Retrieved January 3, 2006, from http://www.quotationspage.com/quote/26754.html

Flournoy, E., Turner, G., & Combs, D. (2001). Critical care: Read the writing on the wall. *Nursing, 31*(3), 8–10.

Flowers, J. (2001). The value of humor in technology education. *Technology Teacher, 60*, 10–13.

Girdlefanny, S. (2004). Using humor in the classroom. *Techniques: Connecting Education & Careers, 79*(3), 22–26.

Hillman, S. M. (2001). Humor in the classroom: Facilitating the learning process. In A. J. Lowenstein & M. J. Bradshaw (Eds.), *Fuszard's innovative teaching strategies in nursing* (3rd ed., pp. 54–62). Sudbury, MA: Jones & Bartlett.

James, D. (2004). Commentary: A need for humor in online courses. *College Teaching, 52*(3), 93–94.

Kathwohl, D. R., Bloom, B. S., & Masia, B. B. (1964). *Taxonomy of educational objectives.* New York: David McKay.

Kronenberger, L. (1972). *A mania for magnificence.* Boston: Little, Brown. Retrieved January 3, 2006, from http://www.poemhunter.com/quotations/funny/page-9

Kuiper, N. A., Grimshaw, M., Leite, C., & Kirsh, G. (2004). Humor is not always the best medicine: Specific components of sense of humor and psychological well-being. *Humor, 17*, 135–168.

Martin, R. A., Puhlik-Doris, P., Larsen, G., Gray, J., & Weir, K. (2003). Individual differences in uses of humor and their relation to psychological well-being: Development of the humor styles questionnaire. *Journal of Research in Personality, 37*, 28–75.

McMorris, R. F., Boothroyd, R. A., & Pietrangelo, D. J. (1997). Humor in educational testing: A review and discussion. *Applied Measurement in Education, 10*(3), 269–297.

Richmond, V. P., Wrench, J. S., & Gorham, J. (2001). *Communication, affect, and learning in the classroom.* Acton, MA: Tapestry Press.

Provine, R. R. (2000). *Laughter: A scientific investigation.* New York: Viking Penguin.

Shibles, W. (n.d.). *Humor reference guide.* Retrieved January 3, 2006, from http://facstaff.uww.edu/shiblesw/humorbook

Southam, M., & Schwartz, K. B. (2004). Laugh and learn: Humor as a teaching strategy in occupational therapy education. *Occupational Therapy in Health Care, 18*, 57–70.

Sultanoff, S. (1995). "What is humor?" Retrieved January 3, 2006, from http://www.aath.org/articles/art_sultanoff01.html

Thorne, B. M. (1999). Using irony in teaching the history of psychology. *Teaching of Psychology, 26*(3), 222–224.

Torok, S. E., McMorris, R. F., & Lin, W-C. (2004). Is humor an appreciated teaching tool? Perceptions of professors' teaching styles and use of humor. *College Teaching, 52*, 14–20.

Wanzer, M. B., & Frymier, A. B. (1999). The relationship between student perceptions of instructor humor and students' reports of learning. *Communication Education, 48*, 48–62.

Weaver, R. L., & Cotrell, H. W. (2001). Ten specific techniques for developing humor in the classroom. *Education, 108*(2), 167–179.

Weber, A. (2000). Playful writing for critical thinking. *Journal of Adolescent & Adult Literacy*, *43*(6), 562–568.

White, G. W. (2001). Teachers' report of how they used humor with students perceived use of such humor. *Education*, *122*(2), 337–347.

Wrench, J., & McCroskey, J. (2001). A temperamental understanding of humor communication and exhilaratability. *Communication Quarterly*, *49*, 142–159.

Yura-Petro, H. (1991). Humor: A research and practice tool for nurse scholar-supervisors, practitioners, and educators. *Health Care Supervisor*, *9*(4), 1–8.

Ziegler, J. B. (1998). Use of humour in medical teaching. *Medical Teacher*, *20*(4), 341–348.

RECOMMENDED READING

Frymier, A. B. (1994). A model of immediacy in the classroom. *Communication Quarterly*, *42*(2), 133–144.

Ziv, A. (2001). The effect of humor on aggression catharsis in the classroom. *Journal of Psychology*, *12*(4), 359–364.

APPENDIX A   Richmond Humor Assessment Instrument

The Richmond Humor Assessment Instrument (RHAI) was designed to be a self-report measure of an individual's use of humor in communication. Unlike some other similar measures, this instrument does not focus on a particular kind of humor (such as story telling). Alpha reliability estimates for this measure have been near 0.90.

Directions: The following statements apply to how people communicate humor when relating to others. Indicate the degree to which each of these statements applies to you by filling in the number of your response in the blank before each item:

5 = Strongly agree; 4 = Agree; 3 = Undecided; 2 = Disagree; 1 = Strongly disagree

_____   1. I regularly communicate with others by joking with them.

_____   2. People usually laugh when I make a humorous remark.

_____   3. I am not funny or humorous.

_____   4. I can be amusing or humorous without having to tell a joke.

_____   5. Being humorous is a natural communication orientation for me.

_____   6. I cannot relate an amusing idea well.

_____   7. My friends would say that I am a humorous or funny person.

_____   8. People don't seem to pay close attention when I am being funny.

_____   9. Even funny ideas and stories seem dull when I tell them.

_____ 10. I can easily relate funny or humorous ideas to the class.

_____ 11. I would say that I am not a humorous person.

_____ 12. I cannot be funny, even when asked to do so.

_____ 13. I relate amusing stories, jokes, and funny things very well to others.

_____ 14. Of all the people I know, I am one of the "least" amusing or funny persons.

_____ 15. I use humor to communicate in a variety of situations.

_____ 16. On a regular basis, I do not communicate with others by being humorous or entertaining.

Scoring: To compute your scores, add your scores for each item as indicated below:

Recode items 3, 6, 8, 9, 11, 12, 14, and 16 with the following format:

$1 = 5$

$2 = 4$

$3 = 3$

$4 = 2$

$5 = 1$

After you have recoded the previous questions, add all of the numbers together to get your composite RHAI score.

Your score should be between 16 and 80. Scores of 60 and above indicate high degrees of humor usage; scores of 30 and below indicate low degrees of humor usage; scores between 30 and 60 indicate moderate degrees of humor usage.

SOURCES

Richmond, V. P., Wrench, J. S., & Gorham, J. (2001). *Communication, affect, and learning in the classroom.* Acton, MA: Tapestry Press.

Wrench, J. S., & McCroskey, J. C. (2001). A temperamental understanding of humor communication and exhilaratability. *Communication Quarterly, 49,* 170–183.

"Richmond Humor Assessment Instrument." Retrieved May 10, 2006, from http://www.as.wvu.edu/~richmond/measures/rhai.pdf

CHAPTER 7

Teaching Value-Sensitive Subjects

Kathy Lee Dunham Hakala

INTRODUCTION

The diverse and global community of today's health care arena is permeated with an array of deeply ingrained cultural values and beliefs that can affect behavior and often bias an individual's attitudes and feelings. Each health care provider, as well as each client who seeks health care, needs an opportunity to recognize and explore value-sensitive beliefs that could adversely bias attitudes or feelings to the point of negatively affecting client outcomes. This chapter will identify teaching techniques to help students recognize and address predisposed value-sensitive attitudes within themselves and/or their clients that could potentially contribute to biased and unfavorable health care.

DEFINITION AND PURPOSES

Value-sensitive subjects are intricately entwined in each individual's own long-standing cultural values and beliefs that are, by their very nature, often heavily laden with unwavering attitudes and passionate feelings (Stuart & Laraia, 2005). Because these values may be basic to one's identity as a member of a culture, individuals often hold these personal values as truths. When people believe that their values are truths, they are reluctant to question the validity of these values; however, the questioning of one's values can lead to critical thinking and ultimately to a change in one's personal basic concepts and resultant behavior. Such change is crucial to the education process and, therefore, imperative for all involved in providing health care.

Although there is general agreement among the nursing profession that holistic care is integral to nursing practice, there may be some health care providers in nursing, as well as other health disciplines, that still find it difficult to address with their clients those value-sensitive areas that are so closely associated with one's own cultural traditions and values. Common examples of value-sensitive areas that the student may find difficult to address with clients and colleagues are listed in **Table 7-1.**

Even though the discussion of such topics is often essential in providing holistic health care, many students and some licensed health care providers may continue to be reluctant to address value-sensitive topics with clients in the clinical setting because of the discomfort that it is likely to cause for either the client and/or the health care provider. However, providers must be equipped to recognize and competently manage value-sensitive subjects in their own lives, as well as assisting clients to do the same (Mohr, 2006). Thus, educational activities that allow students in health care disciplines an opportunity to discover their own values, as well as those of their clients, can be an important tool of empowerment in effecting client change through the delivery of holistic care.

THEORETICAL FOUNDATIONS

The provision of accurate and relevant information is an important component of helping students exploring personal beliefs, values, behaviors, and attitudes.

Table 7-1   Examples of Value-Sensitive Areas in the Health Care Setting

1. Reporting a colleague to a peer assistance program
2. Taking a detailed sexual history from a client (e.g., including information on sexual preferences, practices, and toys)
3. Health care professionals who acquire tattoos
4. Providing care to a client with pedophilia
5. Helping to deliver the baby of a rape/incest victim
6. Witnessing and/or praying with a client
7. The use of marijuana for medicinal purposes
8. Mutual masturbation among teens as an alternative to sexual intercourse
9. Amniocentesis for genetic testing
10. The use of spanking a child as a form of discipline
11. Rationing of health care
12. When parents refuse to consent to treatment for children
13. Euthanasia of the elderly
14. Providing care to a client undergoing an elective abortion
15. Stem cell research
16. Clients who are uncomfortable with a male nurse
17. Providing care to a client with AIDS
18. Providing care to a never-been-married, teenage mother
19. Experiencing racism/ethnicity as a health care provider
20. The appropriate time to tell a client he or she is dying

Such teaching incorporates the behavioral, cognitive, and affective domains of knowledge and promotes critical thinking on the part of the student. The examination of oneself and environment serves as the motivation for the change of values. A student may, indeed, discover uncomfortable feelings when having to assess in detail the sexual history of a client. Teachers then need to provide these students with a classroom milieu in which they can develop trust, communication skills, self-exploration, and confidence to achieve those professional expectations and acquire those skills that are required in the clinical setting.

As students begin to encounter clients, they may discover client-held values that seem odd or eccentric. However, because personally held values can affect one's health behaviors, the student must not only learn to assess those client-held values, but also determine whether he/she, the student, harbors any personally held biases that could negatively affect the delivery of care.

Traditionally held values of a client may be found to interfere with healthy behaviors. For example, cultural beliefs may discount the importance of daily bathing, obtaining routine dental checkups, or being compliant with childhood immunization schedules. Cultural values may contribute to the delay of seeking health care until one is ill. Magical thinking and/or denial may prevent some clients from engaging in healthier behaviors that would potentially enhance the quality of their life. The sense of traditionally held values for the sake of tradition begins to crumble when students are provided with information as well as an opportunity to safely express negative feelings associated with such tradition. As the student begins to develop increased self-knowledge and self-awareness, personal values that are more satisfying and healthy can be adopted.

Affective learning is enhanced when an atmosphere of trust has been built among the classroom participants. Students will be more willing to reveal and discuss their emerging thoughts and feelings within a group setting if the environment feels emotionally safe. Thus, to promote continued self-discovery among group participants, it is important for the teacher to assist students in giving feedback to one another in a nonthreatening and nonjudgmental manner (Yalom, 2000). The teacher must be aware of this vulnerability and provide a safe atmosphere among the group members as they explore and communicate their thoughts and feelings to one another.

The classroom is the environment in which such affective and critical thinking begins. The wise student takes new thoughts, opinions, and feelings to other areas of his or her life and tests them on family and friends to help gain further insights. "Theoretical, empirical, and experiential evidence all indicate that the cognitive, affective, and behavioral domains work in consort to affect one's behavior and that dealing with any domain in isolation significantly reduces the impact of the learning experience" (Koch, 1992). Such multidimensional and holistic learning experiences are important for any educational setting. Academic curriculum and clinical experiences provide the student with an array of opportunities in which further values clarification can take place. Unfortunately, the teacher may find it difficult to evaluate the student's affective learning curve in the classroom since value change is an ongoing process that continues into later experiences. **Table 7-2** identifies early indicators that may be seen by the teacher as the process of affective learning begins.

TYPES OF LEARNERS

All health care students should be provided an opportunity to address value-sensitive subjects as a part of their total affective educational experience. Affective education differs from purely cognitive learning in that it requires the students to become reflective and introspective of their own lives. The students, themselves, become the basis of knowledge. Such introspection requires a certain level of maturity on the part of the student, as well as a willingness to explore one's existing values and beliefs. The student whose life's experiences have been widely varied may be more agreeable to exploring his/her values and beliefs than the student whose life's experiences have been intolerant of and without diversity.

Cognitive learning is concerned with the accumulation and understanding of facts and rarely is concerned with the individual students' feelings or attitudes. Without an understanding of one's own beliefs and values, it is difficult to change unhealthy behaviors. Thus, the clinical arena remains an amazing setting for students in the health care field to not only clarify their own values, but to also assist clients in the exploration of their health care beliefs that potentially impede health. Health care educators would do well to incorporate affective education into theory and clinical courses in an effort to clearly establish that value-sensitive subjects are critical to the holistic care and prevention strategies of clients.

Students and teachers must begin with a basic agreement on health values because such values can clearly be in conflict by well-meaning people. **Table 7-3** identifies both basic health values and beliefs that interfere with basic health (American Hospital Association, 2003). The teacher must encourage the learner

---

Table 7-2   Early Indicators of Affective Learning

1. A willingness to engage in a discussion of the value-sensitive topic *or* to listen as others vocalize their opinions
2. Verbal responses become less defensive and/or less argumentative
3. A desire to independently review available literature regarding both sides of the argument
4. Ability to laugh at one's former position and/or entertain a different position

Table 7-3　Basic Health Values and Beliefs that Interfere with Basic Health

Basic health values for all clients	Beliefs that interfere with basic health
1. Right to obtain health care	1. Only those who can pay for services deserve health care.
2. Right to refuse health care	2. Only health care providers can make sound medical decisions that will determine the client's course of care.
3. Right to decide what course their health care shall take	3. A physician will tell a person what care he or she must receive.
4. Right to be respected by health care workers	4. Health care providers have the right to refuse care for certain groups of people.
5. Right to be protected from communicable disease	5. Children should not receive sex education.
6. Right to receive care in a safe and confidential environment	6. Abusive family members who care for their elderly parents should be given information as to the location of their victim.

AHA, 1990.

to analyze, evaluate, and synthesize in order to operate at a higher level of abstraction to build a strong concept of health. Beyond accepting a set of health values, the student must then be guided to learn how personal cultural values may conflict with these health values.

CONDITIONS FOR LEARNING

> "Family faces are magic mirrors. Looking at people who belong to us, we see the past, present and future."
> *Gail Lumet Buckley*

When teaching value-sensitive topics, the educator's role is to facilitate self-exploration within the student. Thus the teacher's personal values must not be imposed, lest the student's educational process of self-exploration be impeded.

When a student's personal values conflict with basic health values, the teacher may need to help the student further explore his values in order to prevent them from becoming an obstacle to further learning and/or change. Educators must realize that the real obstacle to learning about values is often cultural, not intellectual. Thus, the student may need to change traditional truths.

The teacher must also know how to pose the right questions and guide the student to thoughtful and introspective responses. The teacher's task is to help students transform cultural values that are harmful into more helpful values. In a trusting, comfortable classroom, the student learns through the example of the teacher how to confront unhealthy values. Students need to build a culture that regards the value of health if they are going to help their clients promote better health. Values can and do change over time. If students and professor agree from the outset that basic health values are important, then students are more willing to change those values that inhibit health care and promotion. The same process is true for clients. The student learns that giving information may not, by itself, be the most effective means to changing client behaviors. Rather, self-exploration by the client, in addition to information, may better facilitate the changing of unhealthy values to those that are more healthful.

RESOURCES

The classroom is best arranged in a circular fashion so students face each other while discussing issues with their classmates. Sufficient time must be provided to discuss facts as well as the experiences and emotions that are evoked during the discussion. The facilitation of group process by the teacher, as well as the use of therapeutic communication by all students is essential in building the trust and confidence needed for class members to openly disclose and discuss personal opinions regarding value-sensitive subjects.

USING THE METHOD

The following demonstrates how to help students explore the contradictory and ambivalent feelings they might experience when trying to determine whether or not to report a well-liked colleague suspected of illicit drug use to a peer assistance program. First, the students could be given an assignment in which they are to identify the benefits of a peer review program for both the public and for the colleague suspected of drug use. Following the completion of this assignment, the students could be asked to participate in a group activity in which one group member would be designated as the impaired health care provider.

The other group members would then be asked to discuss the experience of having to report this colleague to a peer assistance program. The designated impaired provider could also provide feedback to the group as to how he/she felt about being reported.

Most students could intellectually agree that public safety is an important role expectation of their profession. However, affectively, the decision to report the colleague may be thwarted by their own personal feelings of guilt as if one were tattling on a colleague. Thus, we see an example of how it is possible for students to intellectually adhere to one value, but at the same time be reluctant to do what is morally, ethically, professionally, and legally correct.

Group process is a useful means of addressing feelings related to value-sensitive areas. Students may at first be surprised that the class, as a whole, holds so many feelings associated with the sensitive subject being discussed. However, as the discussions proceed, students are often relieved to have the opportunity to openly discuss feelings that have long bothered them personally. Self-analysis and values clarification can be an enlightening experience!

POTENTIAL PROBLEMS

Because personal values are often heavily laden with passionate feelings, group discussions may become heated. Thus, it may first be necessary to assist students in developing (or at least reviewing) basic principles of group dynamics, as well as therapeutic communication skills. Like licensed health care professionals, students often have a difficult time communicating with colleagues and other disciplines because of fear of confrontation and difficulty handling conflict. Thus, students initially need to have an opportunity to explore and verbalize their own feelings and values within a safe and structured group setting in which all participants are expected to communicate therapeutically.

Individuals and groups often avoid engaging in honest and direct communication because of lack of experience in providing constructive criticism, fear of confrontation, and/or hurting someone's feelings. Cultural or gender taboos may make it difficult for both the group leader and group members, to share negative or sensitive information in a constructive way. Instead, an emphasis on politeness distorts reality and prevents trust from being developed within the group. Constructive criticism conveys truth in a way that is intended to be objective and productive, not hurtful or vindictive. If the leader discusses and demonstrates how to provide constructive criticism, the group will have the basis for practicing therapeutic confrontation skills. Growth in this area may be rapid or painfully slow, depending upon the background and values of the group.

To help ensure a positive group experience, the leader should take time at the first meeting to clearly identify the purpose of the discussion, as well as the time frame and expected group rules. Although rules/expectations may vary from group to group, examples are given in **Table 7-4.**

The following additional strategies are offered to help teachers address common problems encountered in group situations when discussing value-sensitive subjects.

Breaking the Ice

If students are new to one another, the group will be in the initial stage of the group process. Because members are in the process of establishing trust and determining their role(s), some students may be hesitant to participate. However, the longer a student sits in a group without verbally participating, the harder it can be to finally participate. Therefore, during the initial stage of the group, the leader might want to offer initial activities that direct members to verbally participate to some degree. These activities can be done in a round-robin fashion, or the leader may ask one member to begin the exercise and then ask that person to call upon the next participant. To encourage participation and enhance the initial development of trust, the leader may want to introduce activities that would not require members to put themselves in vulnerable positions of disclosure with other group members.

As the semester continues and the group begins to develop a deeper level of trust, students may become more comfortable with disclosing their thoughts,

---

Table 7-4   Group Rules/Expectations

1. The Role of the Group Leader
   - facilitate group discussion
   - model professional behavior and communication
   - act as a professional resource
2. The Role of Group Members
   - maintain confidentiality
   - be prepared to verbally participate
   - be respectful of each other
   - don't interrupt when another member is speaking
   - use active listening skills
   - refrain from all cross-talking
   - provide constructive criticism
   - accept responsibility for personal behavior

feelings, and values within the group setting to provide an arena of mutual learning for themselves and their fellow group members.

Seating Arrangement

Seating arrangement greatly influences group process. Encourage students to sit in a one-layer circular pattern. This arrangement provides an opportunity for members to have direct eye contact with one another. It also discourages reticent students from disappearing into the woodwork by sitting/hiding behind another student.

Some settings may offer tables at which the students sit. Although some activities may be enhanced by the use of tables on which students can write, the leader needs to keep in mind that any furniture between group members can act as a psychological/physical barrier. The leader may want to have students initially sit in a circular setting without tables to enhance a feeling of openness.

Silence Among Group Members

Group facilitators must resist the urge to rescue by filling in or breaking the silence. Although the silence may be uncomfortable for both the facilitator and the students, allowing the silence to continue for a brief period usually encourages group member participation.

Note: People commonly overestimate the time that silence actually exists. Although the period of silence may seem like a lifetime, the facilitator may want to surreptitiously time the silence in an effort to identify how much time has actually passed. This realization may help the facilitator become more comfortable with silence.

Keep in mind that group silence may be a reflection of group anger and/or a passive-aggressive need for control based upon anger. If you suspect that anger is the problem, help the group verbalize their anger by a statement such as, "I notice that the group is quiet. What's going on?" or "I feel a lot of anger among the group. It would be helpful for us to talk about that." For example, students may resist your open invitation to discuss a particular topic. Again, you might state, "I sense there is some resistance to participation. What is the problem? What do we need to do to get things started?" Remember to focus on open-ended questions and direct eye contact to facilitate communication.

Silence by individual group members may be due to intimidation by the teacher or other group members, shyness, anger, lack of preparation for participation, illness, and/or personal problems. The approach to each of the above would depend upon the identified situation. If the teacher suspects intimidation, ask to speak to the individual outside the group setting to validate the accuracy of the assessment and attempt to foster trust. For example, the teacher might say, "I notice that it seems difficult for you to participate in group. What can be done to help facilitate your participation?"

If shyness is a problem, try to draw out the student by initially offering close-ended questions and/or asking the student to comment on what others have just said. If anger prevents the student from participating, offer an opportunity for the student to express his/her feelings. This could be done either in or outside of the group setting. Statements to facilitate discussion might include: "You seem angry," or "You seem quiet. What do you need from the group?"

Illness can preclude a student from participating in group dynamics. If illness is validated, acknowledge the issue with the student and express interest in his/her participation the next time the group meets. This is also a good opportunity for you to teach and for students to learn personal boundaries and give themselves permission to provide appropriate self-care.

Students often bring many personal problems into the clinical setting. These problems may be exacerbated by and/or carry over into the discussion of value-sensitive subjects. If this is the case, offer a time to meet with them individually after the discussion is over and make necessary referrals as needed (e.g., to Student Services or the academic dean). However, students need to understand that the existence of personal problems is not an excuse for an ongoing lack of participation in group.

Lack of preparation for participation might be addressed by reiterating the purpose of the group meeting and emphasizing the expectation. If the teacher includes points for verbal participation, he or she must be sure to have useful criteria by which to gauge participation. Failure to provide criteria may put the teacher on a slippery slope in terms of grading for quality and quantity of participation.

Be patient. Some groups have more difficulty than others in building dynamics. Despite the facilitator's level of expertise, some groups will never gel. This may have nothing to do with the skills of the facilitator; rather it is a reflection of the group's personality and/or lack of investment in the activity. However, if the teacher is consistently having difficulty with group process, he/she may want to ask a colleague to observe your class and offer you feedback.

Avoidance

Avoidance is a word label that can refer to a number of group process issues, including silence, changing the subject, absenteeism, and scapegoating. If the group facilitator suspects that avoidance is occurring in the group, he or she must first assess the underlying cause(s). For example, when discussing euthanasia, a student who changes the subject, seems uncomfortable, or deflects attention to another student may be dealing with her own issues of unresolved grief. This behavior should be addressed by the leader with the student outside of the group in a supportive manner.

If the entire group is avoiding a topic, the leader needs to confront the group as a whole to explore the reason for the behavior. Some prompting may be necessary by the leader to shatter the avoidance. Acknowledge in the group that discomfort may exist. However, when group members openly discuss difficult issues within the confines of a safe group, resolution and change can occur.

Side Talking

Side talking occurs when two or more individuals carry on private conversations within the group setting, thus excluding/ignoring other group members. This behavior can be very tempting, especially when members are personal friends outside of the group. Side talking may be so insidious that members are not aware of their behavior or its effects on others in the group. However, side talking not only disrupts the group but can prevent group trust from developing because other group members may feel that they are the topic of side conversations. When the group first meets, the leader needs to outline the group rules, including the group's purpose and rationale for each rule. As the group session gets under way, the leader needs to be prepared to confront side talking. This may initially be done within the group by directly confronting the individuals in a nonhostile way. If, however, the behavior continues, the leader may need to meet with the individuals outside the group to discuss why this behavior continues and/or to simply set limits with consequences outlined should the behavior continue.

Lack of Confidentiality

Trust is a fundamental concept to group process. Each member of the group needs to know that *what is shared in the group stays in the group*, whether it is personal or client information. The importance of this should be discussed in the first group meeting. For example, if one group member shares a personal history of abuse with the group that is discussing incest, any further discussion of that topic outside of the group is prohibited unless that group member brings it up. Likewise, when information regarding a client(s) is discussed among healthcare students in an educational group setting, client confidentiality must be maintained according to both the institution's policies and the American Health Insurance Portability and Accountability Act of 1996 (HIPAA). Thus, the teacher should clarify these rules of confidentiality with all group members prior to the discussion of client information (Hakala & Pappas, 2003).

If the teacher suspects that confidentiality is breached, he/she needs to intervene immediately by confronting the issue within the group. If the identity of the individual(s) who violated confidentiality is known, the group leader may want to confront them either inside or outside of the group, depending on his/her comfort level and the circumstances. When individuals are confronted outside of the group, some follow-through is necessary to bring the issue back to the group. The leader needs to facilitate a discussion of the breach within the group in order to restore trust. When managed with discretion, this adverse event can serve as a learning experience for all group members. The sooner the breach can be addressed, the easier it is to restore trust (Hakala, Dunham, & Pappas, 2003).

CONCLUSION

Cultural values and beliefs can bias the attitudes and feelings of health care providers and, subsequently, interfere with client care. Often, students in the health care arena know how they *should feel* or what they *should do* in regard to sensitive topics, but they struggle with their feelings of ambivalence. Affective education provides students an opportunity to openly explore their own values, beliefs, and feelings in a safe and structured environment in order to begin to change those values and beliefs, that could adversely affect the care they provide to clients.

APPLIED EXAMPLE
Providing Care to a Client With Pedophilia

A group of health care students is given a case study and members are asked to discuss their thoughts and feelings about having to provide in-patient health care to a 56-year-old male pedophile who has registered with the local law enforcement agency as a sex offender. The client, who has suffered a mild stroke with right-sided weakness, will require hospitalization for a few days until he is stable enough to return to his residence in the community. At present, he is unable to ambulate and requires assistance with his ADL's (activities of daily living). In preparation for the discussion, the students are asked in advance to research the subject of pedophilia in regard to diagnostic features, possible causes, prevalence, and prognosis.

The students, who are divided into groups of 8–12, are seated in a circular fashion to facilitate communication and visual contact among group members. The teacher (self-appointed group leader) clarifies the purpose of the activity, as well as the rules and expectations of the group members. To begin the discussion and to allow all members an initial opportunity to verbally participate, the teacher asks each student to state one word that he or she thinks would best describe a pedophile. Not only is this a good way to break the ice as it promotes a limited, but initial participation by all group members; but it can also build a sense of universality, camaraderie, and/or trust among group members if similar descriptive words are disclosed. Students are then invited to discuss how such words or labels, if held by health care professionals, could negatively or positively affect the care provided to the client in the case study.

Students are asked to discuss how, if any, their feelings toward pedophiles were changed after researching and reading objective data about pedophilia. Students are also encouraged to identify personal feelings they have in regard to providing care for a pedophile and how those feelings could prevent them from providing the same efficacious care to the perpetrator as they would to the victim of the perpetrator.

Next, the group is subdivided into two groups. Collectively, Group A represents the person with pedophilia and identifies potential feelings that might result as being a client who receives care from health care professionals who know that he is a registered sex offender. Group B will identify the potential feelings that the health care provider might have in regard to caring for a pedophile and how to appropriately handle those feelings in such a way as to exhibit professional and efficacious care. Groups A and B will then share and discuss their findings with each other. Throughout these discussions, the teacher will be attentive not only to any of the potential problems previously addressed in this chapter, but also any of the previously identified early indicators that affective learning is occurring.

REFERENCES

American Hospital Association (AHA). (2003). *The patient care partnership: Understanding expectations, rights, and responsibilities.* Chicago: Author.

Buckley, G. L. (1988). In Simpson, J. B. (Ed.), *Simpson's contemporary quotations.* Boston: Houghton Mifflin. Retrieved February 7, 2006, from http://www.bartleby.com/63/48/3748.html

Hakala, K. L. Dunham, & Pappas, A. (2003). *Group processes for post conference.* Unpublished manuscript, Louise Herrington School of Nursing, Baylor University at Waco, Texas.

Koch, P. B. (1992). Integrating cognitive, affective, and behavioral approaches into learning experiences for sexuality education. In J. T. Sears (Ed.), *Sexuality and the curriculum: The politics and practices of sexuality education* (pp. 256). New York: Teachers College Press.

Mohr, W. K. (2006). *Psychiatric-mental health nursing* (6th ed.). Philadelphia: Lippincott Williams & Wilkins.

Stuart, G. W., & Laraia, M. T. (2005). *Principles and practice of psychiatric nursing* (8th ed.). St. Louis: Mosby.

Yalom, I. (2000). *The theory and practice of group psychotherapy.* New York: Basic Books.

RESOURCES

The following organizations provide information regarding sensitive subjects:

American Association of Sex Educators, Counselors, and Therapists (AASECT)

P.O. Box 1960

Ashland, VA 23005-1960

Telephone: 1-804-752-0056

www.aasect.org

The Jason Foundation, Inc.

181 East Main Street

Jefferson Bldg., Suite 5

Hendersonville, TN 37075

Telephone: 1-888-881-2323

www.jasonfoundation.com

National Mental Health Services

Knowledge Exchange Network, Center for Mental Health Services—KEN

P.O. Box 42490

Washington, DC 20015

Telephone: 1-800-789-2647

ken@mentalhealth.org   or   www.mentalhealth.org

Sexuality Information and Education Council of the U.S. (SIECUS)

130 West 42nd Street, Suite 350

New York, NY 10036-7802

Telephone: 1-212-819-9770

www.siecus.org

Human Rights Education Associates

P.O. Box 382396

Cambridge, MA 02238

Telephone: 1-978-341-0200

www.hrea.org

TEACHING IN STRUCTURED SETTINGS

Section II presents concept-based topics that are applicable in a myriad of situations, regardless of the level of the learner, the topic, or the class size. The universal concepts evident in each chapter include the importance of planning and preparation on the part of the teacher, the manner in which information is conveyed, and the importance of active student involvement and responsibility for learning.

The principles presented in Section I, the Introduction, are used in the traditional classroom environments addressed in these chapters. Application of teaching and learning theories and planned activities directed toward critical thinking are apparent. Educators can use creative innovations with time-honored strategies, such as lecture, to bring a refreshing approach to teaching.

CHAPTER 8

Lecture Is Not a Four-Letter Word!

Barbara C. Woodring and Richard C. Woodring

"A common characteristic found in all great teachers is a love of their subject, an obvious satisfaction found in arousing this love in their students, and an ability to convince them that what they are being taught is deadly serious."
J. Epstein

INTRODUCTION

The authors of the various chapters in this text provide an introduction to creative and innovative teaching strategies that are currently in use in higher education. The 1990s saw the evolution and development of these newer strategies, and the lecture that had been the educational gold standard for centuries appeared to be relegated to the status of a second-class citizen. It has become trendy to "lecture bash," to describe colleagues who openly espouse the use of lecture techniques as old-fashioned and out of step with educational trends. To many educators, the term lecture has been added to their list of unspeakable four-letter words. But a lecture is only a means to an end. Intrinsically, it is neither good nor bad; its success depends upon how it is delivered. In practice, however, the lecture format is alive and well regardless of the negative overtones that may be attributed by some people. The lecture remains one of the most frequently utilized teaching methods in the repertoire of postsecondary educators. When the objective is to communicate basic facts, introduce initial concepts or convey passion about a topic, a well prepared lecture is very useful (Germano, 2003; Gleitman, 2006). In this chapter, the reasons for the long-term popularity of this teaching strategy, how to improve its utilization, and how to become a better lecturer are explored.

DEFINITION AND PURPOSES

By definition, the lecture is one method of presenting information to an audience. Prior to the invention of the printing press, when only scholars had access to handwritten information sources, the lecture was the primary means of transmitting knowledge. Learners would gather around the master/teacher and take notes related to what was said. The lecture remained the common mode of disseminating information until printed resources and technological advancements became more available and affordable.

It would appear that when students were able to purchase their own textbooks and computers, methods of presenting information would have changed. Interestingly, change has occurred slowly. Today, with textbooks, computers, and study guides galore, the lecture remains a commonly used technique. It is suggested that there are two major reasons for this longevity: (1) most current educators learned via the lecture, and it is well known that individuals teach as they were taught unless they make a specific effort to alter their approaches; and (2) the lecture is the safest and easiest teaching method, allowing the educator the most control within the classroom. Some of the common advantages and disadvantages of using the lecture method are listed in **Table 8-1.** Whatever the rationale, positive outcomes can still be achieved by using the lecture, especially when the lecture and lecturer are well prepared.

THEORETICAL RATIONALE

Few lecturers take time to contemplate the theoretical basis of this practice, but the lack of a theoretical or organizational framework may be one reason that learners perceive some lecturers to be disorganized and/or difficult to follow. The teacher may derive a basis for lecturing from a variety of philosophical and theoretical processes. Three common approaches are communication, cognitive learning, and pedagogical/andragogical theories. The theories supporting effective communications should be common knowledge to all health care providers; therefore, they are not discussed here. Health educators should also have an understanding of cognitive learning theory because it is the underpinning of developmental concepts found in most health-related courses. Pedagogical/andragogical theories are not as well understood and are addressed briefly.

Over the past few decades, graduate education for many health professionals has emphasized disciplinary skills. Nursing, for instance, has focused on advanced nursing practice (clinical specialization and nurse practitioners) rather than on educational processes. This change has resulted in limited numbers of younger faculty members who have strong backgrounds in curricular design and learning theory. Pedagogy, a portion of learning theory, loosely refers to educating the chronologically or experientially young or immature. A major tenet of pedagogy lies within the fact that someone external to the learner decides what, when, where, how, and by whom information will be taught; the learner becomes a passive recipient of knowledge. Historically, health-related content

Table 8-1   Advantages and Disadvantages of Using Lectures As a Teaching Strategy

Advantages of a lecture
+ Permits maximum teacher control
+ Presents minimal threats to students or teacher
+ Enables lecturer to enliven facts and ideas that seem tedious in text
+ Enables lecturer to clarify confusing/intricate points
+ Teacher knows what has been presented
+ Lecture material can become basis of publication
+ Students are provided with a common core of content
+ Able to accommodate larger numbers of listeners at one setting
+ Cost-effective student:teacher ratio 200+:1
+ Economy of time:teacher can present content in much less time than to elicit from student or text
+ Teacher controls the pace of presentation
+ Reward for teacher: become known as an expert in specific topic
+ Encourages and allows deductive reasoning
+ Enthusiasm of teacher (role model) motivates students to participate and learn more
+ Lecturer can add the newest information on a moment's notice
+ Permits auditory learners to receive succinct information quickly
+ Enables integration of pro and con aspects of topic
+ Teacher can model kind of thinking desired for student
+ Produces better immediate recall of information

Table 8-1   Advantages and Disadvantages of Using Lectures As a Teaching Strategy (*continued*)

Disadvantages of a lecture
– Teacher may attempt to cover too much material in given time
– An easy teaching method, but a far less effective learning strategy
– About 80% of lecture information forgotten one day later and 80% of remainder fades in one month
– Presumes that all students learn at the same rate
– Not suited to higher levels of thinking
– Classes tend to be too large for personalized instruction
– Creates passive learners
– Provides little feedback to learners
– Student attention wavers in less than 30 minutes
– Teacher attempts to teach all that he or she has learned in a lifetime about a subject in one hour
– Inhibits development of inductive reasoning
– Poorly delivered lecture acts as a disincentive for learning
– Viewed by students as a complete learning experience; think lecturer presents all they need to know
– Affective learning seldom occurs
– If lecture is not written out, information may not be delivered accurately—if it is written out, why not allow students to read the material?

Source: Adapted from Woodring, B. (2001). Lecture is not a four-letter word. In A. J. Lowenstein & M. J. Bradshaw, *Fuszard's innovative teaching strategies in nursing* (3rd ed., p. 67). Gaithersburg, MD: Aspen Publishers, Inc.

and practice, especially that of nursing, has been taught from a framework based on the medical model; pedagogical principles have worked well. Within the pedagogical context, the lecture strategy establishes the teacher as the one in command, the authority from whom answers come. This approach may provide a rationale for lecturing being viewed as traditional and out of step with innovation and creativity in the academic process.

In recent years, both the age and experiential backgrounds of traditional college students have shifted, causing scholars to question the appropriateness of the previously used pedagogical methods. In response, educators such as Knowles (1970), Kidd (1973), and Cross (1986) introduced and refined the concept of *andragogy*. The principles previously utilized in teaching the young (pedagogy) were adapted and applied to mature learners (andragogy).

Those educators who ascribe to andragogical theory treat the learner as an adult who brings a variety of rich, valuable experiences to every learning situation. The who, what, when, and where of learning emanate from within the learner. **Table 8-2** illustrates the comparison of andragogy and pedagogy within the educational process.

Types of Learners

The information included in Table 8-2 emphasizes that the teacher must know as much as possible about both the learners and the topic before deciding on a specific teaching strategy. The concept of know thy student has always been important; however, today it is not only important, it is critical. Many classrooms are filled with students born after 1980 (generations referred to as "millennials," "Gen-X," or "wired") who have been raised in the technology age—whereas the faculty may still be uncomfortable responding via email. This means that in order to bridge this generation gap, the teacher must understand and acknowledge that the new learner has a very short attention span, has an arsenal of electronic devices at her fingertips (and in the classroom), is used to multitasking (answering text messages and listening to electro-tunes while reading about neuroanatomy), and is used to handling a rapid barrage of information (Carlson, 2005). In order to address these different learning needs, the proficient teacher will accompany the lecture with other adjuncts, such as games, video clips, lecture-discussion (discussed later in this chapter) or lecture enhanced with questions/answers, to accommodate the new and/or adult learner.

A lecture can be used effectively with learners who represent a variety of developmental and cognitive levels. In fact, that adaptability is one of the most positive aspects of this method. A teacher may, at a moment's notice, alter the teaching style, depth, sophistication, and level of the material being presented.

Table 8-2 Comparison of Characteristics: Andragogy vs. Pedagogy

Characteristic	Pedagogy	Andragogy
Concept of learner	• Dependent • Passive • Needs someone outside self to make decisions about what, when, and how to learn	• Independent/autonomous • Self-directed • Wants to participate in decisions related to own learning • Will increase effort if rewarded rather than punished
Roles of learner's experiences	• Past experiences given little attention • Narrow, focused interest • Focuses on imitation	• Wide range of experience, not just in nursing, which impacts life/learning • Broad interests—likes to share previous experience with others • Focus on originality

115

Readiness to learn	• Determined by someone else (society, teachers) • Students' focus is on what is needed to survive and achieve • Students tend to respond impulsively	• Students are usually in the educational process because they have chosen to be • Students want to assist in setting the learning agenda • Students tend to respond rationally
Orientation of teaching/learning	• Students look to teacher to identify what should be learned and to provide the information/process to learn • Students focus on particulars concerned with the superficial aspects of learning (grades, due dates) • Evaluation of learning done by teacher or society (grades, certificates) • Students need clarity/specificity	• Teachers are facilitators, providing resources and supports for self-directed learners • Students like challenging, independent assignments that are reality based • Evaluation is done jointly by teacher, learner, and/or peers • Students tolerate ambiguity

Source: Adapted from Woodring, B. (2001). Lecture is not a four-letter word. In A. J. Lowenstein & M. J. Bradshaw, *Fuszard's innovative teaching strategies in nursing* (3rd ed., p. 69). Gaithersburg, MD: Aspen Publishers, Inc.

These alterations can be made based on the needs, interests, and/or responses of the learners, new scientific revelations, or breaking news from the media. The assumption is made that the lecturer has a sufficient command of the subject matter, as well as the presence of mind and flexibility to alter the content and teaching plan (these assumptions may not be accurate with novice educators or when material is being presented the first time).

Combining the lecture with pedagogical approaches to teaching/learning is especially useful in basic and/or beginning courses in a sequence, as well as in orientation to new clinical areas or agencies. Novice learners of any age tend to prefer the structure of pedagogy, rather than andragogy; however, the more mature and secure teachers and learners become, the more they enjoy the flexibility and challenge of integrating andragogical concepts into the lecture format.

Types of Lecturers

Lectures survive because, like bullfights and masterpiece theater, they satisfy the need for dramatic spectacle and offer an interpersonal arena in which important psychological needs are met (Lowman, 1995). A teacher may vary a lecture from a very formal presentation to a much less formal monologue. Lowman described three types of lectures commonly used: formal, expository, and provocative. The *formal lecture* is sometimes referred to as an oral essay. In the formal setting, the lecturer delivers a well-organized, tightly constructed, highly polished presentation. The information provided primarily supports a specific point and usually is backed by theory and research. The presentation may be written and read to the audience, although recent data indicates that most learners do not like lecture materials to be read to them (Masie, 2006). Preparation of a formal lecture is time consuming; therefore, this method probably would not be used for every class period during a school term. It may, however, be appropriate to tie things together either at the beginning and/or end of a course, or for a specified topical area. One of the major problems with a formal lecture is that it ignores the interactive dimension and sometimes fails to motivate learners.

A variation on the formal lecture is *lecture-recitation*. This process is integrated into the formal lecture: the lecturer stops and asks a student to respond to a particular point or idea by reading/presenting materials he or she had prepared. An example of this approach may be a formal lecture related to the pathophysiology of sickle cell anemia (SCA), followed by a student-presented case study about a patient with SCA.

The *expository lecture* is considered the most typical type of lecture. It is much less elaborate than the formal oral essay. Although the lecturer does most of the talking, questions from learners are entertained.

In the *provocative lecture*, the instructor still does most of the talking, but he or she often provokes students' thoughts and challenges their knowledge and values with questions. This type of lecture allows for numerous variations on the theme and is becoming more popular in today's college classrooms. Included in this category are *lecture practice*, in which the instructor uses props to illustrate or demonstrate the subject and may include lectures with simulations or computer or video integration; *lecture-discussion*, during which the instructor speaks for 10 to 15 minutes and then stimulates student discussion around key points presented (the lecturer acts only as a facilitator to clarify and integrate student comments); *punctuated lecture*, in which the presenter asks the students to write down their reflections on lecture points and submit them; and *lecture-lab*, in which the lecture is followed by students conducting experiments, interviews, observations, practicing skills, and so forth during the class period. This lecture method may involve various types of interactive learning activities, where the lecture technique does not stand alone.

Keep in mind that a lecture, in and of itself, is neither a good nor a bad/inappropriate approach to teaching. It may be deemed the best method when dealing with certain groups; however, like any strategy, it is most effective when not used as the singular, exclusive technique. Eble (1982), in *The Craft of Teaching*, suggested that the lecture should be thought of as a discourse—a talk or conversation—not an authoritative speech. As a discourse, the lecture can be viewed as a planned portion of the art or craft of teaching. As such, lecturing becomes a learnable skill that improves with practice.

USING THE METHOD

When presenting an oral essay or formal lecture, preparation must begin well in advance of the presentation date. Planning, organization, and written preparation are essential and time consuming. Less formal forms of lecture may take less time, but their preparation should not be procrastinated. If the lecture is one in a sequence (or within a course), the best time to begin the final preparation of a lecture is at the completion of the preceding one. Significant ideas that need to be reemphasized are still fresh in the presenter's mind, as are the questions that were raised (or should have been raised) by the students. The lecturer can recall the presentation strategies that worked with this group of participants and those that did not. Changes that might have made the lecture more effective can be identified. Most lecturers, however, do not heed this advice, and lecture preparation is often relegated to a brief time immediately prior to the presentation. In order to present an effective lecture, the speaker must invest in preparing for three crucial time segments: the first 5 minutes, the main portion or body of the lecture, and the last 5 minutes.

Lecture Introduction (First 5 Minutes)

During the first 5 minutes of the lecture, two significant things occur: (1) the speaker outlines the objectives, outcomes, and expectations held for the participants; and (2) the audience decides whether to trust the speaker to produce what was promised (objectives) and whether to invest energy in following the presentation.

Some lecturers open with the statement, "There is too much material to be covered within the time allocated, but I'll do the best I can." From a teacher's point of view, this statement is always true, but it should *never* be said to an audience. If a lecturer opens with such a statement, the listener has already been conditioned to expect a less than top-notch presentation. The participant asks himself or herself, "Why should I bother to listen if I can't possibly learn what I need in this hour?" Once this statement has been made, the lecturer will have difficulty regaining the full attention of the listener. So, no matter how tempting it may be to use the statement, eliminate it from your repertoire. Instead, begin by identifying what the learner should gain from the lecture: state the objectives in clear, interesting, pragmatic, and achievable terms. Then, make a solid connection with the listeners by using an example of how the lecture material can be (or has been) used in practice or life in general.

Outline the key concepts that will be addressed, and use your expertise and clinical experience to provide some background and rationale for this lecture. The key points should be limited in number. Research on what is remembered following classes indicated that most students can absorb only three to four major points in a 50-minute lecture and four to five points in a 75-minute presentation (Lowman, 1995). Conclude the introduction by establishing an open atmosphere and describing the "rules of operation" (e.g., "Feel free to ask questions at any time;" or "There will be time at the end of the lecture for questions."). An open atmosphere can be established by posing a question, making a bold statement, using a controversial quote, using humor, or using a visual aid or cartoon. The better one knows the audience, the easier and more successful the introduction becomes.

Body of Lecture

Like the human body, the lecture is divided into specific parts. The main portion, or body, should begin with a definition of concepts or principles that are illustrated by pragmatic, personal/professional experiences. The speaker then conveys the critical information the learner needs to know. The body should be well organized, with smooth transitions between topics. The experienced presenter knows that a lecturer cannot carry the primary responsibility for conveying all information or imparting all skills. Readings or problem-solving assignments must be made to accomplish those goals, and students need to be appraised of this connection. The body of the lecture should contain: (1) general themes that tie together other related topics; (2) topics that are difficult for students to understand (e.g., fluid balance); (3) sufficient depth and complexity to retain the learners' interest; and (4) testimonies (e.g., quotes from cancer survivors), case-specific data (e.g., lab values from unusual patient diagnoses), and exhibits (e.g., charts/graphs of statistics) to support the outcome-related point being made.

The speaker's presentation style is most evident during the body of the lecture. Tips and suggestions made in the Resources section of this chapter will enhance your presentation style.

Lecturer Conclusion (Last 5 Minutes)

The lecture needs a definite stopping point. Closing a notebook, running out of time or simply dismissing the class is not an acceptable conclusion. An effective communicator knows that any interaction deserves closure—a lecture is no exception to that rule. By focusing the learners' attention during the last 5 minutes of class, the lecturer is able to establish finality and make a link between what was taught and what the learner will be able to use in life or practice. A good conclusion ties the introduction and the body together in a manner similar to that of an abstract that precedes a well-written manuscript.

The objectives and outcomes statements that were used as a portion of the introduction should be reiterated, assuming they have been accomplished. The conclusion should also contain a review of the key points or topics covered and allow time for elaboration, amplification and/or clarification of issues presented. Offering suggestions related to the application and transfer of knowledge may be helpful to the participants and the use of summative take-home points may provide additional reinforcement. Using this approach allows the learner to quickly rethink the content, stimulate continued interest, and consider further action. The participants will leave the lecture hall feeling a sense of accomplishment because they can summarize what has been learned. Thus, each lecture should be carefully planned and presented with an introduction (first 5 minutes), a well-organized body, and a meaningful conclusion (last 5 minutes) (Woodring, 2001).

RESOURCES

The major resource needed to utilize the lecture techniques effectively is *you*, the lecturer. Presenting an informative and interesting lecture is a craft and a learnable skill. Because the speaker is the key element for this strategy, the following points are presented to help polish your presentation skills . . . and remember participants want to believe that you are smart, interesting, and a good speaker (Germano, 2003)!

- ***Conveying enthusiasm is the key element in presenting an effective lecture.*** Enthusiasm is contagious and is demonstrated by facial expressions, excitement in the voice, gestures, and body language. A lack of enthusiasm on the part of the speaker is interpreted by the listener as a lack of self-confidence, lack of knowledge, a disinterest in the learner, and/or disinterest in the topic. If you do not have an effusive personality, practice adding a smile and small hand gestures to each lecture. Once these movements are comfortable, add other interactive methods.
- ***Know the content.*** Even a written, formal lecture will not hide the insecurity of being unprepared or underprepared.
- ***Use notes.*** The use of notes is generally the option of the speaker; however, to avoid the distress of losing your train of thought or incorrectly presenting complex information, the use of some type of notes is highly recommended. For ease of handling, record the notes all on the same size paper or card ($4'' \times 6''$ or $5'' \times 7''$ note cards or $8 \ 1/2'' \times 11''$ sheets of paper work well). Sequentially number each card or page; this task is a great asset should you drop or have a breeze, fan, or air conditioner blow away your notes. If you are using PowerPoint slides to accompany the lecture, you may wish to operationalize the notation section and have your lecture notes or outline appear on the computer screen in front of you, while remaining out of the sight of the participants. The depth and content of lecture notes should fit the lecturer's comfort level; use of anything from a skeletal outline to a full manuscript is acceptable. Notes should be prepared leaving white space that is easy for the eye to follow. This layout can be accomplished by handwriting or typing in a double spaced, large font format. Major points should be highlighted so the eye can easily pick up a cue when scanning a page. Although the use of notes is perfectly acceptable, the verbatim reading of notes is *not* acceptable. Rehearse your presentation as long and as often as needed so the lecture will appear spontaneous and enthusiastic and will be completed within the allotted time frame.
- ***Speak to an audience of 200 as if they were a single student.*** Speak clearly and loudly enough to be heard in the back of the room. The use of a microphone may be necessary if you are presenting in a large room or auditorium. Always use the microphone if there is any doubt that your voice will not be heard in the last row. It is sometimes helpful to have a friend sit in the back and signal if your voice is not being heard during the presentation. A small clip-on type microphone is preferable to using a hand-held or stationary microphone because it allows the speaker to move away

from the podium and frees one's hands to handle notes and/or gesture. If a microphone is to be used, the speaker should arrive in the assigned room early enough to try the equipment and to regulate microphone position and sound levels. If the lecture is being transmitted to multiple sites, as in distance/distributive education or videoconferencing settings, be certain to test the sound levels at all sites prior to beginning the lecture.

- *Make eye contact.* Select a participant at each corner of the room with whom you plan to make eye contact. Slowly scan the audience until you have seen each of the designated participants. Smile at familiar faces. If needed, review information related to the process of group dynamics. If the lecture is being transmitted to multiple sites, be certain to look directly into the cameras for the benefit of participants in the distant sites. You may wish to make a concerted effort to look into each monitor as you visually scan the lecture hall and address participants at each site.
- *Use creative movement.* Movements of the speaker's head and hands in gesturing should appear natural, not forced. Be careful when standing behind a podium; do not grip the sides tightly with your hands or lock your (shaky?) knees. This action produces a circulatory response that could cause you to faint. Occasionally step away from the podium and toward the listeners, which conveys an attitude of warmth and acceptance. Avoid distracting mannerisms such as pacing, wringing your hands, clearing your throat, or jamming your hands into pockets and jingling change.
- ***The use of a stage or podium places an automatic barrier between the speaker and the listeners.*** This gulf needs to be bridged early and often during the lecture. Suggestions for bridging the gulf include: (1) use notecards rather than a manuscript because they are more portable and allow freedom to move away from the podium on occasion; (2) step out from behind the podium, especially if you are short in stature. The audience does not wish to see a "talking head"; (3) walk toward the listeners, which is interpreted as a sign of warmth and reaching out to the audience; (4) address the right half of the audience, the left half of the audience, and then the audience at each distant site (each monitor). Do not turn your back to either side of the audience or to transmitting cameras; (5) call on at least one participant in the audience and at each distant site by name; (6) use hand gestures to accentuate words, but be careful not to overdo this action (this is especially important if the lecture is being transmitted to multiple sites because large hand gestures are more distracting when seen on a monitor than when viewed in person); and (7) if given the opportunity to be seated on a stage/platform, be aware of the eye level of the audience. Should speakers seated on a platform feel the need to cross their legs, they should cross them at the ankles.

- *Create a change of pace.* An astute lecturer constantly assesses the audience and reads participants' signals. Facial cues indicate agreement/disagreement with what has been said and may express understanding/misunderstanding of content. Another signal is given when listeners begin having side conversations or squirm in their seats. These signals call for intervention, response, or a change of pace by the speaker. The change of pace can be as simple as turning off the overhead projector or shifting to a new slide (the sound and changing light pattern will cause the listener to refocus attention on the speaker or back to the visual); shifting the focus from the speaker to a handout; using a humorous example; altering the tone or inflection of your voice; requesting written or verbal feedback from participants; dividing into small groups for a brief discussion; or allowing students to stand and stretch or take a break for a few minutes. Keep this rule of thumb in mind: an individual's optimal attention span is roughly 1 minute per year of age up to the approximate age of 45 (e.g., a 5-year-old has a 5-minute attention span; a 25-year-old, 25 minutes), and decreases among the younger, digitally minded. Therefore, plan a change of pace or break according to the average age of your audience. "The mind can only absorb as much as the seat can endure" is a fairly valid guideline.
- *Distribute a skeletal outline only if it will help the learners to identify key points.* Emphasize principles and concepts. Do not copy charts, graphs, and materials that are found in the learners' texts. Handout information should supplement the lecture. The lecture should not be a rehash of basic information from the learners' textbook. If handouts are used, they should be clear and contain a limited amount of information so the learners are not overwhelmed. Handouts printed on colored paper stand out and are more likely to be read than those printed on white paper. The reproduction of handouts of the PowerPoint slides used during a lecture is a well debated topic. Germano (2003) declares technology to be a tool, but notes that tools are not friends and are often rivals. The distribution of full-text class notes, slides that contain a significant proportion of the lecture content, etc. truly discourage class attendance (Stewart, 2006), so consider their dissemination carefully.

Several publications that may be of assistance in keeping the lecture process fresh are: *The Teaching Professor, Change, The National Teaching & Learning Forum,* and *Survival Skills for Scholars* series. In addition, web sites maintained by a number of universities offer assistance. These include: University of Chicago (http://teaching.uchicago.edu/handbook/tac06.html); University of Toledo (http://education.utoledo.edu/par/Adults.html); and Towson State University (http://www.new.towson.edu/facultyonline/ISD/lectures.htm). Numerous online journals and Listservs also can provide rapid access to information related to specific topics of interest.

POTENTIAL PROBLEMS

Nothing is perfect. As with any method or technique, some problems exist with the use of the lecture as a teaching strategy. A key question to be answered is: "What makes lectures and lecturers unsuccessful?" Over the past decade, graduate nursing students have responded to that question, and each year student responses were consistent. The most frequently repeated negative characteristics of lectures/ lecturers focused on the person doing the presenting, *not* the method (Woodring, 2000). Examples of these negatives and some suggestions for improvement are found in **Table 8-3.** The remainder of this section is devoted to dealing with negative perceptions, which are more generic than the characteristics in Table 8-3.

Student Boredom

Educators today face challenges that our predecessors did not even dream about! How can one obtain and retain the attention of the Game Boy and Pod generation? This generation of learners is accustomed to fast-paced, action-packed, colorized entertainment at the flick of a switch. To compensate for this situational dilemma and still utilize the lecture technique effectively, the teacher should experiment with combining advanced technologies and the lecture within the classroom. Some examples include: in-class use of a textbook on CD/DVD with capabilities of adding supplementary information during the lecture; the use of a computer-linked electronic blackboard to transfer information from an e-blackboard to individual students' laptop monitors; the appropriate and creative integration of PowerPoint-type visuals during the lecture or integration of text/ reference materials via a PDA format. These electronic capabilities allow the lecturer to interject computer-generated charts, graphs, diagrams, student input, and up-to-the-minute research findings into the lecture. Luck and Laurence (2005) validated the use of videoconferencing technology used to present a lecture series for beginning college students. The lecture/videoconference was evaluated by the learners as encouraging positive active participation and allowing prompt feedback.

Additionally, assignment of out-of class computer-assisted instructional programs (such as ADAM/EVE, simulations or patient/disease-specific learning packages), communication packages (e.g., WebCrossings), and/or electronic/ Internet-based assignments to complement the lecture will assist in gaining and maintaining the interest of more technologically suave students.

Table 8-3   The Perceived Negative Factors Related to Lecturing

Negatives	Suggestions for improvement
• Material is disorganized or hard to follow • Lack of outline or outline too detailed	• Prepare and follow brief outline for each lecture.
• Speaker wears distracting clothing • Speaker lacks professional appearance	• Dress as a professional role model. If you don't care about wearing stripes and plaids together, enlist the help of a colleague who you consider to be a professional.
• Lack of facial expression by speaker • Speaker has monotone voice (nervous, shaky voice) • Lack of enthusiasm by speaker	• Audio- and/or videotape one of your lectures and analyze it; establish some goals for improvement; then view it with a friend or colleague to support your decisions for change.
• Speaker won't take eyes off notes • Speaker reads the lecture material	• Practice your lecture in front of a mirror or videotape it. • Practice until you know the main points by memory. Use only as many written notes as are absolutely essential. Place cues in the margin for yourself (smile, walk, and relax).
• Speaker often sits behind podium to lecture (referred to as the "talking head" because that is all that students see!)	• Don't stand behind a podium unless you are 6 feet tall. • Ask for a shorter, lower lectern or table.
• Uses no visual aids or visuals of poor quality	• Don't put too much information in small print on slides and overhead transparencies. • Ask librarian, media center, or learning center personnel for assistance in preparing visuals.
• Too many PowerPoint slides	• Use visuals to support, not replace content.

Table 8-3   The Perceived Negative Factors Related to Lecturing (*continued*)

Negatives	Suggestions for improvement
• Doesn't acknowledge that adult learners like to participate	• Review techniques for keeping adult learners engaged. • See references by Cross, Kidd, and Knowles.
• Inconsiderate of learners' needs	• Implement planned change-of-pace activities.
• Distracting habits of characteristics: pacing; staring out windows; playing with objects (paper clips, rubber bands, change); using nonwords (ah, um) and repetitious phrases (you know, like, well, uh)	• Use a videotape of your lecture to identify repetitive habits. • Repositioning hands or holding notecards may help the "nervous hands" problem. • Make a list of alternate words that could be substituted for the frequently repeated pet phrases. • Become aware of the use of nonwords, which are a verbalization that allows your speech to catch up to what your brain is thinking. This may or may not be all you need to eliminate them; when they occur, stop, take a deep breath, and then go on.

Source: Reprinted from Woodring, B. (2001). Lecture is not a four-letter word. In A. J. Lowenstein & M. J. Bradshaw, *Fuszard's innovative teaching strategies in nursing* (3rd ed., pp. 76–77). Gaithersburg, MD: Aspen Publishers, Inc.

Institutional Barriers

Physical, political, and situational barriers exist within every institution, any or all of which may contribute to dissatisfaction with any given instructional approach. The timing of a class offering cannot be overlooked. Traditionally, teachers have disliked teaching, and students have disliked attending classes offered at 7 a.m. or 9 p.m. No one likes getting up that early or staying in class that late! Classes taught immediately after meal time are considered sleepers because blood leaves the brain and moves to the gastrointestinal tract, making everyone sluggish. Classes taught late in the afternoon or early evening are bad because the students and teachers are tired. Try as one might, short of one-on-one teaching, or totally online/asynchronous education, the perfect time to hold a class will probably never be found. Speakers must make their presentations stimulating and motivating at any time of the day!

Another institutional barrier to be considered is the number of students proportional to the size of the classroom and the number of students in proportion to the number of faculty (student-to-faculty ratio). Lecturers are often placed in small, crowded classrooms with large numbers of students or large, cavernous classrooms with smaller numbers of students. Often, geographical relocation of desks/tables could ease the space configuration and provide a more positive learning atmosphere. Should the lecturer have the option, it is most ideal to be able to clearly see and make eye contact with each participant. This may be accomplished by arranging seating in a semicircle around the lectern or angling tables. But if seating is fixed within the classroom, then it becomes the responsibility of the speaker to move and make eye contact as often as possible.

The large student-to-faculty ratio within classes will probably not decrease in postsecondary education in the near future. Large classes, especially at the freshman and sophomore levels, are very cost-effective. The bottom line will continue to impose restrictions that are exacerbated by the increase in distance and multisite class sessions and faculty shortage in many health-related professions. This disproportionate student-to-faculty ratio will require lecturers to implement the tips list under the previous Resources section, as well as utilize technological support, teaching assistants for smaller group interactions, and other creative strategies to enhance student learning for material presented in large lecture sections.

Negative Comments

The faculty member who consistently lectures may be subjected to student-generated negative comments, such as, "This class is so boring—all he does is lecture"; "It's awful, she reads to us right out of her book"; or "I can't learn to think critically if all she does is lecture!" It is generally not the method but the teacher who is at fault if such comments are disseminated. It is often said that lecturing is a poor teaching method, a kind of last resort for instruction. Many lecturers, in fact, do not know how to impart information or stimulate interest effectively; consequently, their lectures are often poorly presented, badly organized, dull, and uninspiring (Gleitman, 2006). In order to correct or prevent negative comments, plan ahead, organize the content and introduce at least one additional teaching method (e.g., discussion, video, question-and-answer, small group interaction, role playing) into each lecture session. This approach will increase student interaction and should increase student satisfaction. In addition, if you tell the students how you are attempting to improve the lecture setting, you will gain the participants' respect because you have acknowledged their feelings and made an overt effort to respond to them.

Knowledge Retention

The problem of retaining information gained from a lecture should be acknowledged and addressed. Although those educators who enjoy using the lecture method hate to admit it, research conducted in the 1990s found that 80% of information gained by lecture alone can not be recalled by students 1 day later, and that 80% of the remainder fades in a month. Since additional research has not been done to alter that perception, one must still heed the results. Educational data is available to indicate that the more a learner's senses (taste, touch, smell, sight, and hearing) are involved in the learning activity, the longer and the higher the volume of knowledge is retained. Therefore, if certain types of equipment were used to illustrate a point (utilizing touch and/or sight), a video clip was inserted into the midst of the lecture (using sight and/or hearing), or any other active learning process (gaming) were introduced, the students' knowledge retention would increase.

In recent years, the use of *punctuated lectures* has also been viewed as a method to increase retention of information. The punctuated lecture requires students and teachers to go through five steps: (1) listen (to a portion of a lecture); (2) stop; (3) reflect (on what they were doing, thinking, and feeling during that portion of the lecture); (4) write (what they were doing, thinking, and feeling during that portion of the lecture); and (5) give (the written feedback to the lecturer) (Cross & Steadman, 1996). This approach provides the lecturer and the students with an opportunity to become engaged with the learning process, as well as to self-monitor their in-class behaviors. In addition, Brookfield (2002) reminds us that students cannot read the lecturer's mind. Students cannot be expected to know what teachers expect, stand for, or wish them to value unless it is explicitly and vigorously communicated to them. The reflective teacher, according to Brookfield, must build a continual case for learning, action, and practice instead of assuming that students see the self-evident value of what we are telling them.

Implementing the suggestions just given should enhance knowledge retention emanating from a lecture.

EVALUATION

An evaluation of the lecture/lecturer must be completed in a timely manner. The most useful time to obtain this data is at the completion of an individual lecture. Obtaining this information need not be laborious. Ask the listeners to respond to a few specific questions, and then allow them to provide additional comments in an anonymous format. This type of feedback is especially helpful for the novice lecturer. The evaluation process should aim to provide constructive criticism and comments for improvement. The author utilizes this technique. The students may make any comments they wish; however, a negative comment cannot be made without offering a suggestion for its resolution. When this evaluation technique is used routinely, the learners become accustomed to it. The process can be completed in 5 minutes or less. Often, teachers are so interested in assessing whether the course objectives have been met that they forget to evaluate the means by which they were met. Lecturers will not improve without suggested change, and suggested change can best be obtained via the use of a planned evaluation tool/method that is completed by peers and/or class participants. The evaluation of a lecture or lecturer should not occur in isolation; it must be viewed as a portion of an overall evaluation plan, and should be conducted only when there are plans for growth, follow-up, and change.

CONCLUSION

Presenting an effective lecture is more than simply standing in front of a group and verbalizing information. The lecturer must consider the learners' needs, abilities, and learning styles; the cognitive and developmental levels of the learners; the stated objectives and desired outcomes of the class; and the individual objectives of the learners. The lecture should be divided into three major segments: introduction (5 minutes), body, and conclusion (5 minutes). Each section should be planned and presented in an organized manner, never off the cuff. The prepared lecturer will be considerate, credible, and in control (not to be mistaken for rigidity and controlling). Several factors enhance the presentation of a lecture, but none is more important than genuine enthusiasm. The lecture should not be considered a secondary teaching strategy. In many situations, it is the most appropriate methodology to be used. To elicit the best results, the lecture should be accompanied by at least one of the other effective strategies discussed in this text.

REFERENCES

Brookfield, S. (2002). Using lenses of critically reflective teaching in the community college classroom. *New Directions for Community Colleges, 18,* 31–38.

Carlson, S. (2005, October 7). The net generation goes to college. *The Chronicle of Higher Education: The Chronicle Review.* Retrieved February 27, 2006, from http://chronicle.com/cgi-bin/printable.cgi?article=jttp://chronicle.com/weekly/v52/i07/07a

Cross, K. P. (1986, September). A proposal to improve teaching. *AAHE Bulletin, 39*(1), 9–15.

Cross, K., & Steadman, M. (1996). *Classroom research: Implementing the scholarship of teaching.* San Francisco: Jossey Bass Publishers.

Eble, K. (1982). *The craft of teaching.* San Francisco: Jossey-Bass Publishers.

Germano, W. (2003, November 28). The scholarly lecture: How to stand and deliver. *The Chronicle of Higher Education: The Chronicle Review.* Retrieved February 27, 2006, from http://chronicle.com/cgi-bin/printable.cgi?article=jttp://chronicle.com/weekly/v50/i14/14b

Gleitman, H. (2006). Lecturing: Using a much maligned method of teaching. In *Teaching at Chicago: A Handbook.* Chicago: The University of Chicago Center for Teaching and Learning. Retrieved February 27, 2006, from http://teaching.uchicago.edu/handbook/tac06.html

Kidd, J. R. (1973). *How adults learn.* New York: Association Press.

Knowles, M. (1970). *The modern practice of adult education: Androgogy versus pedagogy.* New York: Association Press.

Lowman, J. (1995). *Mastering the techniques of teaching* (2nd ed.). San Francisco: Jossey-Bass Publishers.

Luck, M., & Laurence, G. (2005). Innovative teaching: Sharing expertise through videoconferencing. *Innovate, 2*(1). Retrieved October 13, 2005, from http://www.innovateonline.info/index.php?view=article&id=59

Masie, E. (2006). *Most common training mistakes: Results of learning TRENDS survey.* New York: The MASIE Center.

Stewart, E. (2006, February 6). Class-conscious: Teachers want tech to enhance—not replace—lectures. Utah *Desert News.* Retrieved February 22, 2006, from http://deseretnews.com/dn/view/0,1249,635181866,00.html

Woodring, B. (2000). Preparing presentations that produce peace of mind. *Journal of Child and Family Nursing, 3*(1), 63–64.

Woodring, B. (2001). *Student evaluation of teaching effectiveness: Process and Outcome.* Unpublished manuscript.

SUGGESTED READING

Bankert, E., & Kozel, V. (2005). Transforming pedagogy in nursing education: A caring learning environment for adult students. *Nursing Education Perspectives, 226*(4), 227–229.

Cramer, R. (1999). Large classes, intimate possibilities. *The National Teaching & Learning Forum, 8*(4), 5–6.

Felder, R. (2005). Understanding student differences. *Journal of Engineering Education, 94*(1), 57–72.

Olmstead, J. (1999). The mid-lecture break: When less is more. *Journal of Chemical Education*, *76*(4), 525–527.

Stern, B. (2004). A comparison of online and face-to-face instruction in an undergraduate foundations of American education course. *Contemporary Issues in Technology and Teacher Education*, *4*(2), 196–213.

Tanner, C. (2002). Learning to teach: An introduction to "Teacher Talk": New pedagogies for nursing. *Journal of Nursing Education*, *41*(3), 95–96.

Veronikas, S., & Shaughnessy, M. (2004, July–August). Teaching and learning in a hybrid world. *Educause*, *39*(4), 51–62.

Young, P., & Dieklemann, N. (2002). Learning to lecture: Exploring the skills, strategies and practices of new teachers in nursing education. *Journal of Nursing Education*, *41*(9), 404–411.

CHAPTER 9

Problem-Based Learning

Patricia Solomon

INTRODUCTION

Problem-based learning (PBL) is an educational process in which learning is centered around problems as opposed to discrete subject-related courses. In small groups, students are presented with patient scenarios or problems, generate learning issues related to what they need to learn in order to understand the problem, engage in independent self-study and return to their groups to apply their new knowledge to the patient problem. PBL is largely acknowledged as starting in the medical school at McMaster University in the mid-1960s in response to an educational environment that emphasized passive learning of large quantities of information that was quickly outdated and often appeared irrelevant. The emphasis is on learning all content in an integrative way through small group, self-directed study of a problem and the assistance of a faculty tutor who is a facilitator of learning rather than an expert lecturer (Walton & Matthews, 1989). While PBL is theoretically more effective in structuring knowledge, the most agreed-upon advantage is that it is more enjoyable than traditional learning methods.

BACKGROUND AND DEFINITIONS

Since being introduced, PBL has been adopted by many health professional programs worldwide. Although many variants of PBL have been described, the essential elements remain: (1) students are presented with a written problem or patient scenario in small groups; (2) there is a change in faculty role from imparter of information to facilitator of learning; (3) there is an emphasis on student responsibility and self-directed learning; and (4) a written problem is the stimulus for learning with students engaging in a problem-solving process as they learn and discuss content related to the problem (Solomon, 1994).

While PBL may be viewed as an educational methodology, it is most often associated with an overall curricular approach. PBL was originally viewed as an all-or-none phenomenon in which an educational program had to commit entirely to the curricular philosophy to attain the most benefits (Barrows & Tamblyn, 1980). Programs that had individual problem-based courses and more traditional courses running concurrently were thought to produce mixed messages in the student and devalue the problem-based components (Walton & Matthews, 1989). While there is still concern that isolated problem-based courses will not be successful (Albanese, 2000), there is certainly greater acceptance of curricula that use mixed or partial PBL approaches.

There have been several attempts to define and classify PBL curricula. Barrows (1986) describes a taxonomy based largely on the problem design and role of the teacher. Charlin, Mann, and Hansen (1998) present an analytic framework to understand and compare PBL curricula, which varies along 10 dimensions such as the purpose of the problem and the nature of the task to be accomplished during study of the problem. Harden and Davis (1998) offer an 11-step continuum of PBL with theoretical learning and an emphasis on traditional lectures and textbooks at one end, and task-based learning (essentially learning in clinical practice settings with real patients), at the other. As one moves along the continuum, there is greater emphasis on the problem, activation of prior knowledge, contextual learning, and discovery learning. Solomon, Binkley, and Stratford (1996) provide a simple distinction between a problem-based curriculum that they describe as fully integrated (with few or no subject-related courses) and a transitional PBL curriculum that uses more traditional curricular elements early in the curriculum and incorporates increasingly larger components of PBL as the students progress through their program.

THEORETICAL FOUNDATIONS

Some of the original theoretical premises for PBL have not found strong support within the literature. Contextual learning was an appealing rationale for the superiority of PBL. The rationale was that by learning all content, including basic, clinical and social sciences, within the context of a problem, a learner would be able to recall information better when he/she encountered a similar patient within the clinical setting. But there is weak empirical support, and this theory is likely too simplistic to integrate the complexities associated with PBL (Colliver, 2000).

The information processing theory (Schmidt, 1983) incorporates aspects of contextual learning theory and provides more comprehensive theoretical support for PBL as it also considers activation of prior knowledge and elaboration of knowledge as core elements (Albanese, 2000). However, one theory may be insufficient support for PBL. Albanese outlines three others which are salient to PBL: cooperative learning theory, self-determination theory, and control theory. Cooperative learning, in which individuals are dependent on other group members to achieve their goals, is used extensively in small group PBL. Self-determination theory identifies controlled, more maladaptive motivators of behavior, and autonomous motivators that the learner finds more interesting and enjoyable (Williams, Saizow, & Ryan, 1999). Controlled motivators, which include external demands under which people act with a sense of pressure and anxiety, are more characteristic of traditional curricula. Autonomous motivators, which involve a sense of volition and choice, would be more characteristic of a PBL curriculum. Control theory states that all behavior is based on satisfying the five basic needs of freedom: power, love and belonging, fun, survival, and reproduction (Glaser, 1985). Instruction can fail if it does not meet these basic needs of the learner. PBL may be superior at meeting these needs. For example, fun, or enjoyment of learning, has been frequently associated with outcomes of PBL (Albanese and Mitchell, 1993).

TYPES OF LEARNERS

PBL has been used extensively in many health professional programs. Health professional students at all levels can benefit from the use of PBL to simulate realistic clinical situations. It is important to note that students accustomed to more traditional ways of learning often experience stress and anxiety when adapting to this new student-centered style of learning (Solomon & Finch, 1998). Supports must be put in place to ease the students' transition to this type of learning.

RESOURCES

PBL requires different resources to support implementation. Contrary to more traditional programs in which one faculty member lectures to large numbers of students, learning occurs in small groups, necessitating additional faculty to support PBL. There is also a need for numerous small group tutorial rooms and extensive library and other learning resources which enable self-directed learning. As elaborated upon in the next section, there is an additional need for faculty who are well trained to assume the role of facilitator.

ROLE OF FACULTY

There has been significant debate in the PBL literature as to whether expert or nonexpert tutors are preferable. Content experts are thought to be more likely to revert to lecture type of behaviors and be less facilitatory. Although some debate remains (e.g., Kaufman & Holmes, 1998), it is generally recognized that a combination of content and process expertise is preferable.

Dolmans, Wolfhagen, Scherpbier, and Van Der Vleuten (2001) provide an excellent summary of issues related to tutor expertise. Not surprisingly, they conclude that tutors initiate activities with which they are most familiar. Hence content experts use their expertise to direct tutorial performance and noncontent experts use their process facilitation skills to direct group dynamics. However, this relationship is not as simple as once believed. A tutor's performance is not likely to be stable and is influenced by contextual circumstances such as the quality of the written cases, the structure of the course, and students' prior knowledge. Thus, tutor expertise may compensate if the structure of the problem is low and/or the students have little prior knowledge of the case.

While the evidence suggests that it is not a simple distinction between expert and nonexpert tutors, the implications for faculty development are clear; faculty require training to assume more facilitative roles. Hitchcock and Mylona (2000) note that there has been little systematic study on effective ways to train faculty to assume PBL roles, although there have been many descriptions in the literature. They emphasize that while the most obvious training is in tutor facilitation skills, there are many other roles and skills that need to be developed. They emphasize Irby's (1996) sequence of steps of skill development: (1) challenging assumptions and developing understanding of PBL; (2) experiencing and valuing the tutorial process; (3) acquiring general tutor skills; (4) developing content-specific tutor knowledge and skills; (5) acquiring advanced knowledge and skills; (6) developing leadership and scholarship skills; and (7) creating organizational vitality.

It is clear that faculty who possess a level of content expertise in the area under study are the preferred small group facilitators. However, there is an equally important need for faculty who are well trained in PBL and the tutorial process. The skills needed to facilitate and evaluate small group process, to promote metacognitive skills such as self-monitoring of one's reasoning and decision-making skills, to design curriculum, and to develop problems and other instructional materials to support self-directed learning are very different than those skills required in a traditional curriculum and require long-term faculty development initiatives.

USING PBL METHODS

There appears to be no one best way to implement PBL. Although some maintain that fully integrated PBL is preferable, this curricular design may not be feasible for many institutions. Diversity in curricular design and approach is to be expected as different institutional structures and philosophies and faculty knowledge and skill development will influence the extent to which PBL can be incorporated into the curriculum.

Typically, the process is as follows. Students are presented with a written problem as a stimulus for learning. Problems are carefully designed to facilitate discussion related to specific learning objectives. In groups of six to eight, students read the problem (either aloud or to themselves) and brainstorm around what they need to learn in order to better understand the problem or hypothesize around potential causes of the problem. During this initial process, students generate learning issues or questions for self-study. Learning issues can range from factual knowledge (e.g., What nerves innovate the upper extremity?), to more complex physiological questions (e.g., What is the process of inflammation?), to questions that include broader psychosocial issues (e.g., How would I apply a model of ethical decision making to this patient?), or questions that require evaluation of the literature and integration of evidence based practice (e.g., What is the effectiveness of ultrasound in the treatment of lateral epicondylitis?). The process of developing a high quality, learning issue which is researchable may be quite time consuming for the learner who is new to PBL. Generation of the final list of learning issues that will be researched and discussed at the next tutorial constitutes the end of the first stage of the PBL process. Students can choose to independently research all learning issues that have been generated for that session or to divide up the learning issues amongst themselves for self-study. When students return for the next tutorial they discuss their findings and the implications for patient care. At the end of the tutorial, students engage in a structured evaluation of the tutorial process and their performance. Each student provides a verbal self-evaluation of their performance that day and their peers and the faculty tutor provide feedback.

During the tutorial the faculty tutor does not provide expert content information. Rather, his/her role is to establish the climate for learning, encourage problem solving, and promote debate and discussion within the group. The tutor also role models effective self-evaluation and provision of feedback. Barrows (1988) describes the faculty tutoring role as going through three stages: (1) *modeling* the thinking process for the students by questioning and challenging them; (2) as the group becomes more comfortable with the process the faculty role shifts to one of *coaching* when the students are off track or confused; and (3) as students progress further and develop into a well functioning and effective learning group, the role of the tutor *fades*, leaving the group to work more independently. Barrows suggests that groups should meet for at least eight weeks to allow for progression of these three stages.

POTENTIAL PROBLEMS

The costs associated with the number of faculty required to deliver education in small groups is a key concern and potential barrier to implementation (Albanese & Mitchell, 1993). Other costs related to space requirements for small group tutorial rooms and development of self-directed learning resources may also pose barriers (Solomon, 1994). Without institutional support for curricular change, many programs may find it difficult to engage successfully in curriculum reform.

An additional barrier to the implementation of innovative problem-based curricula relates to the lack of rigorous, long-term data which demonstrate significant differences between more traditional and PBL curricula. The lack of evidence reinforces the concerns of critics who ask, "Why bother?" Some argue that PBL is worth implementing even if the only benefit is its more personal, humane, and enjoyable approach. Federman (1999) noted advantages of PBL that are not amenable to measurement and relate more to the personal and interpersonal aspects of practice. Even the most ardent of critics would agree that these are desirable in health professional education. Some of these include: (1) the person-to-person contact inherent in a small group tutorial process; (2) the positive regard that is fostered by the respect afforded to the beginning student; (3) the focus on patients, which promotes relevancy of the curriculum from early days; (4) increased opportunities to discuss moral and ethical issues and for the tutor to share his or her values; and (5) the positive effect on lectures, as with only a few lectures in the timetable, students are more committed to lectures, and this, in turn, has a stimulating effect on the faculty.

Recently, with the rise in popularity of online and web-based learning, there has been an interest in doing PBL online. Increased accessibility and opportunities for asynchronous learning are obvious advantages for distance and continuing education courses. In health professional educational programs, PBL online has inherent appeal as the number of facilitators required could be reduced, thus making it possible to implement in programs without sufficient resources to do face-to-face PBL. Although there have been a few descriptive articles (e.g., Bresnitz, 1996), few have examined the effectiveness of computer-based PBL. Some of the characteristics of PBL, such as using patient problems, sharing learning, promoting integration of knowledge, and self-directed learning are relatively easy to transfer to online formats. However, the advantage of flexibility, related to the ability to access the course in an asynchronous manner, might not be realized in an intensive, integrated professional curricula in which the students' timetables are more restricted. Face-to-face PBL allows for the development of communication and verbal skills related to the ability to clearly articulate and present information, provide feedback to others, and develop and evaluate group skills. The communication skills that are central to professional practice would clearly not be developed in the same way as they would in a small group face-to-face PBL as opposed to online PBL.

CONCLUSION

PBL is an increasingly popular teaching and learning strategy within the health professions. The clinical relevance, small group interactions, and active learning provided make PBL an appealing curricular alternative. Faculty training and expertise are essential for successful outcomes.

APPLIED EXAMPLE

An Interprofessional Problem-Based Learning Course on Rehabilitation Issues in HIV

Problem-based learning (PBL) was chosen as the educational model for an interprofessional course for teaching health profession students about rehabilitation issues in HIV/AIDS. PBL was determined to be ideal for promoting appreciation and respect for the roles of other professions. In this course, students from occupational therapy, physiotherapy, medical, nursing, and social work programs participated in an 8-week tutorial course. Students met once weekly for a 3-hour session. The objectives of the course were broad and included:

1. understanding the basic principles of the biology of HIV disease, its progression, and its transmission from person to person
2. becoming familiar with the types of medical and nonmedical interventions commonly used to maintain health in people living with HIV
3. understanding the management of HIV as a chronic—as opposed to terminal—illness
4. understanding how models of rehabilitation may be applied to the management of clients with HIV
5. developing an appreciation of the psychological, social, political, and ethical issues that have an influence on the experiences of a person living with HIV
6. understanding the various roles and contributions of health care and social service professionals in the rehabilitation of clients at different stages of HIV disease
7. developing skills in communicating, planning, and decision making with an interprofessional group of health professional students

In PBL, the learning stems from a problem itself. Students are expected to learn all content related to the stated objectives within the context of the health care problem. Typically, students are provided with a patient problem that is written; however, the problem may take the form of a standardized patient, a video, or other formats. In this course, students were provided with written patient problems. Students were directed to discuss their previous knowledge related to the patient problem. After students discussed their background knowledge and specific professional perspective, they then proceeded to a discussion on what would be a priority for learning in order to better understand the patient scenario. The learning issues were diverse, reflecting a range of content areas. For example, within the context of one problem, students' learning issues ranged from physiological issues (How is HIV transmitted?), to social issues (What are government and private options for short-term and long-term disability?), to ethical issues (What is the health professional's role in encouraging a newly diagnosed HIV-positive person to inform his/her partner about his/her status?). An important step was for the students to refine the learning issues or learning questions for further study. Neophytes to PBL often struggle with this portion of the process and need guidance to articulate a question that is clear and researchable. Students then engaged in self-directed study, sought appropriate resources to address the learning issues, and then returned to share their findings within the group setting.

Typically in PBL, students will choose to engage in self-directed study around all the learning issues that are generated by the group. This is important because if students select separate and individual learning issues, there can be a tendency for them to present their information in a didactic way when they return to the second tutorial session. If each student pursues all learning issues for self-study, the tutorial discussion is much richer and interactive as students share resources, challenge each other, and debate their findings. In this course, there was an additional individual learning issue related to students having to share their professional perspective. The complexities and interdisciplinary nature of HIV/AIDS provided the basis for diverse and broad-based discussions.

After engaging in self-study during the week, students returned to the tutorial and discussed and debated their findings. Students consulted both personal and written resources, which included texts, videos, journal articles, and web sites. Students then related the information back to the patient problem and provided their perspective on what their professional role would entail (e.g., What would be the priority for the social worker in this scenario? Is there a role for the occupational therapist? What would be the role of the nurse in community care of the patient?). The final stage was evaluation of the tutorial process, the interprofessional learning that occurred, and the performance of the group members. The interprofessional makeup of the tutorial groups simulated a health care team environment. The course was designed with the hope that the sharing of information, discussion, and debate that occurred in the tutorial would promote understanding of roles and teamwork. This element was evaluated weekly by the tutorial group members.

PROBLEM DESIGN

Problem design is an important element of the overall PBL process. Problems are not simply a restatement of all salient clinical information. Rather, the problems are carefully designed to elicit discussion and lead to student identification of the learning issues for which the problem was designed. There is evidence that even small changes to a problem can influence the students' discussions (Solomon, Blumberg, & Shehata, 1992). For example, in this course a change in the gender or sexual orientation of the person living with HIV can lead to very different learning issues. If the problem was based on a heterosexual woman living with HIV, students might generate issues related to the prevalence of HIV in women, the differing risk factors and manifestations in women, and the influence of HIV on gender-related roles. In contrast, if the problem centered around a gay man, students might have discussions related to their values, beliefs, and prejudices.

EVALUATION

Students evaluated this course very positively. In addition to gaining factual knowledge related to HIV/AIDS, students gained increased knowledge and understanding of the roles of other disciplines. They also recognized that they came to the table with preconceived ideas and stereotypes of other professions and were able to gain a greater respect and appreciation of the contribution of others to their tutorial course. Through their discussion, students became aware of the increased breadth of learning that occurs when interacting with students from other disciplines. In having to explain and advocate for their role, students also learn more about what their particular profession could offer to the emerging need for rehabilitation in persons living with HIV/AIDS.

REFERENCES

Albanese, M. (2000). Problem-based learning: Why curricula are likely to show little effect on knowledge and clinical skills. *Medical Education, 34,* 729–738.

Albanese, M. A., & Mitchell, S. (1993). Problem-based learning: A review of literature on its outcomes and implementation issues. *Academic Medicine, 68,* 52–81.

Barrows, H. S. (1986). A taxonomy of problem-based learning methods. *Medical Education, 20,* 481–486.

Barrows, H. S. (1988). *The tutorial process.* Springfield: Southern Illinois University of Medicine.

Barrows, H. S., & Tamblyn, R. (1980). *Problem-based learning.* New York: Springer.

Bresnitz, E. (1996). Computer-based learning in PBL. *Academic Medicine, 71*(5), 540.

Charlin, B., Mann, K., & Hansen, P. (1998). The many faces of problem-based learning: A framework for understanding and comparison. *Medical Teacher, 20,* 323–330.

Colliver, J. A. (2000). Effectiveness of problem-based learning: Research and theory. *Academic Medicine, 75,* 259–266.

Dolmans, D., Wolfhagen, I., Scherpbier, A., & Van Der Vleuten, C. (2001). Relationship of tutors' group-dynamics skills to their performance ratings in problem-based learning. *Academic Medicine, 76,* 473–476.

Federman, D. D. (1999). Little-heralded advantages of problem-based learning. *Academic Medicine, 74,* 93–94.

Glaser, R. (1985). *Control theory in the classroom.* New York: Harper and Row.

Harden, R. M., & Davis, M. H. (1998). The continuum of problem-based learning. *Medical Teacher, 20,* 317–322.

Hitchcock, M. A., & Mylona, Z. (2000). Teaching faculty to conduct problem-based learning. *Teaching and Learning in Medicine, 12,* 52–57.

Irby, D. M. (1996). Models of faculty development for problem-based learning. *Advances in Health Sciences Education, 1,* 69–81.

Kaufman, D. M., & Holmes, D. B. (1998). The relationship of tutors' content expertise to interventions and perceptions in a PBL medical curriculum. *Medical Education, 32,* 255–261.

Schmidt, H. (1983). Problem-based learning: Rationale and description. *Medical Education, 17,* 11–16.

Solomon, P. (1994). Problem-based learning: A direction for physical therapy education? *Physiotherapy Theory and Practice, 10,* 45–52.

Solomon, P., Binkley, J., & Stratford, P. (1996). A descriptive study of learning processes and outcomes in two problem-based curriculum designs. *Journal of Physical Therapy Education, 10,* 72–76.

Solomon, P., Blumberg, P., & Shehata, A. (1992). The influence of patient age on problem-based learning discussion. *Academic Medicine, 67*(10), 531–533.

Solomon, P., & Finch, E. (1998). A qualitative study identifying stressors associated with adapting to problem-based learning. *Teaching and Learning in Medicine, 10,* 58–64.

Walton, H., & Matthews, M. (1989). Essentials of problem-based learning. *Journal of Medical Education, 23,* 542–558.

Williams, G., Saizow, R., & Ryan, R. (1999). The importance of self determination theory for medical education. *Academic Medicine, 74,* 992–995.

CHAPTER 10

Reflective Practice

Hollie T. Noveletsky

INTRODUCTION

This chapter will discuss the application of Johns's model of structured reflection to health professions education. Johns's model provides a framework for clinical discourse that allows for the discovery of the knowledge necessary in the provision of care.

DEFINITION AND PURPOSE

Reflective practice is the process of examining one's own practice in order to uncover those factors that one brings to provider-patient or provider-colleague interactions that either hinder or enhance one's ability to interact therapeutically. Johns (Johns & Freshwater, 1998) refers to reflective practice as the process of exposing the contradictions in practice. In exposing the contradictions, the health professional must first come to understand what he or she defines as ideal practice. Then he/she examines the multiplicity of factors within the clinical interaction that either hindered or enhanced his or her ability to achieve ideal practice. Johns developed a model of structured reflection to aid health professionals in identifying and understanding the complexities of factors within clinical interactions so that they may develop and access their own tacit knowledge.

Benner (1984) identifies expert practitioners as those practitioners who are able to immediately grasp the whole of a situation. The expert is able to understand the multiplicity of factors at play within a given situation. In order for a practitioner to develop this expert knowledge, he or she must first develop and access his or her own tacit knowledge. The process of reflection gives access to the tacit knowledge gained in clinical practice. Boud, Keogh, and Walker (1985) outline three stages in the process of reflection. In the first stage, one identifies and describes a significant event or interaction. In the second stage, one evaluates the event or interaction in order to identify factors that either hindered or

141

enhanced one's learning. In the third stage, one integrates the knowledge gained with his or her past experiences in order to access one's own tacit knowledge. Thus, the reflective process allows practitioners the ability to uncover knowledge embedded in clinical experience.

Schon (1983) described two types of reflection. The first is reflection *in* action, and the second is reflection *on* action. Reflection in action is the process of analyzing or thinking about one's actions while carrying out the action. Reflection on action is the process of retrospective analysis of one's action. For the novice practitioner, reflection in action is difficult. As a novice, the practitioner is still trying to gain theoretical knowledge and mastery of psychomotor skills. At this level, reflection in action is mainly focused on applying appropriate theoretical knowledge within a given clinical situation; however, reflection on action provides the novice with the opportunity for retrospective analysis of clinical situations in order to gain a deeper understanding of the multiplicity of factors involved within the clinical situation. This deeper understanding allows the novice to begin to develop his or her own tacit knowledge for clinical practice and to identify ways to bring his or her practice closer to a defined ideal practice level.

THEORETICAL RATIONALE

According to Habermas, there are three types of knowledge: empirical, interpretive, and critical (Taylor, 1998). Taylor equates Habermas's typology of knowledge with technical, practical, and emancipatory knowledge, respectively. Empirical or technical knowledge is generated through scientific inquiry and allows for the description, prediction, and control of phenomena. Interpretive or practical knowledge is knowledge that is relative and context dependent. Interpretive knowledge is generated through new insight that may allow for evolution or change in perception. Critical or emancipatory knowledge is also knowledge that is relative and context dependent; however, critical knowledge is generated with the specific intent to bring about change. Taylor states that "reflection creates interpretive knowledge for generating meaning and change through raised awareness" (Taylor, p. 138) and critical knowledge for intentional change that enables the health professional to move his or her practice closer to ideal practice.

TYPES OF LEARNERS

Because reflective practice is an evolving process, there are no standardized prerequisites or outcome measures. Growth is measured individually. Therefore, reflective practice is appropriate for all levels and types of students, including undergraduate, graduate, and doctoral students. Because the focus of the reflection is on clinical interactions, however, all participants should be concurrently in a clinical placement.

In addition, reflective practice is an effective method of staff development. In staff development, a novice health professional would be paired with an expert practitioner or would participate in a weekly seminar where the focus of the experience was to critically reflect on significant clinical interactions. This method would provide the novice with a safe environment within which to develop his or her own tacit knowledge.

Expert health professionals can benefit from the use of reflective practice. As contexts of patients' lives continue to change and evolve as society evolves, practitioners need to be able to adapt to the ever changing contexts of health and the provision of care. Expert practitioners, either in pairs or small groups, can use reflective practice to examine their own personal and nursing knowledge needs as they strive to meet the evolving needs of society and the individual.

CONDITIONS FOR LEARNING

Reflective practice as a teaching method requires the development of a safe environment for disclosure. Therefore, reflective practice is appropriate for small group seminars or one-on-one conferencing. Group members need to be encouraged to participate fully and to work toward the development of a safe and respectful environment that allows for disclosure and free discourse.

In addition, students need to develop an understanding of the process of reflection. Foundational readings on Johns's (Johns & Freshwater, 1998) model of structured reflection are necessary to establish a framework from which to process clinical interactions. The facilitator is essential to the process of reflection. The facilitator encourages the students to move beyond superficial examination of interactions toward a level of critical reflection in order to develop their own tacit knowledge. Johns (1998) developed reflective cues and eight framing perspectives to assist the students in examining the interaction from multiple perspectives in order to gain a fuller understanding of the complex dynamics of the interaction. The reflective cues center on the five types of knowledge: aesthetics, personal, ethics, empirics, and reflexivity. These reflective cues take the form of questions that facilitate the student in examining the interaction from different perspectives. The framing perspectives provide different angles from which to examine the interaction in order to gain a deeper understanding of the dynamics. These framing perspectives include framing the development of effectiveness, philosophical framing, role framing, theoretical framing, parallel pattern framing, problem framing, reality perspective framing, and temporal framing.

RESOURCES

The seminar facilitator is an important resource. The facilitator needs to be expert in both theoretical and clinical knowledge and should be competent in the process of reflection. The facilitator does not necessarily need to have expert knowledge within a specific clinical area, however. The role of facilitator is to assist the student in the reflective process through the use of Johns's reflective cues.

The setting of the seminar needs to provide a sense of privacy so that safe disclosure can occur. In addition, the room should be arranged so that all group members are facing one another in order to help foster a sense of group and equality.

USING THE METHOD

Seminar groups should meet weekly for approximately 2 hours per session. Seminar expectations are reviewed during the first class. Expectations include: (1) each student is expected to participate in the group discussion, and (2) each student is expected to work toward the development of a safe and respectful environment that allows for disclosure and free discourse. In addition, each student is to keep a weekly reflective journal. At least one entry per week will examine a clinical encounter with a patient, family, or colleague that the student wishes to further understand. Students are instructed to write a narrative describing the experience. Then, using Johns's model of structured reflection and the reflective cues, students are encouraged to examine those factors that the student brings and those factors that the other brings to the interaction that either hinder or enhance the student's ability to interact therapeutically. The facilitator reviews the journals on a weekly basis, and written feedback is provided regarding the students' insights.

Each student is expected to share three journal entries with the group over the course of the seminar. The student presents the narrative of the interaction and his or her reflective thoughts on the nature of the interaction. This presentation provides a starting point for group reflection on the dynamics of the interaction. This process affords each student the opportunity to gain knowledge vicariously and students the chance to facilitate each other's learning.

At the completion of the seminar course, students are instructed to reflect back on the course by reviewing their weekly journal entries. Students are instructed to write a final reflective paper that examines their own process and product of the seminar experience. This exercise allows the students to realize their growth and the usefulness of reflective practice within their professional lives. The final reflective paper also provides the facilitator with an individualized measure of each student's development.

POTENTIAL PROBLEMS

The most significant potential problem associated with reflective practice as a teaching method is related to the development of a safe environment for disclosure. If the seminar group is unable to bond together in a cohesive, supportive group, individuals will not feel safe to disclose personal feelings and reflections. Group discussion will be stifled. Addressing this issue with the group may help to raise individuals' awareness of the group's dynamics. Because individuals within the group will be at various levels of self-knowing, however, raising the individuals' awareness may not bring them collectively to a point of enough awareness to develop a sense of group cohesiveness. If the group is not able to develop a sense of cohesiveness, then the reflective process will have to be carried out mainly through the use of the reflective journals.

Another potential problem is students who have difficulty expressing themselves publicly. Despite the development of a safe environment, some students are reluctant to openly express their personal reflections. Again, the reflective journals provide a safe avenue for exploration of both the clinical interactions and the students' inability to reflect within the group setting. Reflective discourse between the student and seminar facilitator can occur through the reflective journals. This discourse increases the facilitator's awareness of the individual's needs while assisting the student to reflect on both clinical interactions and his or her personal growth potential.

Finally, the process of facilitating a seminar group using the teaching method of reflective practice requires a high level of personal commitment among the group members. As the group dynamics evolve over time, the group members develop a stronger sense of cohesiveness and commitment to the group. The facilitator, as a member of the group, also develops a strong sense of cohesiveness and commitment. As a result, termination of the group becomes difficult. Some time must be devoted to preparing the group for termination. One strategy to assist in termination is that of identifying alternate methods of continued group cohesiveness. For example, an Internet Listserve can be developed as a means to continue the group after termination. In addition, the facilitator needs time to reflect on the experience in order to process the loss of the group before starting another group. If this process of reflection is not performed, then a sense of loss may interfere with the ability to adequately facilitate the subsequent group.

CONCLUSION

Johns's model of structured reflection provides a useful framework for examining clinical interactions. The structure of the model assists the students in sorting out multiple, competing factors that impact their daily practice while acknowledging the constraints of reality. This model allows the students to critically reflect without assuming unwarranted blame or guilt. One student noted:

> Through the development of reflective thinking in practice, I was reminded of the meaning and value of being truly present. Although it is my habit to examine situations in a reflective way, I realize that it was previously with the motive of fault-finding, usually my own, as if when things went wrong that was proof that I was somehow not good enough, did not measure up, was not able for the task at hand. This semester, reflective practice took on new meaning. Rather than searching for fault and using that as an excuse to give up, I could search for a reason, an explanation, and use it as a springboard to improve . . . Repeatedly asking the questions, "What do I bring to the table?" and "How does my presence change things?" made me realize that there is always an answer to those questions. The assumptions underlying the questions are that I do bring something to the table, and my presence does change things. To be aware of those questions makes it possible to change the answers if need be. It makes the answers purposeful rather than inadvertent (Noveletsky-Rosenthal & Solomon, 1999).

This statement underscores the role of reflection in the development of interpretive and critical knowledge. Students then use this knowledge to change their practice to more closely approximate ideal practice. Through the process of reflective practice, students are able to develop tacit knowledge embedded in clinical practice and to begin the journey from novice to expert practitioner.

TEACHING EXAMPLE

Student Use of Reflective Practice Journal

Using the format for clinical supervision outlined earlier in the Using the Method section, a student submitted a journal entry for discussion in seminar. The journal topic was her clinical encounter with a woman regarding a sexual health issue. The student was aware of a barrier between herself and the client but was unable to identify the origins of the barrier. In the reflective process of describing the encounter in writing, the student started to uncover a reoccurring theme for herself. The student noted that the large age discrepancy between the client and the client's significant other had been an issue for the student.

The writing process gave the student the time and context in which to sort and organize her thoughts regarding the experience in order to be able to present them in a systematic manner. This in turn helped the student to uncover the reoccurring issue of age discrepancy that kept surfacing during her reflections. Once the underlying issue of age discrepancy was identified, the seminar leader was able to direct the group discussion around the student's knowledge, personal beliefs, and feelings concerning age discrepancies within intimate relationships. The student's and the other seminar participants' personal experiences and views were shared and examined using Johns's framing perspectives and reflective cues.

As a result of the discussion, the student became more aware of her own biases regarding age discrepancies within intimate relationships. She was able to identify some misconceptions and identify some beliefs and values that were important to her. There was a shift in the student's level of acceptance of such relationships without a complete revision of her underlying belief system. The shift was related to her becoming more aware of her own personal biases and the impact that they had on her interactions rather than a shift in her own personal value system. However, awareness of one's biases and being able to partially or completely bracket them off within the context of an interaction may represent a subtle shift in the intensity of one's value system with regard to the issue at hand.

REFERENCES

Benner, P. (1984). *From novice to expert*. Menlo, CA: Addison-Wesley,

Boud, D., Keogh, R., & Walker, D. (1985). *Reflection: turning experience into learning*. London: Kogan Page.

Johns, C. (1998). Opening the doors of perception. In C. Johns & D. Freshwater (Eds.), *Transforming nursing through reflective practice* (pp. 1–20). Malden, MA: Blackwell Science.

Johns, C., & Freshwater, D. (Eds.). (1998). *Transforming nursing through reflective practice*. Malden, MA: Blackwell Science.

Noveletsky-Rosenthal, H. T., & Solomon, K. (1999, June). *The use of Johns' model of structured reflection in graduate nursing education*. Paper presented at the meeting of the Fifth Reflective Practice Conference, Cambridge, England.

Schon, D. A. (1983). *The reflective practitioner: How professionals think in action*. New York: Basic Books.

Taylor, B. (1998). Locating a phenomenological perspective of reflective nursing and midwifery practice by contrasting interpretive and critical reflection. In C. Johns & D. Freshwater (Eds.), *Transforming nursing through reflective practice* (pp. 134–150). Malden, MA: Blackwell Science.

RECOMMENDED READING

Hallet, C. E. (1997). Learning through reflection in the community: The relevance of Schon's theories of coaching to nursing education. *International Journal of Nursing Studies, 34*(2), 103–110.

Johns, C. (1997). Reflective practice and clinical supervision—Part I: The reflective turn. *European Nurse, 2*(2), 87–97.

Johns, C. (1997). Reflective practice and clinical supervision—Part II: Guiding learning through reflection to structure the supervision 'space.' *European Nurse, 2*(3), 192–204.

Johns, C. (2002). *Guided reflection: Advancing practice*. Malden, MA: Blackwell Science.

Johns, C. (2004). *Becoming a reflective practitioner* (2nd ed.). Malden, MA: Blackwell Science.

Johns, C., & Freshwater, D. (Eds.). (1998). *Transforming nursing through reflective practice*. Malden, MA: Blackwell Science.

Johns, C., & Freshwater, D. (Eds.). (2005). *Transforming nursing through reflective practice* (2nd ed.). Malden, MA: Blackwell Science.

Kember, D. (Ed.). (2001). *Reflective teaching and learning in the health professions*. Malden, MA: Blackwell Science.

Marland, G., & McSherry, W. (1997). The reflective diary: An aid to practice-based learning. *Nursing Standard, 12*(13-5), 49–52.

Riley-Doucet, C., & Wilson, S. (1997). A three-step method of self-reflection using reflective journal writing. *Journal of Advanced Nursing, 25*(5), 964–968.

Wong, F. K., Kember, D., Chung, L. Y., & Yan, L. (1995). Assessing the level of student reflection from reflective journals. *Journal of Advanced Nursing, 22*(1), 48–57.

SECTION III

SIMULATION AND IMAGINATION

The teaching-learning strategies presented in Section III promote the use of imagination as a way of encouraging students to stretch their thinking and explore their understanding of concepts in different ways. Simulation and imagination techniques encourage students to avoid being locked in to one solution to a problem and provide an opportunity to learn to develop different approaches to the problems they face. Effective learning requires active participation. When students use their imagination to play a role, take an opposing viewpoint to their held views, or learn to express themselves in new and different ways, they become involved in their learning. The role of faculty is a facilitating one, helping students interact with each other to bring out other possibilities, to reinforce learning objectives, and, in a safe, less stressful setting, help students develop insight into the translation of classroom to the clinical environment.

Clinical experience has been a mainstay of health professions education. However, it is more and more difficult to find student clinical experiences in today's managed care world, when providers are under the gun to reduce patient length of stay and restrict the time and amount of ambulatory care visits. The requirement for increased provider productivity does not allow time for teaching. In addition, the informed healthcare consumers of today may or may not be willing to allow neophyte students to practice their skills.

Students can be encouraged to use simulation and imagination to learn how to adapt their clinical knowledge to the practical world. Simulation allows students to problem solve in a safe environment. They can learn to make clinical decisions and correct their mistakes without causing injury to a patient. Participation in simulation activities can make learning a fun, enjoyable, and memorable learning experience. Through simulation, they can be prepared to gain experience that may not be available in the immediate clinical area, but will be part of their practice in the real world of health care.

CHAPTER 11

Debate As a Teaching Strategy

Martha J. Bradshaw and Arlene J. Lowenstein

The debate is a strategy long recognized as a means by which to address a topic in which there may be more than one viewpoint. The value of a debate is not necessarily in the resolution of a topic or persuasive results, but the value as a teaching strategy lies more in the process and presentation of the viewpoints.

DEFINITION AND PURPOSES

A traditional view of debate may be that of argument for the purpose of persuading the audience toward a clearly identified position. To debate an issue is to consider or discuss it from opposing positions or arguments (Berube & DeVinne, 1982). Political debates are used as opportunities for candidates to make their perspectives known on key issues. This form of structured argument has long been used in philosophy, theology, law, and the sciences (Tumposky, 2004). Debate has been defined as "a systematic contest of speakers in which two points of view of a proposition are advanced with proof" (Barnhart, 1966, pg. 311). Based on this definition, debate becomes a useful teaching strategy.

Debate provides opportunities for students to analyze an issue or problem in depth and to reach an informed, unbiased conclusion or resolution. Debate encourages participants to identify quickly the essential nature of the issue as substantiated by evidence, to establish criteria for judging its successful resolution, and to weigh, compare, and contrast the merits of alternative strategies for resolution (Simonneaux, 2002). The analytical process can enhance critical thinking in students (Law, 1998; Walker, 2003). In addition, presentation of the debate allows students to practice oral communication skills, express professional opinions, and gain experience in speaking to groups.

THEORETICAL RATIONALE

Two important components of the professional role are the analysis of significant issues and the ability to communicate in efficient and effective ways. Professional communication is seen in many forms; scholarly publication, oral presentations, and electronic networking are a few examples. Similar to other skills, the development of effective communication skills must be fostered by faculty. The ability to communicate one's thoughts clearly and concisely evolves from the formulation of a perspective on a topic, analysis of that perspective and other views, and development of sound conclusions. Debate enables students to participate actively in a meaningful communication exercise.

DeYoung differentiates debate from general discussion by pointing out that general discussion is based on open-mindedness and a free flow of ideas. Discussion usually aims toward some sort of conclusion and often is a cooperative compromise. Debate, on the other hand, is argumentative, with each team competing to establish its position as the most correct one or the one that should be upheld (1990).

One of the purposes of debate is for the learner to go beyond merely identifying an issue. Learners must analyze the issue: What are its key elements? What historical precedents have contributed to the issue? Who are the key proponents and opponents of the issue? What is the future of the issue? Students can learn how personal values or emotions influence thinking and responses to issues. Students also can identify what factors influence their thinking, such as the views of news analysts, popular literature, or peers (Simonneaux, 2002). Analysis on this level leads to powerful learning, calling for the use of reasoning and other forms of higher-order thinking. The learner first becomes more aware of his own thinking, then broadens and purposefully adapts his thinking (Tumposky, 2004).

CONDITIONS FOR LEARNING

Debate is most useful as part of a course or seminar in professional and academic settings. Because of the nature of this strategy, it should be employed in a course that centers upon issues or topics that raise debatable questions. This strategy can be used to facilitate students' ability to implement analytical skills, to systematically research and critique an issue, to arrive at salient points, and to demonstrate more professional development related to group process (Candela, Michael, & Mitchell, 2003). Furthermore, the learner may be placed in a situation in which she or he explores an issue or evaluates a position opposing to the one held in self (Law, 1998).

The learning goals for the debate strategy include improving oral communication and library skills, structuring and presenting an argument, and exercising analytical skills. The process for formulating and presenting the debate should facilitate these goals as much as possible; therefore, the faculty should provide as much freedom as possible for the students to reach these learning goals independently. Students should be given enough structure or direction to help them plan and organize their work, but they also should understand the responsibility they must take for researching debate positions, analyzing key issues, and practicing speaking skills. In the debate strategy described by Lowenstein and Bradshaw (1989), students were encouraged to take the viewpoint opposite the one they (personally) held. This approach promoted an understanding of existing oppositional perspectives and enhanced the ability to respond to opposing views (Lowenstein & Bradshaw).

Preparation for the debate should begin early in the course to provide adequate opportunity for library research and exploration of issues. Faculty facilitation is an essential part of the learning process. Conditions central to use of debate as an effective strategy include the following:

- Students need to be introduced to key issues in the course and have been able to identify controversial points suitable for debate.
- Students need to be familiar with one another in order to form working groups.
- Students need knowledge of existing resources to use in formulating debate. This includes increased familiarity with the faculty member(s) as a source of support and information.

TYPES OF LEARNERS

Debate can be used with all levels or types of learners, including undergraduate students, graduate students, and practitioners, because the learning goals of debate are suitable for all groups. Lowenstein and Bradshaw (1989) used debate with registered nurse students who were completing their BSN courses. Debate is a particularly successful strategy with this group because these students combine personal experience with actual patient or practice problems with the need to refine communication and analytical skills. Thus, debate provides a true opportunity for professional growth in this type of student. By immersing in the topic, students have a better understanding of it than they would through other means of study.

By creating the need to objectively analyze an issue, debate is useful for a student who is strongly influenced by personal values or certain work experiences.

An undergraduate who has not formed a worldview about sensitive ethical dilemmas, for example, can have the opportunity to examine the issues and how decisions are made. A practitioner who has been receiving negative influence in the work environment has the opportunity for objective analysis of the situation.

RESOURCES

Faculty members serve as an important resource by assuming the role of facilitator. Formal debate questions and positions can emerge from class discussion about important issues. Faculty members can assist students in formulating the debate question and can direct them to resources related to the issue. Clinical experiences and current issues in health care offer a wide range of debate topics. Faculty may wish to prepare the students early in the course by encouraging them to be alert to ethical dilemmas or patient care problems that are suitable for debate (Candela, Michael, & Mitchell, 2003).

The library offers many resources for debate preparation. By using the professional literature to support the debate position, students are introduced to a wide range of journals, books, and other printed material. Electronic information systems are extremely helpful to students as they identify debate issues and develop related positions. Database searches enable students to consider related topics, which may generate additional support for a position. The electronic media access most current information, which may be particularly helpful for students who have timely political topics. Electronic bulletin boards and other communication networks provide students with the opportunity to interact with individuals outside their own institution who are involved with the issue.

The debate can be presented in any planned classroom setting. The environment should be such that the debate teams can be seen and heard by the audience.

USING THE METHOD

In the Lowenstein and Bradshaw method, faculty members define broad (topical) areas from the course outline and identify an advisor for each area. Students choose the general area in which they are interested and form groups of four or five members. At least one group is formed for each topical area to guarantee that course objectives or topics are addressed. Depending on student interest and enrollment, a second group may be formed in certain areas. For example, two groups may choose to address the area of professional roles and responsibilities. Specific debate questions are formulated by the group in keeping with the objectives or broad topics of the course and personal interests of group members. Many of the topics are those currently being debated by our colleagues in all levels of nursing. Healthcare reform, nursing care delivery systems, genetic screening, and euthanasia are a few examples (Lowenstein & Bradshaw, 1989).

Each group should meet with the faculty advisor as needed to organize the debate presentation, gain insight into the points being presented, and receive assistance with resources. Students are guided to consider the perspectives of all individuals or interest groups (Simonneaux, 2002). For each debate group, two students select the affirmative position, two select the negative, and the fifth serves as moderator. In groups of four, the faculty advisor serves as moderator. Each group develops a reading list of significant articles related to the issue under debate. The list is circulated to the entire class at least one week prior to the debate. Students not involved in the presentation are expected to be prepared to discuss the issues under consideration.

The debate consists of opening remarks by a moderator, two affirmative and two negative presentations, rebuttal, and summary. Following the presentation, the floor is opened to the class for discussion. Questions and comments based on the presentations and readings are generated by the class. The debate moderator facilitates discussion and provides a final summary of the issues and discussion. In most situations, the burden of supporting the affirmative view is the more difficult position to hold (Law, 1998). With some issues, it may be appropriate to develop a resolution plan upon conclusion of the formal debate. This plan can incorporate some ideas from both positions to encourage win-win negotiation. This process gives students experience in developing workable solutions to practice-related issues.

Class members not participating in the debate are asked to evaluate each presenter based on a rating scale. Students evaluate the analysis of the issue, the evidence presented, supporting resources, organization of the presentation, the argument presented, interaction with the audience and opponents, and response to questions **(Exhibit 11-1)**. An overall effectiveness score is given, and the evaluators indicate if their stand on the issue changed as a result of the debate. All faculty members participating in the seminar also evaluate the presenters. Debate grades are based on preparation, individual performance, and group efforts that were reflected in the effectiveness of the debate.

To reinforce the learning from the debate, students may be asked to write a formal paper on one of the professional issues discussed in the course. The paper can be evaluated on the presentation of the issue, arguments for both sides of the issue supported by literature, the student's position and rationale for selection of the position, application of ideas to practice, and use of references and format.

EXHIBIT 11-1

Grading Tool: Debate

Date: _____   Subject/topic: _____

Evaluate each speaker using the following scale:

Superior = 5; Excellent = 4; Good = 3; Fair = 2; Below standard = 1

Team A		Team B
1 2 3 4 5	Bibliography (4 max)	1 2 3 4 5
	Overview of problem (1–2)	
1 2 3 4 5	Representing side of debate (1–2)	1 2 3 4 5
	Opening remarks	
_____		_____
Debater		*Debater*
1 2 3 4 5		1 2 3 4 5
_____	Resolution plan	_____
Debater		*Debater*
1 2 3 4 5		1 2 3 4 5
_____	Response to opposing team	_____
Debater		*Debater*
1 2 3 4 5		1 2 3 4 5
_____	Concluding statement	_____

POTENTIAL PROBLEMS

The debate strategy calls for significant student responsibility and preparation, for both debaters and the audience. Debaters are required to thoroughly research the issue and the position taken for the argument. From this preparation, they formulate a succinct and effective presentation. Debaters are expected to practice speaking skills and to prepare supporting materials for the oral presentation. The debate group provides an appropriate reading list for the other class members. Those students take the responsibility to read about the issue prior to the presentation in order to understand the issue and participate effectively in discussion. Lack of preparation leads to inadequate presentation of the issue and superficial discussion.

The debate causes students to clearly classify an issue as one that is right or wrong, or answered "yes" or "no." Many topics have no conclusions or answers, and thus may impose a false dualism (Tumposky, 2004). Students may have to defend a position to which they are not clearly committed. Students with strong moral beliefs about an issue may have difficulty defending a specified position or accepting the views of others. Faculty may have difficulty presenting a neutral position when moderating the debate and guiding discussion (Simonneaux, 2002). At some point during the presentations, it must be made very clear that there is no right or singular answer to most issues.

Nervousness about speaking in public can be a major concern. Some students have had little or no public speaking experience, or they may have had negative experiences that generated anxiety. Tumposky (2004) asserts that female students may be more uncomfortable with the adversarial nature of this strategy than are the male peers. In addition, students of certain cultural groups may have difficulty with open debate as a way to learn. Students need encouragement and need to view the debate as an opportunity to speak to an open, receptive group in order to gain experience. What some students look upon with apprehension often results in being uplifting and beneficial. For example, one student was timid about speaking in groups and was extremely nervous before and during her debate presentation. Her nervousness was manifested in physical symptoms, such as sweating, flushed face, tremulous voice, shaking hands, and rapid blinking. She received appropriate support from faculty and students, which encouraged her to work on this problem during the rest of her academic work. Three years later, she successfully defended her master's project in a dignified and professional manner. Her public speaking skills have now advanced to the point that she is able to address both groups and individuals effectively in her current employment as a clinical specialist.

The argumentative or confrontational nature of the debate may create anxiety. In addition, debate or public speaking may be a new strategy on which students are graded, thus heightening anxiety. Faculty and students must continually place emphasis on the debate as a learning experience. The excitement of defending a position, stressing key points, and deriving a workable solution should be presented as positive outcomes of the debate. Faculty members should stress that students will not be condemned or inappropriately criticized for taking unpopular viewpoints during the debate. Faculty members are prepared to handle strong emotional viewpoints and to help students understand that there is room for conflicting opinions in our society. In using debate as a teaching strategy, Candela, Michael, and Mitchell (2003) discovered that students liked the strategy and found it challenging, but did not see how they would use the skill or strategy in their professional careers. It is possible that, as novices, students are not aware of potential situations in which there will be a need to defend a position regarding health care. Students also need to be encouraged to see the benefit of the opportunity to practice speaking skills, research skills, and group work. As a teaching strategy, Tumposky (2004) points out that use of debate is widespread despite lack of evidence to validate its effectiveness.

CONCLUSION

Debate is a strategy that promotes student interaction and involvement in course topics. There are many advantages to using this strategy. Debate expands the student's perspective on a given issue, creates doubt about the existence of one clear answer, and requires much thought and further evidence before deriving a solution. Debate also increases awareness of opposing viewpoints. As an interactive strategy, debate develops techniques of persuasion, serves as a means by which students confront a controversial issue, and promotes collaborative efforts and negotiation skills among peers. This strategy promotes independence and participation in the decision-making process, as well as enhancing writing and organizational skills. Debate allows for examination of broad issues that influence professional practice. Critical thinking is enhanced by the scrutiny of more than one position on the issue. Debate allows the student a wider forum than writing a paper does, and it may give a greater sense of accomplishment (DeYoung, 1990).

Selection of debate as a teaching strategy requires a strong commitment to preparation and guidance from faculty. Faculty members will have to deal with emotions that can be elicited by the arguments. Faculty members will need to provide support for students who take minority or unpopular positions and for those who have limited public speaking skills. Following the debate, those students whose ideas are not accepted by the majority should be encouraged to recognize those parts of their work that were of value, even if others disagreed with their position. Those students whose ideas reflected the majority view should also recognize that public consensus can change quickly, and, as more information becomes available, opinions may be swayed. Finally, faculty members can help students to recognize that the debate is just a start to exploration of professional issues. Students will need to be encouraged to incorporate their newly learned and practiced skills into their professional practice.

REFERENCES

Barnhart, C. L. (Ed.). (1966). *The American college dictionary.* New York: Random House.

Berube, M. S., & DeVinne, P. B. (Eds). (1982). *The American heritage dictionary.* Boston: Houghton Mifflin.

Candela, L., Michael, S. R., & Mitchell, S. (2003). Ethical debates: Enhancing critical thinking in nursing students. *Nurse Educator, 28*, 37–39.

DeYoung, S. (1990). *Teaching Nursing.* Redwood City, CA: Addison-Wesley.

Law, C. F. (1998). Using argumentation to teach literature. *Exercise Exchange, 43*, 10–11.

Lowenstein, A. J., & Bradshaw, M. J. (1989). Seminar methods for RN to BSN students. *Nurse Educator, 14*(5), 27–31.

Simonneaux, L. (2002). Analysis of classroom debating strategies. *The Journal of Biological Education, 37*, 9–12.

Tumposky, N. R. (2004). The debate debate. *Clearing House, 78*, 52–55.

Walker, S. (2003). Active learning strategies to promote critical thinking. *Journal of Athletic Training, 38*, 263–268.

CHAPTER 12

Games Amplify Motivation in Education

Lynn Jaffe

"Games are one of the things that make us distinctively human."
Betsy Van der Veer Martens, 1998

Throughout our lives, games are enjoyable, goal-directed activities through which we learn or reinforce learning. We learned colors with Candyland; matching with Go Fish; money management and deal making with Monopoly; strategies with chess; and that we are older than we want to admit through Trivial Pursuit. Today's college students and adult learners seek more from academics and in-service training than lecture formats. It seems that mass media has fostered reduced attention spans and increased the need for innovation and novelty to sustain interest in learning situations. Games can fulfill this need because they are experiential. Today's learners also have a consumer orientation to education. College students have expectations about what they believe they need or deserve in their educational process, and seek supportive, frequent feedback. Instructional games are a motivating way to fulfill this need, reinforce skills, and foster collaboration. While there is an extensive literature on games theory in multiple disciplines, this chapter is an introduction to the use of games as a learning tool within the classroom or clinical setting. After some definitions and a brief literature review, the types of learning that will fit most easily within the various game structures will be described, as will the limitations of game use within the educational or clinical environment.

DEFINITION AND PURPOSE

Games are classified in multiple ways. One author divides them into entertainment, educational, experimental, research, operational research, and operational categories. The genres are also split by the focus of action: interaction games refer to the roles of the players, and transaction games refer to the rules of play (Van der Veer Martens, 1998). Educationally, they fall into three categories: games, simulations, and simulation games. Simulations are discussed in a separate chapter. A game is an activity governed by precise rules that involve varying degrees of chance or luck, and one or more players who cooperate or compete (with oneself, the game, one another, or a computer) through the use of knowledge or skill in an attempt to reach a specified goal (de Tornyay & Thompson, 1987; Ellington, Gordon, & Fowlie, 1998). Educational or instructional games expect benefits for all participants that last beyond the game itself. Simulation games are contrived, reality-based conflicts that must be resolved within the constraints of the game rules (Thiagarajan & Stolovitch, 1978). Debriefing is an important aspect of gaming that occurs after the game. It is a discussion about the concepts, generalizations, and applications of the topics covered within the game (Gifford, 2001; Hillman, 2001; Randel, Morris, Wetzel, & Whitehill, 1992; Van der Veer Martens, 1998). Effective debriefing requires a good deal of skill and experience in the facilitator. This process assists learners in recognizing the learning that has occurred with the fun experience of the game, and contributes to the learner's ability to use self-reflection.

Most educational games are derived from *frame games*, which are familiar formats that provide frameworks for inserting content and creating learning activities (Cowen & Tesh, 2002; Stolovitch & Thiagarajan, 1980). These games typically involve a set of rules for player moves and termination criteria so that winners may be determined. The frameworks are easily adaptable to a wide variety of instructional objectives and content. Some authors break frame games into categories, such as board games, television games, and educator-created games (Lewis, Saydak, Mierzwa, & Robinson, 1989). Typical frame games include bingo, Jeopardy, Trivial Pursuit, Monopoly, and Who Wants to Be a Millionaire? The simulation game is a hybrid, involving the best of each approach, and is represented by Monopoly and chess (Ellington et al., 1998).

THEORETICAL FOUNDATIONS

The use of games for educational purposes is a very old idea. The earliest recorded use was for war games 3,000 years ago in China, in the 18th century in Europe, and within this century by the U.S. military (Ellington et al., 1998; Van der Veer Martens, 1998). Game use was brought to the business community by ex-officers to provide training in problem solving and decision making. It was considered a bridge between academic instruction and on-the-job training (Ellington et al.). In the 1950s and 1960s, as the theoretical focus of learning shifted from the instructor to the student, experience-based learning became prominent and games were used to meet this goal, especially in America (Ellington et al.; Keys & Wolfe, 1990). In health-related areas, psychologists and nurses have made numerous contributions to the literature on game use in both academic and clinical education.

Game use falls under the theoretical umbrellas of active learning strategies and cooperative learning described in Chapter 1. The focus is upon engagement with the educational material and classmates. Educators must appreciate the different maturational stages students pass through and the particular needs of adult learners to engage meaningfully with the content and apply it in a variety of methods. Chickering and Gamson (1987) have a classic list of seven best educational practices (see **Figure 12-1**) that can be accomplished through the interactive, immediate, and diverse format of gaming.

One review of the literature on the instructional effectiveness of games compared to conventional classroom instruction in liberal arts subjects during the 1963 to 1991 period found most of the evaluations had been anecdotal, descriptive, or judgmental (Randel et al., 1992). However, the formal evidence in the health care and social science fields has been flourishing in the past 2 decades, and outcomes are primarily positive regarding the effectiveness of games upon motivation, attention, and attendance at in-service training (Berrenberg & Prosser, 1991; Gibson, 1991; Keutzer, 1993). Studies have shown game use to positively affect motivational factors such as confidence and satisfaction (see reviews by Keys & Wolfe, 1990; Kuhn, 1995; or Henry, 1997). One study found that game use increased knowledge retention significantly, corresponding to a letter grade difference, in a nursing class on cardiovascular dysfunction (Cowen & Tesh, 2002). There have been a number of dissertations in the field of nursing regarding the use of games on such attributes as student achievement and retention (Anderson, 1998; Montpas, 2004; Sprengel, 1992), empathic communication (Regan, 2000), and diagnosis skills (Weber, 1992). In each case, gaming was described as beneficial academically and preferred by the students.

Figure 12-1   Seven principles for good practice in undergraduate education.

1. Encourages contact between students and faculty.
2. Develops reciprocity and cooperation among students.
3. Encourages active learning.
4. Gives prompt feedback.
5. Emphasizes time on task.
6. Communicates high expectations.
7. Respects diverse talents and ways of learning.

Source: Chickering & Gamson, 1987.

TYPES OF LEARNERS

Games are being used throughout the educational continuum, from nursery school through graduate education. As just mentioned, they can be used for students who like to compete or for those who prefer to cooperate. They are used to review facts or reinforce or test knowledge, understanding, and application. Games motivate learners with achievement needs through the competitiveness inherent in many games. Games may also be motivating for those with strong affiliation needs because games can require team play and cooperation for completion.

Games are one vehicle for developing interdisciplinary approaches to problem solving and empathy with clients. They require a degree of flexibility on the part of the student in order to adapt to changing circumstances within the game (Cessario, 1987). Finally, games and simulations provide the practice necessary for a clinical field in times when clinical placements are being overloaded. However, reading of class assignments has been shown to have the strongest positive effect on test performance (Klein & Freitag, 1991; Randel et al., 1992).

CONDITIONS FOR LEARNING

Games can be used to address all levels of cognitive objectives, from reinforcing the learning of basic facts, through developing application and analysis skills, and culminating in promoting synthesis and evaluation. They do this through the promotion of initiative, creative thought, and affective components within a safe forum for listening to others (Ellington et al., 1998). Games are credited with encouraging application of information, supplementing rote memorization, providing useful organization of material, and providing comic relief from the otherwise anxiety-provoking task of preparing for exams (Keutzer, 1993). Games are inherently student-centered and interactive, generating enthusiasm, excitement, and enjoyment (Klein & Freitag, 1991). An experiential learning method, such as gaming, creates an environment that requires a participant to be involved in a personally meaningful activity. In addition, learning has greater impact when it has an element of emotional arousal, takes place within a safe environment, and has a period of debriefing to provide a cognitive map for understanding the experience (Keys & Wolfe, 1990). Additionally, when new students are asked what their preferred learning style is, the predominant answer is always hands on—experiential. Getting a match between teaching strategies and student needs is one of the key factors in effective education.

Games tend to be most appropriate for skill-based knowledge and practice in the cognitive domain (Keys & Wolfe, 1990), though they easily tap decision making. Jeopardy and Trivial Pursuit are quite popular in many disciplines for reviewing course information in such subjects as abnormal psychology and research methods. In health care, both would lend themselves to reviews in human development, clinical conditions, or other primary knowledge topics. Games can also be created for the psychomotor domain: speed of manipulation, safety in transfers, and knowledge of intervention techniques could all be addressed through a game format that would reward an individual or a team. Crossword puzzles, word searches, and bingo-style games have been used in nursing in-service training to review required materials as well as increase staff attendance and compliance (Lewis et al., 1989). Simulation games are another way of teaching problem solving. Problem solving is best taught through practice and evaluation (Kues et al., 1992) and within the format of the simulation game there is a bit more structure for repetition.

In addition, there is one description in the literature of using a game as part of student evaluation: in the "Create-a-Game Exam," students were assigned to not only develop questions and categories, but to determine the difficulty of the questions as related to points offered for correct answers (Berrenberg & Prosser, 1991). The authors found that the number of questions prepared usually exceeded the number that would be on an exam, and the process stimulated thought about the organization of material.

RESOURCES

Creating games for the classroom usually takes time, imagination, and desire. The rewards can be great, though in our productivity-driven age the trade-offs must be considered. As has been described, the quickest resources are based on those games that are currently available in toy stores or on television. Using the frames of these games requires loading in course material and the games are then easy to introduce to the students because of their familiarity with the format. A more challenging approach is developing the entire game from your imagination, although if you engage small groups from a class to create the game using some of the guiding principles in **Figure 12-2,** this may become more doable.

Using crossword puzzles or word games has become quicker thanks to computer software (for example, see Crossword Puzzles at http://www.cross word-puzzles.co.uk). Articles describing gaming used in classroom education and in-service training, predominantly in nursing, though representing various disciplines, are listed in Recommended Readings at the end of this chapter. Some articles specifically target a greater use of technology, such as computer or web-based games. Some of the references that describe active learning and cooperative learning are excellent background information for the new academician and are available online.

Figure 12-2   Criteria for game development.

- It should have specific objectives and provide immediate feedback to the participants. These objectives may parallel and/or facilitate the course objectives.
- It should fit within the curriculum and the environment. Are the concepts relevant? Is there adequate functional space for implementation?
- It must meet the needs of the students. Does the game help organize the course material? Is it a reliable measure of their comprehension, or will it mislead them? Does the game encourage the players to laugh with as opposed to laugh at one another? Is it inclusive in nature?
- It should involve conflict; whether this is a time limit, competition between teams, or competition with manager will depend upon the objectives. Does it provide a just-right challenge?
- It should have easily communicated rules of play and criterion for closure. Will it be competitive or cooperative? Will there be a single winner, or will everyone win?
- It should have a mechanism (such as pretesting and posttesting) that allows measurement of learning. A game pulled out of nowhere, just to be novel, will have no effect upon the performance outcome measurement.
- It must be field tested to eliminate bugs.

Adapted from Cessario, 1987; de Tornyay & Thompson, 1987; Hillman, 2001; Lewis et al., 1989).

USING THE METHOD: BASIC HOW TO

Many authors have described the methodology behind using games in the classroom and their advice is summarized in Figure 12-2. In essence, the educator must determine the content area, statement of the problem, and objectives of the game. After this, she must determine the game format, number of players, time frame, and rules. If using a frame game, the generic rules already exist and can be adapted for the topic within health care. Next, the instructor must decide what roles players will assume and scenarios in which play occurs. These can be simple adaptations for frame games, or they can be more complex if setting up a simulation game of a clinic. The scoring system and physical elements of a frame game tend to remain consistent with the original game; for simulation games, they need to be created outright. The media used, whether common materials or specially constructed components, are chosen by the designer based upon available time and resources. The game needs to be piloted, critiqued, and possibly revised. Finally, it is beneficial to the community of healthcare educators if the game is then disseminated (Kuhn, 1995).

Overarching elements that must be considered when using instructional games include the layout and amount of space in the classroom, in order to ensure equal opportunity to play; time to be spent during the game with enough time planned for the debriefing; and rewards for results, whether it be intrinsic or extrinsic. Remember that for best effect, the game must be directly related to the subject and the students must be aware of the rules (Ridley, 2004).

POTENTIAL PROBLEMS

Effective use of games in the classroom can be undermined in the ways most strategies fail: poor preplanning, lack of attention, and lack of follow-up. One example of inappropriate simulation game use stemming from each of these obstacles was the use of a simulation game to evaluate treatment skills. There was a specific scoring sheet to test students on the use of a computer program for cognitive rehabilitation. The students were *therapists* with faculty *clients*. This experience was to provide feedback on the student's knowledge of the computer program, as well as provide valuable lessons on therapist-client interaction and use of the environment; e.g., paying attention to the physical environment even though they were intervening for a cognitive task. The main drawbacks to this experience were neglecting to emphasize the game nature of the simulation to reduce trepidation and having faculty be the clients, which increased anxiety. More preplanning would have improved the introduction of the activity. More faculty attention during the experience may have provided the impetus to revise the format so that there could have been peer *clients*. More knowledge about the use of educational games could have made this a more relaxed and appreciated learning experience.

Other potential pitfalls of game use require the instructor to be aware of:

- **Timing:** Instructors must work out and enforce the timing of games. This includes monitoring play, termination, and transition to the next learning activities. Fun activities can take on a life of their own. Simulations (especially) and games reduce control of the timing of the class period; the instructor must be comfortable with that reduced control or it will not work. While spontaneity and flexibility are admirable, there is also a need for planned sequences of activities and firm timekeeping.
- **Competition:** Motivation may be limited to those who win; losing may produce a failure experience that decreases self-esteem. Be conscious of all class members and monitor the degree of competition and cooperation required to achieve educational goals.
- **Cost:** Developing and running a game may be expensive initially; it is quite time consuming to create or flesh out even a frame game. In some instances, it is no more than developing more test questions (as in a Jeopardy or Trivial Pursuit type game), but that is often easier said than done.

In the case of simulation games, a lot of thought is necessary to create an adequate situation and produce a complete cast of characters with goals and belief systems.

- **Participants' needs:** Needs of all participants may not be met within a simulation or game. Do not depend upon these strategies as solo teaching approaches.
- **Lack of appropriate debriefing:** There is a chance, when students have fun, to lose sight of the educational value of a session. By facilitating appropriate debriefing through addressing the goals that have been met, this can be avoided (de Tornyay & Thompson, 1987; Gardner & Benzing, 1990; Keys & Wolfe, 1990; Klein & Freitag, 1991; Stolovitch & Thiagarajan, 1980).

CONCLUSION

Games are a suitable supplement for a variety of academic and clinical situations. They are a method of helping people recognize how much they know or how much they still need to study. Different types have been described, as has the appropriate usage within the wide variety of instructional objectives and content in healthcare curricula. The choice and time management required may seem daunting, but time and again educators have found the respite from standard practice enjoyed while developing and implementing an educational game is well worth the effort.

APPLIED EXAMPLE(S)
Description of Strategy in Use

The format of Jeopardy lends itself for review of lots of material. One example was for preexam reviews in an undergraduate mental health class for occupational therapy students with categories covering such areas as theories, DSM-IV, defense mechanisms, leadership techniques, and pharmaceuticals. The class was divided into three teams. The regular Jeopardy and Double Jeopardy were employed, although Final Jeopardy was not. Each team had a person designated as the "beeper" and they could collaborate within the team to come up with the question that matched the answer on the overhead (Elmo) projector. Most of the class engaged in the spirit of the game. During the process there was time for discussion and clarification of the topic areas. There were errors made on the exam itself, despite the review, so the game did not lead to the degree of achievement expected. However, it was not formally evaluated nor compared with other methods. The participation and apparent enjoyment of that review class was clear, though.

An example of a simulation game for these same students employed the use of percentage dice rolls that each pair of students used to create families and newborns that would function across the semester to demonstrate typical human development from birth through adolescence. Each newborn had characteristics (motor skill, cognitive level, appearance, longevity, social environment, financial environment, etc.) that would be based upon a limited number of dice rolls. The higher the dice roll, the better the performance or status of the attribute to which it was assigned. The students' first objective was to determine which combination of attributes would lead to the best life outcomes for their children. Was it more important to be very smart or very attractive? Could someone be successful with poor motor skills? After these decisions, there were journaling assignments regarding the development of the children and lots of negotiation between the partners regarding a series of developmental issues, culminating in special dice rolls in adolescence that determined whether the adolescent ended up smoking, involved in violence, engaged in sexual activity, etc. Student feedback on this experiential assignment was mostly positive, although some did report that it was quite time consuming. The expected degree of learning regarding human development was demonstrated in the journals. However, the greater learning experience seemed to be attitudinal change based upon the discussions between partners of differing backgrounds and how they managed to cope with some of the unexpected events of these pretend lives.

REFERENCES

Anderson, K. S. (1998). *Let the games begin: The gaming approach as an alternative paradigm in nursing education.* Unpublished doctoral dissertation, North Carolina State University.

Berrenberg, J. L., & Prosser, A. (1991). The create-a-game exam: A method to facilitate student interest and learning. *Teaching of Psychology, 18*(3), 167–169.

Cessario, L. (1987). Utilization of board gaming for conceptual models of nursing. *Journal of Nursing Education, 26*(4), 167–169.

Chickering, A. W., & Gamson, Z. F. (1987). Seven principles for good practice in undergraduate education. Reprinted from *American Association of Higher Education Bulletin* and retrieved February 7, 2006 from http://honolulu.hawaii.edu/intranet/committees/FacDevCom/guidebk/teachtip/7princip.htm

Cowen, K. J., & Tesh, A. S. (2002). Effects of gaming on nursing students' knowledge of pediatric cardiovascular dysfunction. *Journal of Nursing Education, 41*(11), 507–509.

de Tornyay, R., & Thompson, M. (1987). *Strategies for teaching nursing* (3rd ed.). New York: Wiley.

Ellington, H., Gordon, M., & Fowlie, J. (1998). *Using games and simulations in the classroom.* London: Kogan Page Ltd.

Gardner, D. L., & Benzing, P. (1990). Age-related sensory changes: Using simulations in geriatric education. *Educational Gerontology, 16*, 535–545.

Gibson, B. (1991). Research methods Jeopardy: A tool for involving students and organizing the study session. *Teaching of Psychology, 18*(3), 176–177.

Gifford, K. E. (2001). Using instructional games: A teaching strategy for increasing student participation and retention. *Occupational Therapy in Health Care, 15,* 13–21.

Henry, J. M. (1997). Gaming: A teaching strategy to enhance adult learning. *Journal of Continuing
Education in Nursing, 28*(5), 231–234.

Hillman, S. M. (2001). Humor in the classroom: Facilitating the learning process. In A. J. Lowenstein
& M. J. Bradshaw (Eds.), *Fuszard's innovative teaching strategies in nursing* (3rd ed., pp.
54–62). Sudbury, MA: Jones & Bartlett.

Keutzer, C. S. (1993). Jeopardy in abnormal psychology. *Teaching of Psychology, 20*(1), 45–46.

Keys, B., & Wolfe, J. (1990). The role of management games and simulations in education and research. *Journal of Management, 16*(2), 307–336.

Klein, J. D., & Freitag, E. (1991). Effects of using an instructional game on motivation and performance. *Journal of Educational Research, 84*(5), 303–308.

Kues, J. R., Fitzwater, E., Schwartz, P. J., Braun, D. M., Frederick, K. A., & Greengus, L. B. (1992). The
development and use of gaming in multidisciplinary geriatric education. *Educational Gerontology, 18,* 27–40.

Kuhn, M. A. (1995). Gaming: A technique that adds spice to learning? *Journal of Continuing Education in Nursing, 26*(1), 35–39.

Lewis, D. J., Saydak, S. J., Mierzwa, I. P., & Robinson, J. A. (1989). Gaming: A teaching strategy for
adult learners. *Journal of Continuing Education in Nursing, 20*(2), 80–84.

Montpas, M. M. (2004). *Comparison of "Jeopardy" game versus lecture on associate degree nursing students' achievement and retention of geriatric nursing concepts.* Unpublished doctoral
dissertation, Wayne State University.

Randel, J. M., Morris, B. A., Wetzel, C. D., & Whitehill, B. V. (1992). The effectiveness of games for
educational purposes: A review of recent research. *Simulation & Gaming, 23*(3), 261–276.

Regan, R. (2000). *The effect of gaming on the empathic communication of associate degree nursing students.* Unpublished doctoral dissertation, Widener University School of Nursing.

Ridley, R. T. (2004). Classroom games are COOL: Collaborative opportunities of learning. *Nurse Educator, 29*(2), 47–48.

Sprengel, A. D. (1992). *A study of the attainment of diabetes concepts using a simulation-gaming
instructional strategy.* Unpublished doctoral dissertation, Memphis State University.

Stolovitch, H. D., & Thiagarajan, S. (1980). Frame games. In D. G. Langdon (Series Ed.), *The Instructional Design Library* (Vol. 24, pp. 3–102). Englewood Cliffs, NJ: Educational Technology.

Thiagarajan, S., & Stolovitch, H. D. (1978). Instructional simulation games. In D. G. Langdon (Series Ed.), *The Instructional Design Library* (Vol. 12, pp. 3–76). Englewood Cliffs, NJ: Educational
Technology.

Van der Veer Martens, B. (1998). *Rational and irrational interactions: From role-playing to in-
telligent agents.* Retrieved February 6, 2006, from http://www.theorywatch.com/ist501/games.html

Weber, J. R. (1992). *The effectiveness of a gaming-simulation strategy for teaching nursing diagnosis skills.* Unpublished doctoral dissertation, Memphis State University.

RECOMMENDED READING OF GAME DESCRIPTIONS

Corbett, R. W., & Lee, B. T. (1992). Nutriquest: A fun way to reinforce nutrition knowledge. *Nurse
Educator, 17*(2), 33–35.

Dologite, K. A., Willner, K. C., Klepeiss, D. J., York, S. A., & Cericola, L. M. (2003). Sharpen customer service skills with PCRAFT Pursuit. *Journal for Nurses in Staff Development, 19*(1), 47–51.

Free, K. W. (1997). What if? What else? What then? A critical thinking game. *Nurse Educator, 22*(5), 9–12.

Haddad, A. M. (1988). Teaching ethical analysis in occupational therapy. *American Journal of Occupational Therapy, 42*(5), 300–304.

Hamill, S. B., & Hale, C. (1996). Your lot in life. *Teaching of Psychology, 23*(4), 245–246.

Ingram, C., Ray, K., Landeen, J., & Keane, D. R. (1998). Evaluation of an educational game for health sciences students. *Journal of Nursing Education, 37*(6), 240–246.

Israel, R. D., Dolan, T. A., & Caranasos, G. J. (1992). Gerontopoly: Development and testing of a new game in geriatric education. *Gerontology & Geriatrics Education, 12*(4), 17–30.

Johanson, L. S. (1992). Three games for classroom instruction. *Nurse Educator, 17*(5), 6–9.

Jones, A. G., Jasperson, J., & Gusa, D. (2000). Cranial nerve wheel of competencies. *Journal of Continuing Education in Nursing, 31*(4), 152–154.

Masters, K. (2005). Development and use of an educator-developed community assessment board game. *Nurse Educator, 30*(5), 189–190.

McDougal, J. E. (1992). Bringing electrolytes to life: An imagery game. *Nurse Educator, 17*(6), 8–10.

Morton, P. G., & Tarvin, L. (2001). The pain game: Pain assessment, management, and related JCAHO standards. *Journal of Continuing Education in Nursing, 32*(5), 223–227.

Smith-Stoner, M. (2005, September/October). Innovative use of the Internet and intranets to provide education by adding games. *CIN: Computers, Informatics, Nursing*, 237–241.

Stringer, E. C. (1997). Word games as a cost-effective and innovative inservice method. *Journal of Nursing Staff Development, 13*(3), 155–160.

Terenzi, C. (2000). The triage game. *Journal of Emergency Nursing, 26*(1), 66–69.

Ward, A. K., & O'Brien, H. L. (2005). A gaming adventure. *Journal for Nurses in Staff Development, 21*(1), 37–41.

CHAPTER 13

Role Play

Arlene J. Lowenstein

DEFINITION AND PURPOSES

Role play is a dramatic technique that encourages participants to improvise behaviors that illustrate expected actions of persons involved in defined situations. A scenario is outlined and character roles are assigned. The drama is usually unscripted, relying on spontaneous interplay among characters to provide material about reactions and behaviors for students to analyze following the presentation. Those class members not assigned character roles participate as observers and contribute to the analysis.

Part of the category of simulation, role play allows participants to explore why people behave as they do. Participants can test behaviors and decisions in an environment that allows experimentation without risk. The scenario and behaviors of the actors are analyzed and discussed to provide opportunity to clarify feelings, increase observational skills, provide rationale for potential behaviors, and anticipate reactions to decisions. New behaviors can be suggested and tried in response to the analysis.

Role play is used to enable students to practice interacting with others in certain roles and to afford them an opportunity to experience other people's reactions to actions they have taken. The scenario provides a background for the problem and outlines the constraints that may apply. Defining the important characteristics of the major players establishes role expectations and provides a framework for behaviors and actions to be elicited. The postplay discussion provides opportunity for analysis and new strategy formation.

Although it is a dramatic technique, the focus is on the actions of the characters and not on acting ability. An actor plays to the audience; the role player plays to the characters in the scenario. The audience also has a role, that of observing the interplay among characters and analyzing the dynamics occurring. The instructor's role is that of facilitator rather than director. The impetus for the analysis and discussion belongs with the learners. The instructor's role is more passive, clarifying and gently guiding.

Role play is a particularly effective means for developing decision-making and problem-solving skills (Hess & Gilgannon, 1985). Through role play, the learner can identify the systematic steps in the process of making judgments and decisions. The problem-solving process—identification of the problem, data collection and evaluation of possible outcomes, exploration of alternatives, and arrival at a decision to be implemented—can be analyzed in the context of the role play situation. The scenario can include reactions to the implementation of the decision as well as the evaluation and reformulation process (Alden, 1999; Domazzo & Hanson, 1997). Role play has also been used to increase student cultural awareness, aiding in the development of cultural competence in patient care (Shearer & Davidhizar, 2003).

Role play provides immediate feedback to learners regarding their success in using interpersonal skills as well as decision-making and problem-solving skills. At the same time, role play offers learners an opportunity to become actively involved in the learning experience, but in a nonthreatening environment. Role play is not limited to use in the classroom. Corless et al. (2004) successfully used role play as a student assignment that required the adoption of a persona of a person with HIV who was required to take a number of medications over a specific period of time. Students carried out the role play in their homes, taking placebos in place of medication over a specific time frame. Their experiences in following the HIV regimen was then discussed in class, leading to an awareness of the difficulties patients faced in following the regime. Role play is also being used as a teaching strategy in online courses (Mar, Chabal, Anderson, & Vore, 2003).

THEORETICAL RATIONALE

Role play developed in response to the need to effect attitudinal changes in psychotherapy and counseling (Shaffer & Galinsky, 1974). Psychodrama, a forerunner of role play, was developed by Moreno as a psychotherapy technique. Moreno brought psychodrama to the United States in 1925 and continued to develop it during the 1940s and 1950s (Moreno, 1946). In psychodrama, players may be required to recite specific lines or answer specific questions and may represent themselves, whereas in role play, players are encouraged to express their thoughts and feelings spontaneously, as if they were the persons whose roles they are playing (Sharon & Sharon, 1976).

Psychodrama provided a foundation for further development of role play as an educational technique. Corsini (1957) and other psychotherapists and group dynamicists began using role play to assist patients to clarify people's behavior toward each other. Further development led to the use of role play in sensitivity training, a technique that became popular in the 1970s. Human relations and sensitivity training events share a common educational strategy. The learners in the group are encouraged to become involved in examining their thought patterns, perceptions, feelings, and inadequacies. The training events are also designed to encourage each learner with the support of fellow learners to invent and experiment with different patterns of functioning (Gordon, 1970). Role play can be used to meet those educational objectives and is often used in human relations and sensitivity training but has many other uses as well. DeNeve and Hepner (1997), in a study comparing role play to traditional lectures, found that students believed that the use of role play was stimulating and valuable in comparison to the traditional lecture method, their learning increased, and they remembered what they had learned.

CONDITIONS

Role playing is a versatile technique that can be used in a wide variety of situations. One set of learning objectives might be role play dealing with the practice of skills and techniques, whereas another different group of objectives would use role play to deal with changes in understanding, feelings, and attitudes. Van Ments (1983) points out that role play is conducted differently for these two sets of learning objectives. The role play used for the practice of skills may be planned with the emphasis on outcome and overcoming problems. The second type of objective may be best met with an emphasis on the problems and relationships. This method explores why certain behaviors are exhibited and requires expertise from the instructor in dealing with emotions and human behavior. The teacher is responsible for helping the students to avoid the negative effects that could come from the exploration of their feelings and behaviors.

PLANNING AND MODIFYING

Teachers who are new to the technique need to plan before class, but they should monitor the needs of the group as the experience progresses and be able to modify those plans if necessary. The situation developed should be familiar enough so that learners can understand the roles and their potential responses, but it should not have too direct a relationship to students' own personal problems (McKeachie, 2002). It can also be effective to use two or more presentations of the same situation with different students in the roles if the objective is to point out different responses or solutions to a given problem. When that method is used, the instructor may choose to keep those students involved in the second presentation away from viewing the first presentation, to avoid biasing their reactions. The same role play scenario can be used throughout the semester to allow students to react to changing events within the same scenario (Rabinowitz, 1997).

Role play strategy qualifies as an adult-learning approach because it presents a real-life situation and tries to stimulate the involvement of the student. It has special value because it uses peer evaluation and involves active participation. However, it must be carefully guided to be sure participants have an understanding of the objectives and that feedback received from other players is congruent with outcomes that would exist in the real world (Mann & Corsun, 2002).

TYPES OF LEARNERS

Role play is appropriate for undergraduate and graduate students. It is especially effective in staff development programs because of its association with reality. It is used effectively to reach affective outcomes. Role play can be simple or complex, depending on the learning objectives. Regardless of the simplicity of the play itself, it is important to allow adequate time for planning, preparing the students for the experience, and postplay discussion and analysis. The actual role play may be as brief as 5 minutes, although 10 to 20 minutes is more common. Van Ments (1983) suggests that the technique be broken into three sections: briefing, running, and debriefing. Equal amounts of time may be spent for each session for simple objectives, or a ratio of 1:2:3, with most time spent on the debriefing or analysis, for more complex learning objectives.

RESOURCES

Role play can be used in most settings, although tiered lecture rooms may inhibit the ability of the players to relate to each other and to the observing students. In that setting, the theatricality of the technique is likely to be emphasized over the needed behavioral focus (Van Ments, 1983). Special equipment or props may be simple or not used at all, again depending on the objectives. An instructor may choose to use video or audio taping. This can be especially helpful to review portions of the action during the debriefing and analysis section. Reviewing tapes may also be helpful for participating students who, because of their roles, were not in the room to hear and see some of the interaction that occurred in other role plays.

Outside resources are not usually needed for most role play situations, although additional instructors, trained observers, or specific experts may appropriately be used to meet certain objectives. The technique is best for small groups of students so that those not involved in the character parts can be actively involved in observing and discussing the action in the debriefing or analyzing portion. Van Ments (1983) found role play increasingly unsatisfactory as a technique in groups with more than 20 to 25 students, although there may be exceptions, depending on objectives and strategies for involving the audience.

USING THE METHOD

Planning is crucial to effective use of role play as a learning technique. It may be helpful to pilot the exercise before running it in the class situation to allow the instructor to anticipate potential problems and evaluate if the learning objectives can be met. Discussing critical elements of the role play with colleagues can be useful if full-scale piloting is not feasible. A small amount of time going through the plans with someone else may prevent a critical element from going wrong and disrupting the exercise (Van Ments, 1983).

Selecting a scenario and deciding on character roles is an important part of planning. McKeachie (2002) cautions that situations involving morals or subjects of high emotional significance, such as sexual taboos, are apt to be traumatic to some students. He found that the most interesting situations, and those revealing the greatest differences in responses, are those involving some choice or conflict of motives. Student input into planning can also be effective.

To implement the role play, the scenario and characters need to be described briefly but with enough information to elicit responses that will meet the learning objectives. This planning is extremely important for obtaining good results. Spontaneity should be encouraged, so it is preferable to avoid a script, other than bare outlines of the action. Although spontaneity is valued in character dialogue, students need to have a clear understanding of who their characters are and what their basic attitudes and/or thought patterns are. In some instances, spontaneity in the character description area could compromise the objectives and results, but if students understand the expected character, they can still be spontaneous within the character parameters. Allowing students in the character roles to have a few minutes to warm up and relate to the roles they will be playing is often helpful. Observing students absolutely must be briefed on their role. Enough time must be allotted for discussion and analysis of the action. The debriefing following the role play also allows for evaluation of the success in meeting the learning objectives.

In addition to the development of learning objectives and planning, the instructor is responsible for setting the stage for the role play, monitoring the action, and leading the analysis. Students need a clear understanding of the objectives, the scenario, the characters they are to play, the importance of the role of the observers, and the analysis as a vital part of the process. On occasion, the instructor may take a character role, but usually character roles are given to students.

When planning a role play session, the instructor needs to be concerned with the amount of time students may be excluded from the room while waiting for their turn to participate. This issue is especially important when two or more presentations of the same situation are to be used, or the role play has characters who should not be exposed to the dialogue that occurs before they appear in their roles. It is important to avoid the need for the excluded students to roam the corridors with nothing to do for long periods.

In some instances, it may be appropriate to have students switch roles during the role play. This technique can be useful if the group is large and more students need to be involved in the action. This approach also may provide students with an opportunity to see and feel different reactions to similar situations. Another example of when to use this technique might be when the objective is to learn how to conduct a group. Students may benefit by playing group members and switching to leader or vice versa during the exercise.

The instructor needs to encourage students to respond to interactions in the role play in a spontaneous, natural manner, avoiding melodrama and inappropriate laughing or silliness. Effective use of role play focuses on student participation and interaction. The instructor, as facilitator, channels the discussion to meet the learning objectives but avoids monopolizing the play or discussion. The instructor must also be able to monitor and control the depth of emotional responses to the situation or interplay as needed, terminating the play when the objective has been met or the emotional climate calls for intervention.

Students need to understand the importance of playing the character roles in ways in which they believe those characters would act in a real-life situation (Mann & Corsun, 2002). Students in the observer roles must be strongly encouraged to present their observations and contribute to the discussion and analysis. Students can also take part in the development of role play scenarios, identifying their learning objectives, issues, and problems they feel need to be explored, and scenarios that may provide that exploration.

Role play can be used in the online environment using the same basic principles, but with some differences, since the characters will not be visible to each other or to the audience (Mar et al., 2003). A synchronous environment, in which all parties are online at the same time, will allow for a written dialogue flow between parties, with more similarity to an actual conversation (Phillips, 2005), but an asynchronous environment, in which parties log on at different times, will take longer to carry out the scenario, and may not have as much spontaneity, but can be as effective (Lebaron & Miller, 2005). As in all cases of role play, designing an online role play will depend on the learning objectives.

POTENTIAL PROBLEMS

Van Ments (1983) refers to the hidden agenda and warns that stereotyping may occur as roles are presented, often reflecting the expectations and values of the students or the teacher. This stereotyping may lead to unanticipated learning that can reinforce prejudices and preconceptions. Instructors need to be aware of this possibility and avoid writing in stereotypes. They should describe only functions, powers, and constraints of the role described. Roles should be rotated to avoid overidentification of one student with a specific role. In the debriefing session, the students are invited to question and challenge assumptions.

Students may not always make a distinction between an actor and a role. Criticism of the student playing the role must be avoided, while allowing for critique of the behavior of the role character. The instructor must be aware of the emotional tones involved in the role play and channel the emotions into activities that will lead to successful attainment of the learning objectives.

Planning and learning objectives should determine the course of the role play. Students may take the role play in an unexpected direction, possibly because they have a need to explore another issue or problem. If it is not appropriate to revise the learning objectives to accommodate student needs, then the play can be terminated. In that case, the postplay discussion can be used to assist students in recognizing why the technique was not effective. Students should advise how to improve the role play or develop a different teaching strategy. Repeating a scenario with the same or different characters can sometimes afford a more in-depth examination and add to the experience.

The instructor and students need to be aware that this is not a professional drama. Some students, because of stage fright, shyness, or other reasons, do not like participating (Middleton, 2005; Turner, 2005). Although at times it may be appropriate to change actors if the role play does not seem to be going well, it is important not to blame the students. In most cases, the teaching strategy, rather than the actors, needs changing. If that is understood and addressed, role play can be an effective and creative strategy to provide active student participation to meet specific learning objectives.

Teaching Example
Role Playing with Sensitive Subject Matter
Linda C. Andrist, PhD, RNC, WHNP

Nursing students in our nurse practitioner (NP) program find that counseling patients about sexual and reproductive health issues can be very difficult until they become comfortable in dealing with their own feelings about sensitive subjects. In addition to values clarification exercises, I find that role playing can be a valuable tool in helping them overcome their awkwardness. I ask for two volunteers, one to be the nurse practitioner (NP) and one to be the patient (Pt). Each student is given a script; at several points, I break in to engage the class on the interaction. A sample role play is described below.

A 25-year-old woman presents to the clinic with a sexually transmitted infection. She has been with her current partner for 6 months. The student NP is to counsel the patient on how it was possible for the patient to become infected. The patient is worried that her partner has had other sexual partners but also how to explain that she now has an infection.

NP: So, tell me how you are feeling about this diagnosis.

[*Instructor*: Let me stop you for a minute and ask the class, why was this good way to begin the conversation? *Student 1*: She started with an open-ended question, so the patient can hopefully open up. *Student 2:* A closed question, such as "Are you angry at your partner?" asks that the patient respond with a "yes" or "no." You don't get enough information when asking a "yes" or "no" question. *Instructor*: Good answers, remember that asking open ended questions or reflecting back on what the patient is concerned about will help her open up. You get to the root of the issue that way. Let's continue.]

Pt: Well, frankly, I am very angry that he could give me this. He has obviously been cheating. I don't know what I am going to do, I thought we'd be together a long time.

NP: Let's talk a bit about how this infection is transmitted. (NP goes on to explain that in this particular infection—genital herpes, type 2—the infection could have been dormant in either partner and doesn't necessarily mean he has been with other partners. The patient or her partner may have been infected prior to this current relationship. The patient begins to understand her partner may not have had sex with someone else.

Pt: So now what do I tell him? Maybe he will think I have been cheating.

NP: Why don't you just explain what I have shared with you?

[*Instructor*: Okay, let's pause and reflect on the way you asked that question. Class, any comments? *Student 1:* The NP is kind of telling the patient what to do and I am not sure she picked up on the patient's concern about her possibly cheating. *Instructor*: Good observation. How could the NP follow up on that? *Student 2:* Maybe the NP should inquire about why the patient feels this way? *Instructor:* That's a good start, let's see what happens.]

NP: Tell me why you feel your boyfriend will think you have been with someone else.

Pt: I don't know. This is so complicated; I am not sure how I can explain what you told me. I don't really understand how an infection can be there but you don't have any symptoms for such a long time. [Pt begins to cry]

NP: [touching the Pt on her arm and then handing her tissues] I understand how difficult this seems. [NP allows Pt to calm down for a minute or so].

[*Instructor:* Well done. Anyone want to comment on that interaction? *Student 3:* That was great! The NP demonstrated empathy and validated the patient's concerns. *Instructor:* Yes, I agree. How do you all think the NP should proceed? *Student 1:* She could ask if the patient would like to bring her partner in so they could all have a conversation. *Student 2:* She could explain everything again and give the patient some pamphlets on patient education. *Student3:* There's a great Web site for lay people that has chat rooms and quite a bit of user-friendly information. She and her partner could both log on and learn a lot. *Instructor:* Those are all good ideas. Let's summarize what we've learned.]

Over the course of the semester, each student is able to play both patient and NP. By mid-semester, once students have had enough clinical experience to share clinical anecdotes from their practice, we stop using scripts. Students role play situations that either went well, but they were concerned about ahead of time, or were problematic in the student's mind. The students consult with each other about their interactions with patients and how things could go differently the next time they encounter this issue. I am very rewarded to witness the ways in which students grow by the end of the course

REFERENCES

Alden, D. (1999). Experience with scripted role play in environmental economics. *Journal of Economic Education, 20*(2), 127–132.

Corless, I., Gallagher, D., Borans, R., Crary, E., Dolan, S. E., & Kressy, S. (2004). Understanding patient adherence. In A. J. Lowenstein & M. J. Bradshaw (Eds.), *Fuszard's innovative teaching strategies in nursing* (3rd ed., pp. 128–132). Sudbury, MA: Jones & Bartlett.

Corsini, R. J. (1957). *Methods of group psychotherapy.* New York: McGraw-Hill.

DeNeve, K. M., & Hepner, M. J. (1997). Role play simulations: The assessment of an active learning technique and comparisons with traditional lectures. *Innovative Higher Education, 21,* 231–246.

Domazzo, R., & Hanson, P. (1997). Community health problems, apparent vs. hidden: A classroom exercise to demonstrate prioritization of community health problems for programs. *Journal of Health Education, 28,* 383–385.

Gordon, G. K. (1970). Human relations—sensitivity training. In R. M. Smith, G. F. Aker, & J. R. Kidd (Eds.), *Handbook of adult education* (pp. 427–440). New York: Macmillan.

Hess, C. M., & Gilgannon, N. (1985, April). *Gaming: A curriculum technique for elementary counselors.* Paper presented at the Annual Convention of the American Association for Counseling and Development, Los Angeles, CA (ERIC Document 267327).

Lebaron, J., & Miller, D. (2005). The potential of jigsaw role playing to promote the social construction of knowledge in an online graduate education course. *Teachers College Record, 107*(8), 1652–1674.

Mann, S., & Corsun, D. L. (2002). Charting the experiential territory: Clarifying definitions and uses of computer simulation, games and role play. *The Journal of Management Development, 21*(9, 10), 732–745.

Mar, C. M., Chabal, C., Anderson, R. A., & Vore, A. E. (2003). An interactive computer tutorial to teach pain assessment. *Journal of Health Psychology, 8*(1), 161–174.

McKeachie, W. J. (2002). *McKeachie's teaching tips: Strategies, research, and theory for college and university teachers* (11th ed.). Boston: Houghton Mifflin.

Middleton, J. (2005). Role play is not everyone's scene. *Nursing Standard, 19*(24), 31.

Moreno, J. L. (1946). *Psychodrama* (Vol. 1). Boston: Beacon.

Phillips, J. M. (2005). Syllabus selections: Innovative learning activities. Chat role play as an online learning strategy. *Journal of Nursing Education, 44*(1), 43.

Rabinowitz, F. E. (1997). Teaching counseling through a semester long role play. *Counselor Education and Supervision, 36*, 216–223.

Shaffer, J. B. P., & Galinsky, M. D. (1974). *Models of group therapy and sensitivity training.* Englewood Cliffs, NJ: Prentice-Hall.

Sharon, S., & Sharon, Y. (1976). *Small group teaching.* Englewood Cliffs, NJ: Educational Technology Publications.

Shearer, R., & Davidhizar, R. (2003). Educational innovations: Using role play to develop cultural competence. *Journal of Nursing Education, 42*(6), 273–276.

Turner, T. (2005). Stage fright. *Nursing Standard, 19*(22), 22–23.

Van Ments, M. (1983). *The effective use of role play: A handbook for teachers and trainers.* London: Kogan Page.

RECOMMENDED READING

Alden, D. (1999). Experience with scripted role play in environmental economics. *Journal of Economic Education, 20*(2),127–132.

Ashmore, R., & Banks, D. (2004). Student nurses' use of their interpersonal skills within clinical role plays. *Nurse Education Today, 24*(1), 20–29.

Chester, M., & Fox, R. (1996). *Role playing methods in the classroom.* Chicago: Science Research Associates.

Goldenberg, D., Andrusyszyn, M., & Iwasiw, C. (2005). The effect of classroom simulation on nursing students' self-efficacy related to health teaching. *Journal of Nursing Education, 44*(7), 310–314.

Greenberg, E., & Miller, P. (1991). The player and professor: Theatrical techniques in teaching. *Journal of Management Education, 15*(4), 428–446.

Griggs, K. (2005). A role play for revising style and applying management theories. *Business Communication Quarterly, 68*(1), 60–65.

Kane, M. (2003). Teaching direct practice techniques for work with elders with Alzheimer's disease: A simulated group experience. *Educational Gerontology, 29*, 777–794.

Loprinzi, C. L., Johnson, M. E., & Steer, G. (2003). Doc, how much time do I have? *Journal of Clinical Oncology, 21*(9 Suppl.), 5S–7S.

Northcott, N. (2002). Role play: Proceed with caution! *Nursing Education in Practice 2*(2), 87–91.

Silberman, M. (1996). *Active learning: 101 strategies to teach any subject.* Boston: Allyn & Bacon.

CHAPTER 14

Creative Movement: Embodied Knowledge Integration

Carol Picard and Ellen Landis

DEFINITIONS AND PURPOSES

The education of healthcare practitioners has been enriched by expressive techniques, such as movement, poetry, and art (Byers & Forinash, 2004; Picard, 2000; Picard & Mariolis, 2002; Picard, Sickul, & Natale, 1998). Expressive techniques are activities to assist students in bringing to awareness some aspect of their academic understanding or experience that is grounded in immediate, personal knowing. Embodied learning exists on a continuum of sensory awareness. Emphasis is given to the location of the learning experience, the body, with the mind included as a sensory organ. Embodied knowing is cognition that incorporates information from multiple senses.

Embodied knowing techniques build on customary learning activities within the curriculum such as lecture content, reading assignments, and clinical experiences. Reflection on the models and media used in the experience enhances learning (Benner, Tanner, & Chesla, 1996; Brookfield, 2005; Byers & Forinash, 2004; Levy, 1988; Schon, 1987). Through such a process of expression through movement and reflection, a richer and more complex understanding of the knowledge of the healthcare professions can occur. Interest in embodiment in the healthcare literature highlights the value of student attention to this orientation for themselves, their patients, and their families (Watson, 1999; Wilde, 1999).

Nursing has a rich tradition of reflective practice, pioneered by Orlando (1990) and further advanced by Johns and Freshwater (1997), but the educational activities have been primarily text- and dialogue-based. Within the field of creative arts therapies, an umbrella phrase for the arts in psychotherapy, including dance movement therapy, drama therapy, music therapy, and expressive arts therapy (a multimodal arts-based psychotherapy), expressive techniques are united with reflective practice and built into undergraduate and graduate course work. In the academic setting, students learn how to examine their biases through a combination of creative activities and group dialogue. Bateson and Bateson (1988) addressed embodied learning by suggesting that movement might be a basis for metaphorical thinking through shifting between modes of expression. "Can I, for instance, change my understanding of something by dancing it" (p. 195)? In family therapy, the creative mechanism for reflection is the approach to relational discourse as demonstrated by Hoffman (2002) and White (2004).

In Western culture, movement experiences have been disconnected from reflection and valued knowledge. Although it is a universal mode of expression, modern Western society does not routinely incorporate movement as a mode of expression in academic learning. Dance movement therapy literature has described the transformational potential of movement for insight and understanding. It supports the development of critical new thinking and movement patterns, which foster an experience of unifying mind/body/spirit.

Marcow-Speiser (1998), describes movement as the container or bridge to connecting the inner and outer experience. Yuasa (1987) who explores the modern Western perspective through an Eastern philosophical lens, states:

> The mind-body issue is not simply theoretical speculation, but a practical, lived experience, involving the mustering of one's whole mind and body. The theoretical is only a reflection on this lived experience (p. 18).

This technique for embodied knowing makes use of what Bryner and Markova (1996) call *physical thinking,* or an underused intelligence resource. These authors use movement activities in teaching corporate executives creative strategies for understanding management issues. Movement as an educational technique changes the learning context and shifts perceptions as students move to know curricula content.

Neurologists are beginning to promote the use of embodied care as their research has demonstrated desirable brain activity during movement psychotherapy (van der Kolk, 2004). Yet, many questions remain in the healthcare community about how to teach expressive techniques to future and experienced healthcare practitioners who are not specializing in creative arts therapies. There are limited reports of the use of this teaching strategy in healthcare educational programs. However, in dance movement therapy and drama therapy graduate degree programs, certificate programs for learning body-integrated techniques for psychotherapy flourish. A growing body of literature has arisen from within these disciplines (Fisher & Stark, 1992; Chaiklin, 1998).

Movement experientials may be guided and structured by the teacher, with specific instructions for movement. The activity may also take the form of creative movement, where the invitation is to respond to a particular theme, concept, or issue using student's choice of movement. Words may be added later only to enhance the group understanding of the movement experience. Creative movement is defined as the intentional creative expression of self in dance, gesture, and posture. This form of movement is intended to express meaning and can be considered a form of embodied reflection (Picard, 2000).

The focus of this chapter is the authors' experience with academic learning goals achieved through movement activities incorporated into the classroom. The purpose of movement-integrated classroom learning is to use embodied intelligence to help students understand selected aspects of professional healthcare work. These activities create opportunities for students to (1) enhance awareness of self and other, (2) explore conceptual learning through embodied reflective action, (3) appreciate the multiple dimensions of clinical situations, (4) develop an appreciation of the patient/family experience, and (5) come together in community as students/faculty for this learning.

THEORETICAL RATIONALE

According to Newman (1994), health is expanding consciousness, and the capacity for self-reflection, expression, and pattern recognition are aspects of expanding consciousness. Consciousness evolves toward increasing complexity in one's relationship to the world. Newman emphasizes the process of becoming, the evolutionary nature of consciousness, and the importance of meaning in appreciating pattern. Newman described movement as the fullest expression of consciousness. Through movement, we come to know our world, others, and ourselves. Exploring a mode of expression that supports wholeness can illuminate and uncover aspects of self-knowledge and meaning.

The use of Newman's theory to ground this pedagogical strategy supports the students' growth as part of their own expanding consciousness. Learning through facilitated experiential learning gives students an opportunity to address the issues of embodiment, relationship, and the models employed to examine their experience. Very little time is spent in most healthcare education programs helping the student assess his or her own embodied experiences. It is important to explore the untapped resources in the students' physical being. This rediscovery of the wisdom of the body-mind can support a well-rounded attitude toward others and an enhanced awareness of one's own body potential, as well as being in a mindful relationship with the environment. The use of expressive techniques also provides an opportunity for students to appreciate directly the potential health-promoting effects of expressive techniques for patients (Lane, 2005). Clinical application of expressive techniques needs to be carefully considered, for each intervention has an effect on the patient.

The teacher-student relationship can be a mirror of the student-patient relationship (Picard et al., 1998). In both cases, collaboration leads to an appreciation of the unfolding nature of knowledge of our person/world experience. Using Newman's theory as a ground from which to practice, the goals are awareness of process, appreciation of pattern, relatedness, and transformational change. Each aspect of this exercise can present an opportunity for learning about the whole person.

This technique can also be examined in relation to Carper's (1978) four patterns of knowing: personal, empiric, ethical, and aesthetic. Expressive techniques offer an embodied mode of knowing of all four patterns.

Personal Knowing: Self-Awareness

Through expressive techniques, students have an opportunity to engage in reflection with a sense of immediacy. The exercises provide an opportunity to take knowledge and make it their own. This is an opportunity to reflect on the questions: What aspects of myself do I bring to my practice? How does who I am influence the care given? How do I come to understand the ways I embody my attitudes, feelings, beliefs, and new knowledge?

Empirical Knowing: Integrating Knowledge

Movement experientials provide an opportunity to play with concepts, theories, and clinical knowledge, as is described in the following exercises. These activities create body metaphors, or body-stories, and move out of limited analytic, text-based approaches to understanding. The knowledge gained is then reintegrated with prior learning. Dialogue includes the examination of the theories and models through which the experience takes place.

Ethical Knowing: How Should I Act With This Knowledge?·

Every component of these exercises provides moments to engage the moral imagination of students. For example, if a student chooses to pass on a certain portion of the activity, then the principle of respect for their choice can be discussed, not only in relation to the group but also in relation to patients' choices.

Aesthetic Knowing: How Do I Express My Understanding of This Knowledge?

Exploring movement and other expressive art forms engages participants in questions about what information is valuable. Arts-integrated education helps to balance customary practices that emphasize rational, literal approaches with multisensory awareness. Through expressive techniques, the students have an opportunity to create, in movement or gesture, answers to these questions: How do I express my understanding? What does it mean to me? How will I develop my knowledge for practice? They also have the opportunity to share what they create with classmates. The group component provides a way to practice participating in a community of creation. The process and the outcome of the activity are equally emphasized.

Creative movement with reflective dialogue is an invitation to students to integrate the four ways of knowing grounded in theory, with an emphasis on the student's own expanding cognition.

CONDITIONS

The teacher constructs a general framework of exercises for the students that relate to a particular topic or issue. Examples of issues for embodied activities include the experience of mobility and immobility, self-sufficiency and loss of dominion. Other topics that lend themselves to creative movement are the elements of a relationship: trust, security abandonment, loss, and vulnerability. Every learning situation provides some opportunity for embodied reflection of the relationship between the individual, others, and the environment.

TYPES OF LEARNERS

All types of learners may participate, including both graduate and undergraduate students. All exercises may be adapted for students with physical disabilities. It is helpful to suggest that the student is free to pass on any part of the activity. Creating a safe space will support all learners. Moving in space without any clear expectations may make some students anxious. By framing the exercise with Carper's (1978) ways of knowing, students are invited to reflect on their responses to each part of the process. For example, if a student becomes anxious, she has the opportunity to learn techniques to overcome the anxiety. Each student can reflect on his or her own experiences with anxiety. What does it feel and look like? If you couldn't use words, what would its shape be? How does the experience differ from person to person? Have they met any patients whose anxiety was manifested in movement? The students' integrated embodied knowledge may be utilized later in the clinical arena.

With each part of the movement experience, teachable moments and insights are available to students. The leader simply opens with a question, such as: If we are anxious about moving when all is uncertain, what is it like for the patient in strange surroundings, being asked to do things that seem unnatural in some respect?

RESOURCES

Any space with movable desks is a good site for movement-integrated curricular exercises. In good weather, the use of outdoor space may also be effective; however, if the space is not private, many students may feel uncomfortable with that degree of exposure. In the group with students, teachers may participate, setting the stage for this process as one of full engagement.

Teachers who are interested in professional development might participate in movement improvisation workshops because a direct experience of this process with guidance is helpful. Creative movement workshops are often taught in major cities. Colleges offer arts integrated curriculum design courses. The authors recommend any lesson plan that includes a movement experiential be thoroughly critiqued with a colleague prior to and after the class.

USING THE METHOD

Consider the goals of the experience, keeping in mind to trust the process because insights and developments will arise during the activity and become an important part of shaping the activity. The creative impulse is in each teacher and student. Talk with students ahead of time and give them a brief explanation of the activity. Let them know that the class will involve a movement activity and to dress in comfortable clothes.

With a movement activity, organization of the learning plan is paired with the preparation of the students for experiential learning. Some exercises may be highly structured, whereas others are a less structured form of creative movement. More instructive explanation is best for students who have not had prior experience with such exercises. Less instruction is needed for students who have previously been introduced to arts-integrated learning. Introduction of exploratory movement activities can be tailored to each group's readiness.

First, identify the time parameters for the session. One to two hours is recommended. This time frame allows for the process to unfold. As previously mentioned, an important part of the activity is creating a safe place. In order for students to take a risk with a new mode of academic expression, they must feel safe with the teacher and their peers.

Leventhal's five-part movement session (1980) can be applied to the classroom schema. The five parts are warm-up, release, theme, centering, and closure. These five parts make up each movement session. They can also be brought into designing a course over a semester, with any part being the focus of a number of meetings. There are many ways to address these five parts.

Warm-up: A warm-up provides an opportunity for the individuals in a group to limber their body and voice for the activity of the class. An example of a warm-up is the instructor leads a simple movement for the group to follow, each to the extent that he or she feels comfortable. In demonstrating a simple exercise, such as reaching upwards, while explaining what may feel like a reach up to one person, with arms and elbows extended and to another up may be a movement with hands reaching just above the shoulders. Then the teacher invites students to take turns to lead, introducing a particular movement, which everyone does their own way. Everyone gets a chance to lead and follow.

Another warm-up invites students to walk around the room and greet each person in a unique way using voice and gesture. Emphasize the mutual respect and mindfulness necessary for this exercise. One lesson here is the importance of introductions in the clinical setting. This simple warm-up also supports connectedness among students necessary for continuing experiential learning and collegial rapport.

Release: Release involves letting go of what was on one's mind before the activity in order to focus on the present and upcoming activity. These movements may look like a shaking off, dusting off, washing off, even writing a note to yourself of something you need to return to thinking about later.

Theme: Theme is a selected psychosocial content focus. For instance, a theme of confidence in self and others arises or is planned for the class. Participants can be given pieces of elastic cords to explore weight bearing with each other. Alternatively, participants can stand at a distance from each other with one person's role to stand in one place while one or more participants move towards her. The exploration is to try to sense another's comfort and expectations.

Centering: Centering brings together the physicality and cognition of the thematic material. Centering brings the focus from the thematic material to participants' sensations and the environment of the classroom. It is soothing, calming, even energizing based on the experience of the session. Centering may be facilitated by the instructor asking the participants to bring what they are doing to an end; to breathe deeply into their lungs and belly; to feel their feet on the ground; to notice the sensations in their bodies; to remember them; to identify a word, feeling, or phrase that describes their experience.

Closure: Closure is the opportunity to organize the body-mind experience in a manner that enables one to attend to other tasks that follow this session. It may include changing to a different mode of expression, such as writing or drawing before talking with each other about their findings in small groups or one large group.

POTENTIAL PROBLEMS

Anxiety

Because of the newness of this teaching technique, students may be anxious. The teacher may be anxious! Many students think the movement will be about traditional forms of dance and may feel uncomfortable, particularly if they have had no dance training. It is important to emphasize that this movement is not like other dance forms with which they may be familiar and requires no prior formal training.

Anxiety may be expressed as laughter or overtalkativeness during the experience. Encourage students to center themselves and to talk only when the activity requires it. Silence when moving allows for a heightened awareness of one's sensory information. Attention to the activity is also important for safety reasons. Let students know they will always be invited to engage in a reflective dialogue after the activity.

Simple instructions and an overview of the learning goals may make the new structure seem more familiar. Emphasize that each student's process will be different and deserving of respect. It helps students to hear that self-awareness is the key; that the work will not be graded or judged. By demonstrating a clear design plan and spirit of collaborative inquiry students can approach the exercise with a sense of mastery.

Uncovering Painful Material

When an activity is related to a painful topic such as loss, an embodied approach may put the students in touch with their own experiences, which may be difficult or painful. The instructor must be available to address such content. Students can be surprised and unsettled by their reaction to an activity. Always provide time to debrief students from the experience.

As with any other triggering that might occur for students either in the clinical area or in the classroom, refer the student for assistance as indicated.

Avoidance

If a student feels uncomfortable with some part of the exercise, that student can become the observer of the process. In the authors' experience of working with students in this format, only once did a student find the process so uncomfortable that she could not participate, and only in the creative movement portion of the activity. Students are told that they can pass on any part of the activity.

CONCLUSION

An essential aspect of training in healthcare work is developing one's own range of motion. Whether it is through expanding understanding, emotional capabilities, or movement options, students gain insight as they attune to their sensory experiences. It is often through this process that students gain a more nuanced understanding of their patients and colleagues as well. Building these methods into a healthcare curriculum expands a student's capacity to interact with the knowledge at hand. This, in turn, lays the groundwork for developing healthcare practitioners who are flexible, versatile, and capable of facing challenges in a fully embodied way.

EXAMPLE 1.
Movement Vocabulary

Introducing movement into classroom education opens up a world of kinesthetic language. Although there are well-documented schools of thought for describing movement, such as Laban Analysis and the Kestenberg Movement Profile that offer extensive training in certification programs, these are not necessary for the instructor. When introducing movement awareness for the first time and for a single class, the following activity brings attention to cognitive as well as kinesthetic experience of human movement, or embodied knowing. This exercise makes use of a repetitious structure that employs the use of time to support students and invites exploration.

Divide the class into two groups. Each group is asked to write a list of different kinds of movements that have a relationship to what they are learning in their coursework. The facilitator may start the list for both groups by suggesting terms such as stiff, shaky, bold, grounded, and strong. The facilitator may choose to give movement examples of a few of these different kinds of movements. Each group chooses a scribe—someone to write down the group's movement terms.

After 10 minutes of making the lists, half the class is asked to bring its list to one end of the room, and the other half brings its list to the other end of the room. The instructor asks the groups to carefully observe the movement they see, to witness the differences in how people move and make meaning of the same term. Each group begins by choosing one of their movement terms for the other group to enact. The facilitator acts as a host or moderator for this nonverbal experience. The facilitator invites one group to begin, and after about 30–50 seconds, stops them by saying, "Thank you, that was great," or somesuch.

The two groups switch roles, and the first movement group now chooses a movement term from its list for the other group to enact. Again, the facilitator is the timekeeper, starting and stopping the activity.

This call and response is repeated several times, giving the students an opportunity to get comfortable moving, being seen and observing the differences in how people interpret or experience the same word differently. After they have repeated this process it is interesting to modify the experience by inviting the group that is moving to do it as slowly or quickly, or as small or as large as they can. The activity can be modified again by combining two movement terms. The instructor then asks the moving group to do one kind of movement with their arms and another with their legs, or suggests they try doing one kind of movement with their faces and another with the rest of the body.

Inevitably, laughter occurs at both how difficult it is to try these different movement terms and at how complex and common it is to recognize in others and in ourselves the multiple experiences going on at once in a person. The instructor can remind students that their professional work will often include observation of patients and colleagues. This activity also supports development of compassionate observation skills as well as a willingness to try what it is they will be asking others to do: to be observed.

Discussion following the experiential activity is a chance to hear from each participant. Themes that often arise for groups doing this activity include dispensing of assumptions, as students have witnessed the variety of ways a common concept is interpreted by different people. What is it like to witness another, and be witnessed? What kinds of movement are most comfortable? How did trying movements you rarely do feel?

EXAMPLE 2.

Trust and Safety: A Holding Environment

Baccalaureate nursing students came together to engage in a creative movement reflective dialogue about their new clinical experience as part of a curriculum component called "awareness group." Up until this point, all activities in the group had been discussions. The teacher posed the possibility of a movement activity, and the students agreed.

The students had begun their classroom lectures and reading on topics related to maternal and child health, and on this particular week, they were in the newborn nursery and maternity unit. The students identified care of the new family as the learning of the week. The teacher asked what they thought was the most important thing new parents and infants needed. The group agreed that the baby needed a safe holding environment and that first-time parents needed to feel safe and confident in their new roles. Warm-ups and centering meditative exercises were used to set the stage for the activity. Once the students were able to focus on themselves and their own movement, they were able to begin other exercises that required group activity.

Walking blind: This was a trust exercise as well as an invitation to notice one's body in space while moving. One student led another, whose eyes were closed. Students paired off, switching roles after 3 to 4 minutes. Pairs then changed partners and repeated the exercise until each person walked with everyone in the room. The students reflected on each pairing, leading and not seeing. The students explored insight into their own comfort level with trust and responsibility for others. The variations in their response with different classmates led to insight regarding patients' comfort level with different staff. Dialogue about comfort ensued, and students planned to read Morse and Bottorff's (1995) research on comfort for the following week.

Trust fall: The students were invited to take turns standing rigid in the center of a very narrow circle (like a bowling pin) and give their weight to their classmates. The leader demonstrated how to support the center person's weight while maintaining good body mechanics. At first the circle was very small, so the degree of movement was small. As the group and the person in the center became comfortable, the circle widened. The students were asked to do this in silence. After the exercise was completed, the teacher invited the group to reflect. Creating a holding environment, being supportive, letting go of control, and receiving care were themes brought up by the students. With this group, the compelling issue of trust in the group to support their weight gave an immediacy to a discussion of what it must be like to need the kind of care a newborn needs and how trust might be experienced. Participating gave them insight into the uniqueness of a person's response. Several students shared their individual experiences with newborns in their own families, as well as personal family experiences as new mothers, or with relatives or friends who had newborns. They then related their experience to the class lecture that week.

Rocking in space: To experience a holding environment, students were invited to give their weight to classmates and be rocked in space. One student at a time would lie on the floor, and the nine other students and the teacher would lift the person in silence and rock that person slowly. After 1 to 2 minutes, they were gently lowered to the floor. All of this movement was done in silence. Many students described a feeling of peace and safety. One student passed on this exercise, saying that she could take great risks when she felt in control, such as skydiving, but that she could not bring herself to give up control to be lifted four feet off the ground. Students reflected on this lesson of not assuming what another person would want, but rather asking and responding with what was needed.

Creative movement: Students were invited to go to a spot in the room by themselves and, after doing a centering exercise, to express in movement or gesture what their feelings about this clinical rotation might be. When they were ready, the group came together in a circle and, one by one, shared the creative movement. They then told the group about the movement's meaning, did the movement again, and then the group tried the movement. As each student in sequence shared her movement, the group tried it and then added it to the movement repertoire of the whole. At the end of this exercise, the group had a piece of choreography that spoke to the collective wishes of this clinical cohort. They had also formed a sense of community, appreciated how much they had in common, and how each of them was unique. Some of the movements related to caring, being able to help, learning not to fear, becoming strong, and being knowledgeable. When the creative movement group was over, the students expressed enthusiasm for this model of reflection. Although the group time was over, students stayed in the studio to continue their discussion of what the activities offered.

This expressive technique of using creative movement, movement exercises, and reflective dialogue supported student-embodied knowing. Students reported experiencing a heightened sense of themselves in space and an enthusiasm for understanding concepts in action. They reflected on the knowledge acquired as it related to patients and what should happen in a caring environment. They used the time and activities to form a cohesive group, which would work together most effectively over the course of the semester. Subsequent group meetings also used more expressive techniques generated by the students.

REFERENCES

Bateson, G., & Bateson, M. C. (1988). *Angels fear: Toward an epistemology of the sacred.* New York: Bantam.

Benner, P., Tanner, C., & Chesla, C. (1996). *Expertise in nursing practice.* New York: Springer.

Brookfield, S. (2005). *The power of critical theory: Liberating adult learning and teaching.* San Francisco: Jossey-Bass.

Bryner, A., & Markova, D. (1996). *An unused intelligence.* Berkeley, CA: Conari Press.

Byers, J., & Forinash, M. (Eds.). (2004). *Educators, therapists and artists on reflective practice.* New York: Peter Lang.

Carper, B. (1978). Fundamental patterns of knowing in nursing. *Advances in Nursing Science, 1*(1), 13–23.

Chaiklin, S. (Ed.). (1998). *Dance movement therapy abstract: Doctoral dissertations, master's theses, and special projects 1991–1996.* Columbia, MD: The Marion Chace Foundation.

Fisher, A. C., & Stark, A. (Eds.). (1992). *Dance movement therapy abstract: Doctoral dissertations, master's theses, and special projects through 1990.* Columbia, MD: The Marion Chace Foundation.

Hoffman, L. (2002). *Family therapy: An intimate history.* New York: W. W. Norton.

Johns, C., & Freshwater, D. (1997). *Transforming nursing through reflective practice.* London: Churchill Livingstone.

Lane, M. R. (2005). Creativity and spirituality in nursing. *Holistic Nursing Practice, 19*(3), 122–125.

Leventhal, M. (1980). Dance movement therapy as treatment of choice for the emotionally disturbed and learning disabled child. In S. Fitt & A. Riordan (Eds.), *Focus on dance IX: Dance for the handicapped* (pp. 43–46). Reston, Virginia: American Alliance for Health, Physical Education, Recreation and Dance.

Levy, F. (1988). *Dance/movement therapy: A healing art.* Reston, VA: American Alliance for Health, Physical Education, Recreation, and Dance.

Marcow-Speiser, V. (1998). The use of ritual in expressive therapy. In A. Robbins (Ed.). *Therapeutic Presence: Bridging Expression and Form.* Bristol, PA: Jessica Kingsley.

Newman, M. (1994). *Health as expanding consciousness.* Sudbury, MA: Jones & Bartlett.

Orlando, I. (1990). *The dynamic nurse–patient relationship.* New York: National League for Nursing.

Picard, C. (2000). Uncovering patterns of expanding consciousness in mid-life women: Creative movement and the narrative as modes of expression. *Nursing Science Quarterly, 13*(2), 150–158.

Picard, C., & Mariolis, T. (2002). Praxis as a mirroring process: Teaching psychiatric nursing grounded in Newman's health as expanding consciousness. *Nursing Science Quarterly, 15*(2), 118–122.

Picard, C., Sickul, C., & Natale, S. (1998). Healing reflections: The transformative mirror. *International Journal of Human Caring, 2*(3), 29–37.

Schon, D. (1987). *Educating the reflective practitioner: Toward a new design for teaching and learning in the professions.* San Francisco: Jossey-Bass.

Yuasa, Y. (1987). *The body: Toward an Eastern mind-body theory.* Albany: State University of New York Press.

Watson, J. (1999). *Postmodern nursing and beyond.* New York: Churchill Livingstone.

White, M. (2004). *Narrative practice and exotic lives: Resurrecting diversity in everyday life.* Adelaide, South Australia: Dulwich Centre Publications.

Wilde, M. (1999). Why embodiment now? *Advances in Nursing Science, 22*(2), 25–38.

SUGGESTED READING

Angus, I., & Langsdorf, L. (1993). *The critical turn: Rhetoric and philosophy in postmodern discourse.* Carbondale: Southern Illinois University Press.

Bateson, G. (1979). *Mind in nature: A necessary unity.* New York: Dutton.

Cricket, B., & Keegan, L. (2000). Exercise and creative movement. In B. M. Dossey, L. Keegan, & C. E. Guzzetta (Eds.), *Holistic Nursing* (pp. 453–465). Gaithersburg, MD: Aspen.

Hanna, J. L. (1995). The power of dance: Health and healing. *Journal of Alternative and Complementary Medicine, 1*(4), 323–331.

Hervey, L. W. (2000). *Artistic inquiry in dance/movement therapy: Creative alternatives for research.* Springfield, IL: Charles C. Thomas.

Maturana, H. R. (1992). *The tree of knowledge: The biological roots of human understanding.* Boston: Shambalala.

Morse, J., Bottorff, J., & Hutchinson, S. (1995). The paradox of comfort. *Nursing Research, 41,* 14–19.

Picard, C. (2005). Creative movement and reflective art: Modes of expression for participant and researcher. In C. Picard & C. Jones (Eds.), *Giving voice to what we know: Margaret Newman's theory of health as expanding consciousness in nursing practice, research and education* (pp. 119–130). Sudbury, MA: Jones & Bartlett.

Samuels, M., & Lane, M. (1998). *Creative healing.* San Francisco: Harper.

Shotter, J. (1993). *Cultural politics of everyday life: Social constructionism, rhetoric and knowing of the third kind.* Buffalo, NY: University of Toronto Press.

Varela, F., Thompson, E., & Rosch, E. (1991). *The embodied mind.* Cambridge, MA: MIT Press.

CHAPTER 15

High-Fidelity Patient Simulation

Alfred E. Lupien

Patient simulators have been used by health professional educators for more than 50 years (Rosen, 2004). Computer software may be used to teach anatomy, physiology, pathophysiology, pharmacology, and clinical decision making. Technical skills associated with airway management, vascular catheter insertion, and birthing can be developed using physical part-task trainers. Virtual reality devices combine computer-generated images and haptic (tactile) feedback enabling the learner to refine technical skills. High-fidelity simulators, the focus of this chapter, are life-sized mannequins with complex interrelated multisystem physiological and pharmacological models that generate valid observable responses from the mannequin and allow students to interact with the simulator as they would with an actual patient in the clinical environment.

DEFINITION AND PURPOSES

The first high-fidelity patient simulators were developed in the 1960s, but their use did not become widespread until the early 1990s, when anesthesia educators and researchers began using simulators to improve education and study clinician performance. Since the narrowly focused introduction of patient simulators, a wide variety of healthcare applications have been developed to include procedure training, evaluation of individual response to critical incidents, equipment evaluation, task analysis, and team training (Gaba & De Anda, 1988; Howard, Gaba, Fish, Yang, & Sarnquist, 1992). Common educational applications of simulation include theme-based workshops on ventilation, pharmacology, airway management, conscious sedation, and disaster response; ongoing skills development (such as progressively complex anesthesia techniques); and practicing clinical decision making. The first nursing users of high-fidelity simulators were nurse anesthetists; however, applications of simulation have expanded to include acute care, critical care, perioperative, and emergency nursing.

Features of the simulators include a functioning cardiovascular system with synchronized palpable pulses, heart sounds, measurable blood pressure (by palpation or oscillometry), electrocardiographic waveforms, and invasive parameters such as arterial, central venous, and pulmonary artery pressures. Respiratory system components include self-regulating spontaneous ventilation, measurable exhaled respiratory gases, and breath sounds. Other simulator features include a pharmacological system capable of responding to anesthetic, analgesic, and vasoactive agents; a urologic system; reactive pupils; and the ability to accept defibrillation, needle cricothyroidotomy, jet ventilation, needle thoracocentesis, chest tube insertion, and pericardiocentesis.

This chapter emphasizes highly automated patient simulators such as METI (Medical Education Technologies, Incorporated; Sarasota, Florida) adult Human Patient Simulator, PediaSim, and BabySim products in which the simulator may respond autonomously based on underlying interactive physiological and pharmacological modules; however, other simulators requiring more instructor involvement, including the METI Emergency Care Simulator and Laerdal (Laerdal Medical Corporation; Wappingers Falls, New York) PatSim are also available. The simulator includes four components: a lifelike mannequin, a freestanding enclosure containing many of the simulator's components, a computer to integrate the function of simulator components, and an interface that allows the user (either student or faculty depending on the objectives of the exercise) to control the simulation and modify physiologic parameters (see **Table 15-1**). Many simulators have both a portable interface allowing instructors to control simulations from the bedside and a stationary console that can be positioned away from the mannequin so that changes in the simulation can be made without the knowledge of trainees. To initiate a simulation, the user selects a patient profile (such as healthy adult male or full term parturient). If desired, a clinical scenario (such as anaphylaxis) can be superimposed. Once a simulation has been initiated, the instructor may allow the simulation to run as programmed or make modifications to emphasize specific teaching points.

Through simulation, a predictable environment can be created to allow healthcare providers to practice under realistic conditions in real time using actual clinical supplies. Practical advantages of simulation include the abilities to represent critical or uncommon clinical problems, to allow management errors to develop or multiple treatment options to be explored without injury or discomfort to actual patients, and to manipulate time (compression, expansion, and replication).

Educational advantages of simulation include the opportunities to actively involve the learner, provide relatively consistent experiences for all students, and collect physiologic, video and audio data for use in reflective sessions following the simulation session (Fletcher, 1995; Gaba, 1997). The simulated environment

Table 15-1   Modifiable Parameters of High-Fidelity Patient Simulators[a]

Cardiovascular
Baroreceptor response
Cardiac rhythm
Heart rate (fixed or baseline)
Heart sounds
Hemoglobin
Intravascular volume
Ischemic sensitivity
Pericardial fluid
Pulmonary vascular resistance
Pulses
Systemic vascular resistance
Valve resistance (aortic, mitral, pulmonic, and tricuspid)
Venous return
Venous capacitance
Ventricular contractility (right and left)
Respiratory
Breath sounds
Bronchial resistance (right and left)
Chest wall capacity
Chest wall compliance
Functional residual capacity
Inspiratory:expiratory ratio
Intrapleural volume (right and left)
Lung compliance (right and left)
Oxygen consumption
Partial pressure of venous CO_2
pH (baseline)
Respiratory quotient
Shunt fraction
Other
Chest tube air leak
Chest tube flow
Eyes (open, closed, blinking)
Intracranial pressure
Pupil size (right and left)
Urine output
Temperature
Weight

[a]Not all features are available on every simulator.

may also be used to create a standardized setting for testing critical thinking and decision making.

Disadvantages of simulation include the costs of starting and maintaining a simulation program, extensive faculty time commitment, and a tendency for the simulated environment to induce *hypervigilance*, or exaggerated caution. Moreover, despite a significant amount of human physiologic, pharmacologic, and phenomenonological data, anatomical and physiological models are incomplete and imperfect (Gaba, 1997). Finally, the transfer of learning from the simulated environment to actual clinical practice is not well documented.

THEORETICAL FOUNDATIONS

The landmark Flexner Report to the Carnegie Foundation in 1910 established the dominant paradigm for healthcare education in the 20th century (Papa & Harasym, 1999). Two key components of the model were a university-based scientific curriculum coupled with a clinical practicum.

The scientific curriculum historically featured lecture-based instruction in which students were passive recipients of factual knowledge. Information was imparted by domain experts according to a predetermined timetable. Although the lecture format assured that important educational material was disseminated, the passive/uninvolved student might not develop the conceptual links necessary for effective, long-lasting learning.

By contrast, the clinical practicum involved the student more effectively as an active participant in the learning process as experience was gained in discipline-specific care. Unfortunately, because of the random nature of clinical experiences, it was impossible for educators to construct the comprehensive array of experiences that allowed a student to gain knowledge across the broad spectrum of required activities.

Achieving a successful balance between academic and clinical education has been a challenge for educators as healthcare institutions demand graduates with both broad-based knowledge and improved specialty clinical skills (Manuel & Sorensen, 1995). The result is often competition between classroom learning and clinical experiences with one educational component occurring at the expense of the other (see **Figure 15-1**).

Instead of concentrating on the struggle between classroom and clinical teaching, deconstructing classroom instruction as a *passive-controlled* learning environment and clinical instruction as an *active-random* environment reveals two distinct pedagogical dimensions: learner involvement and content control. New educational classifications become available as these dimensions are maximized. **Figure 15-2** illustrates options within each dimension. Tradi-

Figure 15-1 Traditional concept of nursing education. In the traditional educational model, classroom and clinical education are often in competition for limited student time.

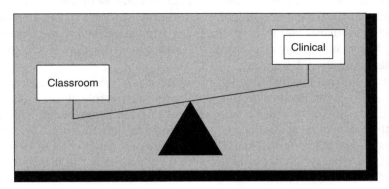

tional lecture and clinical formats are represented as quadrant I and IV activities. In this representation, two additional educational environments become manifest: passive-random and active-controlled. Of particular relevance to this chapter is the active-controlled quadrant, which allows the instructor to control the material to be disseminated, yet encourages active participation by the learner. Educational formats that can be classified within this quadrant include both problem-based learning and high-fidelity simulation. Both of these methods emphasize the central tenet of situated cognition, specifically that information is most useful when it is learned in contextual schema (Brown, Collins, & Duguid, 1989).

Figure 15-2 Two-dimensional concept of nursing education. This representation allows educational activities to be classified according to learner involvement, as well as the instructor's control over content, and it illustrates how simulation can be used to control content while using active learning methods.

	LEARNER	
	PASSIVE	ACTIVE
CONTROLLED	Lecture	Simulation
RANDOM	Journal skimming	Clinical instruction

Critics of situated cognition often focus on the role of the instructor. Tripp (1996) noted that the teacher often was used as a coach rather than master teacher. He argued that the teacher must act as a master of the domain and expose students to the expert abilities of master practitioners rather than assume the role of motivator or critic. Additionally, Tripp suggested that some content is taught more effectively in a controlled classroom setting than in what he characterizes as on-the-job training.

Instruction through high-fidelity simulation can be designed to address these criticisms. The simulated environment can promote the role of teacher as active participant and role model. Because clinical situations may be repeated as desired, the teacher can act initially as a role model by demonstrating a procedure or decision-making process, then allow the student to practice in an identical or similar situation. By contrast, in the actual clinical area, the faculty member who actively models a procedure, such as insertion of an intravenous catheter, often provides the demonstration at the expense of the student, who will not be able to repeat the process. The timing of simulated experiences can be designed so that these *clinical* experiences are introduced to reinforce what has recently been learned in the classroom, with the level of difficulty adjusted to match student capabilities. The ability to create an active learning environment that has been customized for each student is a compelling argument for the addition of high-fidelity simulation to the instructional armamentarium of nurse educators.

TYPES OF LEARNERS

The Russian psychologist Vygotsky (1978) believed that learning was most effective when it occurred within what he termed the "zone of proximal development," where what was to be learned was just beyond the current knowledge level of the student. Each simulation session can be adjusted to the optimal level of difficulty for a particular student or group: from beginner through expert and technical, undergraduate, and graduate by altering the delivery setting, patient history, clinical conditions, and patient sensitivity to therapeutic interventions. For example, beginning emergency and critical care students who are learning to recognize the signs of acute myocardial infarction may be asked to provide care for a patient with a robust cardiovascular system where signs of myocardial ischemia develop gradually without precipitating a cardiac arrest, whereas a more advanced student would be expected to recognize subtle physiologic clues quickly and initiate prompt, effective interventions. Nurse anesthesia, acute care nurse practitioner, respiratory care, or emergency care students who are learning basic principles of airway management can use the simulator as a part-task trainer to refine fundamental skills such as insertion of pharyngeal airways and bag-valve-mask ventilation. As the student's knowledge level increases, he or she may be expected to maintain ventilation in an apneic patient using oxygen saturation and respiratory gas measurements to guide ventilation. Advanced students may be expected to perform sophisticated airway procedures to include tracheal intubation and needle cricothyroidotomy in simulated patients with abnormal airway anatomy.

CONDITIONS FOR LEARNING

Because of the ability to create customized learning scenarios, high-fidelity simulators can be used in a wide variety of situations for all types of students. Simulation can precede, complement, or replace actual clinical experiences.

Prior to clinical experiences, simulation can be used to orient students to an unfamiliar unit. Chatto and Dennis (1997) used high-fidelity simulation to desensitize physical therapy students prior to their first critical care rotation. The simulation laboratory was configured to resemble a surgical intensive care unit. Students were introduced to the types of monitoring equipment, life-support devices, dressings, tubes, and drains that might be encountered during an actual clinical rotation. As students performed physical therapy on the simulator, common events were simulated to include sudden vital sign changes, gradually increasing intracranial pressure, cardiac alarms, and ventilator disconnection. Together with physical therapy and nursing faculty, students implemented safe and effective therapy, identified problems unique to the critical care environment, and practiced collaborative patient care.

In contrast to a one-time orientation session, simulation can also be used to allow students to practice technical skills and decision making before actual clinical experiences. For example, students in an anesthesia nursing program may accrue up to 100 hours of simulation practicing sequences of technical skills and decision making prior to their first clinical experience as a nurse anesthetist (Lupien, 1998; Monti, Wren, Haas, & Lupien, 1998). Students who have practiced using simulation prior to real clinical situations may be received more positively by clinical preceptors and the students receive more efficient and constructive clinical education.

Used concomitantly with clinical practice, simulation provides students and faculty the opportunity to replicate real clinical experiences and then use the simulator for reflection to explore different strategies for managing the situation. Students also have the opportunity to create customized patients based on their knowledge of physiology and pathophysiology and then compare the responses of their simulated patients to actual patients observed in clinical practice (e.g., Register, Graham-Garcia, & Haas, 2003).

Although the fidelity of patient simulators is not developed sufficiently to suggest that training with simulators can replace contact with human patients, simulation can be used to create learning opportunities that are unavailable in the real clinical environment. Students can practice high-risk technical procedures, such as defibrillation, in real time using actual equipment. Beyond technical skills, students can gain experience in critical clinical situations (e.g., cardiac life support or anaphylactic reaction) that might not occur during scheduled clinical times for all students.

Simulation has also been used to develop higher order skills in a fashion that exactly parallels applications of simulation in commercial aviation. Aviation simulation has expanded beyond its use as a teaching/training tool for individual pilots to encompass team training through a program called Crew Resource Management (Helmreich & Foushee, 1993). Similarly, in the field of anesthesiology, programs such as Anesthesia Crisis Resource Management (ACRM) (developed in the United States by Gaba and colleagues) and Team Oriented Medical Simulation (developed in Switzerland by Schaefer and Helmreich) focus on the actions of all members of a healthcare team with the goal of improving team performance (Baker, Gustafson, Beaubien, Salas, & Barach, 2005). Fletcher (1998) extended the concept of ACRM by developing ERR WATCH, a program focused specifically on the role of nurse anesthetists in crisis management.

In addition to its uses as an instructional tool, simulation potentially can be used for both formative and summative evaluation. Techniques for formative evaluation of student skills and abilities include using simulation as a mechanism for providing feedback on current skills and decision-making processes or to observe the progression of a student's abilities. Applications of simulation in summative evaluation are more controversial because the relationship between the performance of students in a simulated environment and actual clinical performance has yet to be demonstrated. Elements of the evaluation puzzle are currently being resolved. Descriptions of the psychometric properties of the actual instruments are limited. Devitt et al. (1998) reported estimates of internal consistency (α) as high as 0.66 with their instrument for evaluation of anesthesiologist performance. Monti, Wren, Haas, and Lupien (1998) described the use of a rudimentary weighted scored checklist to evaluate the performance of beginning students in a limited clinical scenario with moderately high reliability ($r = 0.83$). Devitt et al. (1997) and Gaba et al. (1998) reported excellent indices of inter-rater reliability for instruments to evaluate performance in simulated environments. While these reports describe initial forays into the evaluative use of simulation, there remain considerable limitations. Most notably, the implications of inadequate performance during simulation remain unclear because simulators provide an incomplete representation of a patient to the trainee. The simulation environment may also interfere with accurate assessment of performance. Scenarios based on substandard care may be perceived as improbable, and participants may be overly vigilant or anxious in the simulated environment (Hotchkiss, Biddle, & Fallacaro, 2002).

RESOURCES

Perhaps the most critical aspect of a successful simulation program is the designation of dedicated physical space for the simulator and its support equipment. To accommodate the simulator, instructor, and four to six students requires approximately 250 square feet of floor space. A sample floor plan for a simple simulation room is presented in **Figure 15-3**.

Simulators require both electricity and gas sources. Depending on the type of simulator chosen, there may be requirements for a complete range of respiratory gases including air, oxygen, carbon dioxide, and nitrogen. Nitrous oxide is optional for the simulation of general anesthesia. Electricity requirements include two to four outlets for the simulator plus additional sources of power for patient care equipment.

Patient care equipment depends on the types of simulations involved and may include physiological monitors, infusion pumps, ventilators, anesthesia machines, and a defibrillator. Support equipment includes airway devices, needles and syringes, dressings, chest tubes, urinary catheters, scrub wear, gloves, surgical masks, caps, and gowns.

The efficacy of simulation can be enhanced through the video recording of sessions with subsequent debriefing. Recording systems range from a single video camera to complex recording systems that allow multiple camera views, superimposed physiological waveforms and audio recordings from participants and faculty. Dedicated simulation centers include a debriefing room where the videotapes can be reviewed by students and faculty. The debriefing room may also have the ability to receive live video and audio transmissions from the training room for observation by, or simultaneous instruction of, other students.

Some simulation centers also include a control room adjacent to the training room. One-way glass between the rooms allow individuals in the control room to observe simulation sessions as the operator and faculty communicate via headsets with microphones. A technician or faculty member in the control room is responsible for monitoring the simulator, making adjustments as necessary, and selecting video and audio sources for recording.

Because simulation is so resource intensive, adequate personnel support is essential. Depending on the type of simulators and simulation, key faculty with moderate computer skills may be sufficient to support simulation activities on an as needed basis, although many centers have found it beneficial to designate

Figure 15-3 Sample of floor plan for human simulation laboratory. Representation of human simulation laboratory illustrating location of patient simulator, monitors, and recording devices. Video outputs from the physiological monitor can be recorded with traditional video signals to facilitate scenario review.

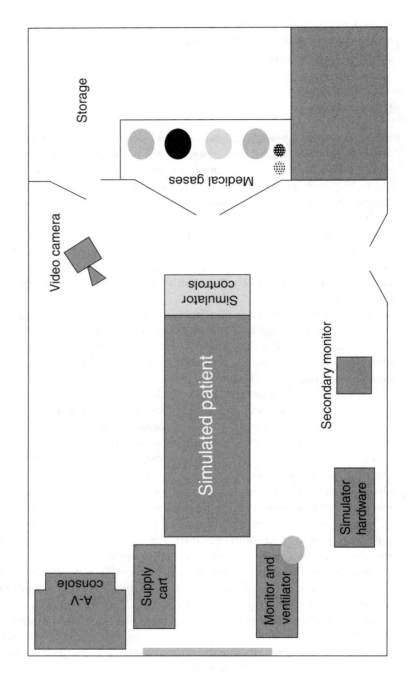

one faculty member or an associate, to coordinate simulation activities and maintain the simulator.

USING THE METHOD

Successful simulation sessions depend on carefully planned scenarios and clearly defined roles for faculty. The primary instructor is responsible for setting the scenario, guiding students through the simulation, providing important information and clinical cues not available through simulator, providing transition cues to the simulator operator, modeling behaviors, monitoring or correcting student performance, and correcting simulator errors. In some situations, the faculty may be assisted by another faculty member or technician serving as the simulator operator. The operator's responsibilities include activating the simulation system, starting patient software, overlaying clinical scenarios, monitoring the progress of a scenario, and adjusting the scenario as dictated by the primary instructor. Depending on the expertise of the faculty, complexity of the scenario, and type of simulator being used, one individual may serve as both the faculty member and operator. Complex scenarios may require not only an instructor and operator, but also other faculty, students, and/or assistants to role-play as members of the healthcare team and family.

To develop and implement a new simulation scenario, the seven-step process listed in **Table 15-2** is recommended.

1. **Determine educational objectives/goals.** Among the considerations for faculty is whether the simulation is intended to promote advancement of technical, cognitive, or behavioral abilities. The instructor should also determine in advance whether the simulation be constrained to unfold in a predetermined sequence or develop spontaneously. The faculty should

---

Table 15-2   Seven-Step Process For the Development of Simulation Session

1. Define educational objectives
2. Construct the clinical scenario
3. Define underlying physiological concepts
4. Modify programmed patients and scenarios, as necessary
5. Assemble required equipment
6. Run program and collect feedback
7. Reiterate steps 2–6 until satisfied

also decide in advance whether the goal of the exercise is to encourage students to focus their thinking or explore and test new ideas.

2. **Construct a clinical scenario to facilitate attainment of the educational objectives.** The scenario should be clinically realistic, customized for the students' current level of expertise, include requirements for decision making by the student, and designed to promote successful progress toward a higher level of functioning (Glavin & Maran, 2003; Zull, 2002).

3. **Define underlying physiological concepts to be manifest throughout the scenario—patient and events.** The primary instructor determines which essential elements of the clinical scenario are represented in the simulation, which are absent and can be overlooked, and which missing elements need to be integrated. For example, as a patient develops a progressive hypoxemia, the development of tachypnea and decreasing hemoglobin saturation, as measured by pulse oximetry, are expected. A real patient will eventually develop cyanosis, but whether the change in skin color is essential for the simulation depends on the educational objectives. When considering the accuracy of clinical situations, it is also essential to decide whether changes need to be technically accurate or sufficiently realistic and prominent to elicit the intended response from the learners.

4. **Modify programmed patients and scenarios, as necessary.** Program modification generally includes specifying the baseline physiology and clinical condition of the underlying patient, preparing the scenario to include optional modifiable states, and defining transitions between states.

5. **Identify required equipment.** The instructor decides whether devices will be displayed prominently or stored (as they might be in a clinical environment), whether learners will have the opportunity to inspect, assemble, and test equipment prior to the exercise; and if the student will have options among multiple devices for use in the simulation. The instructor also determines whether additional personnel will be required to implement the clinical scenario, the qualifications (both actual and role played) of the additional participants, and how primary learners will be able to access/involve the supplemental personnel resources.

6. **Run program and collect feedback.** Prior to use with students, the scenario is run to establish that the simulation unfolds as designed, with the intended levels of instructor and student participation.

7. **Reiterate steps until satisfied.** The simulation scenario is continuously refined until it unfolds as intended, without unintentionally ambiguous details that distract from attaining the educational objectives, and the faculty is able to concentrate on observing and evaluating the student's performance while maintaining a positive effective learning environment.

Once the simulation starts, the instructor has many options in terms of his/her involvement, including whether to serve as role model who demonstrates critical thinking, decision making and therapeutic interventions; a coach who is available to help students when necessary; or a passive bystander observing the scenario with minimal involvement. Regardless of level of participation during the simulation, one of the instructor's key functions is to actively *debrief* the session with students, describing and interpreting the scenario, clarifying learner thoughts and actions, critiquing performance, and generating possible alternative decisions and actions. Depending on the educational goals, the simulation may be repeated to increase the level of student involvement, explore alternative courses or actions, or improve student performance.

POTENTIAL PROBLEMS

Perhaps the most significant potential problem with simulation is its dependency on faculty support. The majority of commercially available simulation scenarios were developed for medical education. Although many of these scenarios are directly applicable beyond physician education, there is also a need for development of uniquely focused scenarios. Scenario writing does not require specialized computer programming skills, but the process of creating and refining scenarios to illustrate specific learning objectives is time intensive. The intimate nature of instruction through simulation also necessitates small group format for instruction, which also extends faculty time.

A second limitation to simulation is its incomplete presentation of reality. Although quite lifelike in representing human beings, simulators do not exhibit a complete range of signs and behaviors. Participants in a simulation session are expected to suspend disbelief and respond to the patient based on what they see. The instructor must provide any missing cues that are necessary for appropriate use of the scenario. Although it is surprisingly easy to engage in a simulation, instructors need to be aware of critical cues that are absent or contradictory with the intended signs.

Another potential problem with simulation is controlling the overgeneralization of findings to the real world. At least two types of generalization errors can occur. The first type is the generalization of an observed response in one situation to all patients. For example, whenever the baseline healthy 70 kg patient receives an intravenous bolus of 20 μg (microgram) epinephrine, the heart rate is raised approximately 20 beats per minute. Caution must be exerted to avoid the generalization that to increase a patient's heart rate by 20 beats, a dose of 20 μg epinephrine can be administered. To overcome this limitation, faculty can create a series of similar-appearing patients with slightly different physiologic parameters such as body weight, oxygen consumption, or baroreceptor responses. By using these similar patients interchangeably, students see variations in drug responses.

The second error of generalization is an incorrect attribution of simulator responses. As an incomplete representation of a human patient, simulators do not present a completely accurate or comprehensive clinical portrait. For example, the simulator patient, when breathing spontaneously, cannot create high negative pressures like a human is capable of generating. Therefore, using the simulator to practice measuring inspiratory effort would lead to inaccurate results. Faculty who understand how the simulator functions will quickly recognize which clinical findings are authentic and which are artifact. Simulation sessions can then be designed to take advantage of areas where the simulator is a reasonable portrayal of a real human and avoid involving students in activities that are different than would be expected under actual clinical conditions.

Finally, participants are often hypervigilant during simulation sessions because they anticipate the onset of a clinical problem. Although hypervigilance cannot be avoided completely, its effect can be minimized by either mixing routine and critical event simulations or developing a series of potential events which evolve from a common scenario stem.

CONCLUSION

Simulation is an exciting application of advanced technology in healthcare professions education. Used correctly, whole-body, high-fidelity patient simulators can effectively bridge the gap between static classroom-based instruction and the dynamic, unpredictable clinical environment. Although the use of simulation in healthcare education was, at one time, limited to anesthesia, critical care, and emergency care; ongoing refinements in simulators, such as the introduction of pediatric models and open architecture for the development of new simulation applications, have gradually allowed the introduction of high-fidelity simulation in settings not imagined even 10 years ago.

APPLIED EXAMPLE

Using High-Fidelity Simulation in an Undergraduate Critical Care Nursing Course

This example[1] illustrates how simulation was used to reinforce concepts of respiratory assessment and nursing care as part of a critical care nursing elective for senior-level undergraduate nursing students. The course included 40 didactic hours and was designed to complement a 200-hour clinical practicum. The course focused on pulmonary, cardiovascular, and neurological critical care; advanced hemodynamic monitoring; and critical care pharmacology. The respiratory care section of the course included lectures on respiratory gas exchange, advanced assessment techniques, arterial blood gas analysis, airway management, and ventilatory support. To complement the lectures, the seven-step process listed in Table 15-2 was used to develop a simulation session.

1. **Determine educational objectives.** The simulation session was designed so that the student would be able to achieve the following objectives:
   - Complete and continuously revise the assessment of a patient who is acutely and dynamically ill.
   - Select appropriate oxygen therapy devices for a specified clinical situation.
   - Collect and prepare the appropriate equipment and medications for emergent tracheal intubation.
   - Administer appropriate medications to facilitate emergent tracheal intubation and assess the drug effects.
   - Perform airway management procedures, as indicated, to include bag-valve-mask ventilation, tracheal intubation, and endotracheal suctioning.
   - Confirm appropriate placement of an endotracheal tube.
   - Prepare an unstable patient for transport from an inpatient unit to a critical care unit.
   - Initiate positive pressure ventilatory support for an acutely ill patient and adjust ventilatory parameters (to include mode, FiO_2, tidal volume, respiratory rate, and positive-end expiratory pressure) as indicated by patient condition, arterial blood gases, capnography, and spirometry.

Although the scenario involved only nursing students, it can be easily expanded to include respiratory and emergency care providers. The instructor was actively involved in session as a coach to students, providing interactive feedback and helping students clarify clinical observations.

2. **Construct a clinical scenario.** Students were told that they were going to evaluate a patient with pneumonia hospitalized on an inpatient medical unit. A brief patient history was provided.

   Students were given the opportunity to assess the patient, including observation of respiratory effort, lung auscultation, estimation of arterial oxygenation

[1]Scenario developed by Beverly George-Gay, MSN, CCRN; Assistant Professor and Coordinator of Distance and Continuing Education; Department of Nurse Anesthesia, Virginia Commonwealth University; Richmond, VA.

by pulse oximetry, and measurement and analysis of arterial blood gases. At the time of initial contact, the patient demonstrated signs of moderate hypoxia to include rapid shallow breathing, mild oxyhemoglobin desaturation, and rales on chest auscultation. Upon a signal from the instructor to the simulator operator, the patient experienced a significant oxyhemoglobin desaturation.

The scenario was designed so that the patient initially would require oxygen therapy, then require more aggressive treatment including tracheal intubation, positive pressure ventilation using a bag-valve device with both face mask and tracheal tube. Once transferred to the critical care unit, ventilatory support using various modes such as assist control, intermittent mandatory ventilation, positive-end expiratory pressure, and pressure support ventilation could be explored.

3. **Define underlying physiological concepts to be manifest through scenario: patient and events.** The physiological concepts underlying pneumonia include decreased lung compliance and increased shunt. Manifestations of these alterations include an adaptive respiratory pattern with increased rate and smaller tidal volume, increased peak inspiratory pressure, hypoxemia, mild hypercarbia, rales, tachycardia, and cardiac dysrhythmias. Patient deterioration within the scenario results from progressive reductions in lung compliance and increases in shunt. For this exercise, it was determined that sufficient physiological changes to induce learner critical thinking, decision making, and action were more important than technical accuracy.

4. **Modify programmed patients and scenarios, as necessary.** A geriatric model developed by faculty and master's level nursing anesthesia students was used.[2] To exhibit signs of pneumonia, rales were introduced, lung compliance was decreased, shunt fraction was increased, and the CO_2 set point was increased slightly (to produce mild hypercarbia). Temperature was increased slightly to reflect an underlying infective process. As a result of these changes, tidal volume decreased automatically and respiratory rate increased to compensate for the reduced tidal volume. Physiologic alterations were also manifest automatically through changes in heart rate and arterial blood gases.

So that the patient would initially appear to be stable and then deteriorate upon the instructor's command, baseline and decompensation states were created. Although an automatic transition could have initiated the decompensation at a predetermined time, a manual transition was selected to assure that the destabilization occurred when intended by the instructor.

5. **Assemble required equipment.** Because the patient is not physically transported from the medical unit to the critical care unit, the simulation lab was originally configured with equipment available to acute care personnel. Items included a resuscitation cart with cardiac monitor and defibrillator, oxygen source, oxygen therapy devices, various airway management devices such as bag-valve-mask device, pharyngeal airways, endotracheal tubes, laryngoscopes, and suction equipment. Once the scenario shifted to the critical care unit, a positive pressure ventilator was also available for student use.

[2]Development of the geriatric model was supported, in part, by a grant from the Division of Nursing, U.S. Department of Health and Human Services Bureau of Health Professions.

6. **Run program and collect feedback.** Prior to use with students, the scenario was run several times to observe the rate of change for physiological variables and the effects of various therapeutic options.
7. **Reiterate steps 2–6 until satisfied.** Physiological parameters were modified incrementally so that the patient would appear stable, but with sufficient respiratory compromise to entice the learner to initiate oxygen therapy. Once the deterioration sequence was initiated, the decompensation needed to be sufficient to warrant more aggressive therapy yet progress at a rate such that novice nurses with limited skills and therapeutic options could stabilize the patient.

To implement the simulation, the instructor selects the customized geriatric patient from the Patient Options menu of the user interface and respiratory exercise from the Scenario Options menu. The simulator immediately begins emulating the pneumonia patient in the stable baseline state. Progression to the decompensation state requires only one additional keystroke or mouse click.

Careful pilot testing of the simulated patient and clinical scenario reduces the likelihood of unanticipated events during the educational session; however, the instructor should be prepared to help students with assembling and using unfamiliar equipment as well in performing advanced technical skills, such as effective bag-valve-mask ventilation and tracheal intubation. Careful coordination with the simulator operator will allow the patient to deteriorate at a rate appropriate for the experience of the learners with pauses in the deterioration, if desired, during specific teaching moments or as technical maneuvers are performed.

For this exercise, evaluation of learner achievement was formative and informal. After the simulated patient's condition was stabilized, the faculty and students reflected on clinical signs observed and how the patient's condition, clinical setting, and events affected decision making and actions; medications, devices, and procedures used to stabilize the patient; and potential alternative solutions that would have led to more rapid or improved outcomes.

REFERENCES

Baker, D. P., Gustafson, S., Beaubien, J. M., Salas, E., & Barach, P. (2005). Medical team training programs in health care. In Agency for Healthcare Research and Quality, Advances in patient safety: From research to implementation (Vol. 4, pp. 253–267). (AHRQ Publication No. 050021-4). Rockville, MD: Author. Retrieved August 8, 2006, from http://www.ahrq.gov/downloads/pub/advances/vol4/Baker.doc

Brown, J. S., Collins, A., & Duguid, P. (1989). Situated cognition in the culture of learning. *Educational Researcher, 18*, 32–42.

Chatto, C., & Dennis, J. K. (1997). Intensive care unit training for physical therapy students: Use of an innovative patient simulator. *Acute Care Perspectives, 5*(4), 7–12.

Devitt, J. H., Kurrek, M. M., Cohen, M. M., Fish, K., Fish, P., Murphy, P. M., et al. (1997). Testing the raters: inter-rater reliability during observation of simulator performance. *Canadian Journal of Anaesthesia, 44*, 925–928.

Devitt, J. H., Kurrek, M. M., Cohen, M. M., Fish, K., Fish, P., Noel, A. G., et al. (1998). Testing internal consistency and construct validity during evaluation of performance in a patient simulator. *Anesthesia and Analgesia, 86*, 1160–1164.

Fletcher, J. L. (1995). Anesthesia simulation: A tool for learning and research. *AANA Journal, 63,* 61–67.

Fletcher, J. L. (1998). ERR watch: Anesthesia crisis resource management from the nurse anesthetist's perspective. *AANA Journal, 66,* 595–602.

Gaba, D. M. (1997). Simulators in anesthesiology. In C. L. Lake, L. J. Rice, & R. J. Sperry (Eds.), *Advances in anesthesia* (Vol. 14, pp. 55–94). St. Louis: Mosby.

Gaba, D. M., & De Anda, A. (1988). A comprehensive anesthesia simulation environment: Recreating the operating room for research and training. *Anesthesiology, 69,* 387–394.

Gaba, D. M., Howard, S. K., Flanagan, B., Smith, B. E., Fish, K. J., & Botney, R. (1998). Assessment of clinical performance during simulated crises using both technical and behavioral ratings. *Anesthesiology, 89,* 8–18.

Glavin, R., & Maran, N. (2003). An introduction to simulation in anaesthesia. In D. Greaves, C. Dodds, C. M. Kumar, & B. Mets (Eds.), *Clinical teaching: A guide to teaching practical anaesthesia* (pp. 197–205). Lisse, Netherlands: Swets & Zeitlinger.

Helmreich, R. L., & Foushee, H. C. (1993). Why crew resource management? Empirical and theoretical bases of human factors training in aviation. In E. L. Weiner, B. G. Kanki, & R. L. Helmreich (Eds.), *Cockpit resource management* (pp. 3–46). London: Academic Press.

Hotchkiss, M. A., Biddle, C., & Fallacaro, M. (2002). Assessing the authenticity of the human simulation experience in anesthesiology. *AANA Journal, 70,* 470–473.

Howard, S. K., Gaba, D. M., Fish, K. J., Yang, G., & Sarnquist, F. H. (1992). Anesthesia crisis resource management: Teaching anesthesiologists to handle critical incidents. *Aviation, Space, and Environmental Medicine, 63,* 763–770.

Lupien, A. E. (1998). Simulation in nursing anesthesia education. In L. C. Henson & A. C. Lee (Eds.), *Simulators in anesthesiology education* (pp. 29–37). New York: Plenum.

Manuel, P., & Sorensen, L. (1995). Changing trends in healthcare: Implications for baccalaureate education, practice, and employment. *Journal of Nursing Education, 34,* 248–253.

Monti, E. J., Wren, K., Haas, R., & Lupien, A. E. (1998). The use of an anesthesia simulator in graduate and undergraduate education. *CRNA: The Clinical Forum for Nurse Anesthetists, 9,* 59–66.

Papa, F. J., & Harasym, P. H. (1999). Medical curriculum reform in North America, 1765 to the present: A cognitive science perspective. *Academic Medicine, 74,* 154–164.

Register, M., Graham-Garcia, J., & Haas, R. (2003). The use of simulation to demonstrate hemodynamic response to varying degrees of intrapulmonary shunt. *AANA Journal, 71,* 277–284.

Rosen, K. R. (2004). The history of medical simulation. In G. E. Loyd, C. L. Lake, & R. B. Greenberg (Eds.), *Practical health care simulations* (pp. 3–26). Philadelphia: Elsevier Mosby.

Tripp, S. D. (1996). Theories, traditions, and situated learning. In H. McLellan (Ed.), *Situated learning perspectives* (pp. 155–165). Englewood Cliffs, NJ: Educational Technology Publications.

Vygotsky, L. S. (1978). *Mind in society: The development of higher psychological processes.* Cambridge, MA: Harvard University Press.

Zull, J. E. (2002). *The art of changing the brain.* Sterling, VA: Stylus.

RECOMMENDED READING

Dunn, W. F. (Ed.). (2004). *Simulators in critical care and beyond.* Chicago: Society of Critical Care Medicine.

Guest, C. B., Regehr, G., & Tiberius, R. G. (2001). The life long challenge of expertise. *Medical Education, 35,* 78–81.

Jeffries, P. R. (2005). A framework for designing, implementing, and evaluating simulations used as teaching strategies in nursing. *Nursing Education Perspectives, 26,* 96–103.

Loyd, G. E., Lake, C. L., & Greenberg, R. B. (Eds.). (2004). *Practical health care simulations.* Philadelphia: Elsevier Mosby.

SECTION IV

TECHNOLOGY AND DISTANCE EDUCATION

Educational technology continues to grow by leaps and bounds and has changed the complexion of the world of education. The technology can be as simple as communicating by e-mail, or as complex as presenting full degree-granting programs by distance learning. Libraries have become accessible to distance learners by use of technology, and full text articles are now available online. The Internet has opened a new and extensive world of information that was not previously available. Teaching in a technological world requires faculty collaboration with information specialists to learn how to use the ever-changing systems, but also to keep abreast of new resources as they become available and provide technological support for students.

The discussion in these chapters provides a look at different ways of utilizing available technologies and discusses strengths of the system and problems that can occur. Technology may be used to assist learning, but it does not replace the instructor. Learning objectives must be the main focus for the decision to use technology. Teaching methods require adaptation to be effective in this new environment and should be evaluated for that effectiveness. The amount of Internet information may be overwhelming, and it is critical that faculty and students learn to cull the material to a reasonable amount, and validate accuracy. The use of educational technologies may require extra time and effort from faculty, but can be very effective in enhancing learning and rewarding for students and faculty alike.

CHAPTER 16

The Use of Video in Health Profession Education

Clive Grainger and Alex Griswold

INTRODUCTION

Video is the strongest medium we can use to reveal interpersonal relationships. Through the use of words alone, it is nearly impossible to fully communicate what may be revealed in a person's eyes, face, and gestures. Video production can be a collaborative or solo venture, but in either case it should be fun.

In this chapter we aim to provide the reader with ideas as to how video might be used in the education of the health professional. Our aim is to offer advice to both faculty and students in order that they acquire greater confidence through the utilization of simple techniques to improve their technical knowledge. We will review some of the uses of video production in education, as well as the process of production in layman's terms. We will highlight some simple tips, learned from many years of video production in the classroom and in the broader field of education. When we use the term *video*, which is technically the visual part of a recording, we are using it in colloquial form meaning sound and picture together.

In addition to improving technical knowledge, we aim to increase the effectiveness of communicating a message without the need to involve technologist specialists in the process. This is not an exhaustive how-to, and our aim is not to swamp the reader with technical language. There are many excellent reference books and web sites to consult about the process of video production, and we suggest you refer to some of these for more in-depth study.

USES FOR VIDEO IN EFFECTIVE TEACHING

As a tool for learning, video is useful for documenting events for later study and/or for communicating with large numbers of people. For example, a lecture can be recorded and made available on the web to people who could not attend in person. Video allows events to be studied in multiple dimensions: a recording of a patient-caregiver interview can be used as a record of the interview. It can also be used for diagnosis or treatment, or in an educational setting.

There are a number of uses that may be considered for the use of videotape in the classroom by both educator and student. **Table 16-1** is by no means an exhaustive list—you may come up with ideas of your own.

Table 16-1   Video Usage

- **Creating clinical records.**
  A video camera can make more useful and comprehensive records of patient progress than a written chart or even a still photograph.

- **Documenting presentations/training sessions.**
  These can be reviewed later in the classroom so that instructors can fill in gaps or offer interpretations. Time can also be shortened—points can be illustrated by fast-forwarding or with judicious editing.

- **Recording interactions between students and patients.**
  Instructors may use the videotape as examples of what went well and what might be improved. Students can use these tapes for study outside the classroom.

- **Communicating case studies for individual or group study.**
  Video case studies enhance traditional print case studies by revealing body language and other subtle clues. As a teaching tool, video can serve to provoke thought and encourage students to express their opinions.

- **Recording clinical or informal interviews.**
  Interviews may be logged and transcribed for later study. Some patients may find it easier to reveal thoughts and feelings to a camera, with no operator, than to talk to a medical professional behind that camera.

- **Revealing patient understanding and misconceptions.**
  Many clinicians are aware of the most commonly held misconceptions about various ailments. Both hearing and seeing patients present their incorrect ideas is far more effective than reading about them. New misconceptions might also be revealed.

- **Comparing and contrasting examples of both good and bad professional interaction.**
  Videotaped interviews may be especially helpful in conveying the interaction between health professional and patient. A little humor might be used to illustrate the wrong way!

Table 16-1   Video Usage (*continued*)

• **Demonstrating clinical procedures.** Those procedures that are not easily demonstrated to groups of students can more effectively be demonstrated in a video. Use of video to present material to a larger group can be very effective—saving the instructor from becoming a sage on the stage.
• **Communicating specific medical information.** Video is an excellent tool for those who may be elderly, face mobility challenges, or are unable to read. It is possible to use alternative audio tracks or subtitles for ESL patients. Such material may also be used for review by the caregivers of such patients.
• **Continuing education.** In-service training is an important part of every medical professional's career. The presentation of development materials via video can be the most convenient way for the busy professional to choose where and when they might study.
• **Evaluating student progress.** Students may be encouraged to produce their own video projects. These may be used to measure how well a sequence of concepts has been understood. Presentation for classroom peer review may also be simplified.

NEW TECHNOLOGY / ACCESS

Videotape has become an almost ubiquitous medium. The use of video materials is integrated into most health professional education college courses. It can be particularly effective when used for distance learning. During the past few years, there has been a revolution in access to affordable video equipment. Many families now own and use relatively sophisticated video cameras. To many students, this technology is not as unfamiliar or expensive as it once was.

One can readily access modestly priced camera equipment along with relatively sophisticated editing software, often bundled with computers. Examples of bundled editing and recording software are Apple's iMovie and iDVD. The reader will find similar Windows-based editing programs such as Windows Movie Maker. Cheap hardware and software have also enabled the creation of CDs and DVDs for the dissemination of materials.

New uses for video are being developed for the web, on cell phones, and even on the ever popular iPod. We are witnessing a merging of technologies such as embedded video into PowerPoint presentations and the use of streaming video where a little goes a long way! Use of innovative multimedia continually increases the effectiveness of educational communication.

With effective use of new technologies come challenges for both the educator and student. Learning to effectively use yet another technology effectively may be daunting. It is possible to lessen any anxiety by researching and leveraging resources that may be available locally, consulting with your technology specialist and discussing concerns with fellow faculty. Many of your colleagues may have or have had similar concerns to your own. It may be possible to sponsor professional development sessions related to the use of emerging technologies.

The term *videotape* may soon be as obsolete as *record*—how many of today's students would know what a 45 rpm record looked like (let alone a 78 rpm record)? Technological development is always in a rapid state of flux, but we are heading into an exciting future with completely unpredictable possibilities.

WHY USE VIDEO? ADVANTAGES AND DISADVANTAGES

The old adage that a picture is worth a thousand words may be true, but the moving image can be worth even more! Try to describe each shot of a short film or even a television advertisement and see how many words it takes.

Video production at the highest levels may appear to be challenging, but many of the techniques used by professionals are within the grasp of those with even the simplest of tools. Classroom viewing of the moving image allows the audience to witness inaccessible events with a sense of immediacy that other media cannot convey. Video may be coupled to other forms of interactive media to produce powerful learning tools.

If there is a choice, the first question you may want to ask is whether video is really the correct medium for the task. Watching video in its simplest form can be a very linear, passive experience—there is a beginning, a middle, and an end—is this the most effective way for you or your students to tell a story or to present material? We have already highlighted many of the ways that video might be used—we recommend that you see the various excellent and innovative examples that may be found on the web.

Perhaps you will want to consider breaking your material into smaller sections, or perhaps an audio-only radio treatment may be a more appropriate (and less time-consuming) choice. Sometimes just listening will help a participant fill in his own visuals, perhaps allowing for a more active or thoughtful participation. Video also has an authority, and many of us are visual learners. Creating a video can also be time consuming—do you really have enough time?

There are many advantages to using video for the right project. Some learners see a lot better than they write—use of a visual and audio medium can help these students overcome potential written communication problems. Sometimes an assignment must be videotaped for presentation.

Video professionals use many terms that may be unfamiliar to the new user but most can be easily deciphered. There are many excellent reference books and web sites that may be used in order to decipher such terms. An example of such a term new videographers may have heard is *streaming video*. Streaming video consists of a sequence of moving images sent in compressed form over the Internet. It is displayed on the viewer's computer as it arrives rather than as a large file that must be fully downloaded in order for it to be viewed (Annenberg Media, 2006).

THE PRODUCTION PROCESS

In order to produce videotaped material, the minimum equipment required includes:

- A camera with plenty of tape and batteries, and/or a wall adapter. There is nothing worse than your tape or batteries running out at an inopportune moment—we've all experienced it and yes, even the most seasoned of producers have, too (but only once).
- A tripod for taping interviews, or at least a pair of steady hands.
- A microphone that is separate from the camera.
- A friend. Though one certainly can tape single-handedly, not having to concentrate on every aspect of the shoot will relieve much stress. It is nice to have someone carry the equipment, write notes for use in editing later, and to listen to one's commiserating should anything just happen to go wrong!

ADAPTING TO THE NEEDS OF YOUR PRODUCTION

We previously listed the many uses for video in teaching and learning. We'll revisit some of those examples, and offer a few tips for each one. The most straightforward shooting is usually preferable. The background should not be distracting and, if necessary for close analysis, it's often useful to incorporate a measured grid or distance scale as part of the backdrop.

Presentations

When there is one speaker at a podium, it's usually quite easy to obtain a clear video image of his or her presentation. Use a tripod, if available. The audio may be more problematic. If there is a public address microphone, there may be a way to tap into the audio directly from the PA amplifier. If not, try to place a microphone on the podium . . . but test it ahead of time, and by all means, try to find out if the speaker wants to walk away from the podium. In that case, a wireless lapel microphone may be your best choice. PowerPoint presentations or other graphics should be either captured with a second dedicated camera or imported directly into the editing system as digital files.

Interviews

There are many types of interviews. One of the most common is the clinical interview, in which a researcher and interviewee sit opposite each other across a table. The camera should be set up at the side, not directly in the interview subject's line of sight. The height of the lens on the tripod is very important. The inexperienced videographer will often set the camera too high, so it looms down on the subject. This creates an impersonal feel to the interview—it's better to adjust the tripod so that the camera lens is level with the top of the interviewer's and interviewee's heads. Adjust the shot so that any objects of interest are included in the frame; if necessary, zoom in on the subject of interest and pan to adjust so that the object of interest is clearly visible. Audio can be captured with a microphone placed unobtrusively on the table, aimed at the interviewee, although if you need to hear the interviewer clearly you may need a second microphone for the interviewer.

Demonstrating Clinical Procedures

The key (perhaps obviously) is to make sure that the area of interest is clearly visible. The use of a tripod is optional; sometimes it is better to have the mobility of a handheld camera. This will help to avoid the area of interest being blocked by the person demonstrating the procedure.

In-service Training

Video used to illustrate a point or trigger a discussion can be very useful in training sessions. These don't have to be too elaborate; often they can be shot with available lighting and in real settings. This is where the reality camera approach could actually make a presentation more believable.

PLAN YOUR VIDEO OR "YOU'RE A PRODUCER NOW . . ."

Planning is a most important part of video production—it requires much preparatory work before any footage is shot. This may seem tedious, but will more than pay for itself in the long run. What goes right or wrong during production is often related to the time spent or not spent in purposeful planning. Careful planning will also help you to consider other issues that you may not have thought about.

SOME DIFFERENCES—PROFESSIONAL VS. AMATEUR VIDEO

Readers of all degrees of expertise are encouraged to read the following descriptions of a few key differences between video produced by the experienced and inexperienced camera operator.

Audio

Audio is critically important—the recording of quality audio is one of the most overlooked elements in successful video production. You may not realize this until you experience the difference between clear and noisily recorded speech recorded in an interview. Remember, the point is to hear what the interviewee is saying. Your pictures may be very pretty, but they are of little use if your audience cannot hear what is being discussed.

A built-in camera microphone is convenient, but unless you are very close to and pointing directly at your subject, it will record noise around the area as well as your subject. If you choose to be distant or a "fly on the wall," the problem is compounded. Use of an external microphone on an extension cable will allow you to record an interview clearly. Use of an external microphone with a little wise positioning will cover many situations. Look at TV reporters—they hold a microphone in their hand, moving it between interviewer and interviewee—you can try that technique if your interviewee is not seated.

Composition

Take a look at holiday snaps, or home video. Compare them to material taken by a professional. What differences do you observe? Quite often the framing of the experienced shooter will be more pleasing; heads are not in the middle of the frame, nor is there an excess of space above the subject. Also the camera will often be closer to the subject, creating a more intimate interview. Unless the action dictates that you do so, avoid shooting too wide.

Always be aware of what is happening in the background of your shot—it is very distracting to see plants growing out of people's heads. Avoid shooting into crowds of people; they can be distracting and have been known to steal the scene by waving at the camera.

The Wobbles

It is helpful to steady your camera when taping to avoid making viewers seasick. The use of a tripod will also help you to step out from behind the camera to deal with matters that you may not be able to attend to otherwise. Scenic shots are easier to record with the use of a tripod.

Lighting

In most clinical situations, it is impossible to set up additional lighting. Ambient lighting is all that can be used. Modern video equipment will record at very low light levels, but the images look best if illuminated at least to the level of a typical office. To avoid silhouetting your subject, do not show the light source (e.g., an exterior window) in the field of view, unless there are other light sources that illuminate the subject. Most video cameras have automatic exposure control. Many experienced users set the exposure on their camera to manual to avoid the overall changes in light levels as the camera pans around the scene.

Transcripts

Although typing an unabridged copy of any spoken word on your tape might seem tedious, there are a number of benefits. A transcript will save you time when you edit interviews; the process will force you to review all of your material making you aware of what was actually said. You may think you know what was recorded but it may be different from the reality; this is sometimes good and sometimes bad. It is possible that you only need or have time to present a taste of the full interview in the version shown to an audience. With a transcript, video makers can distribute a verbatim copy of all or part of an interview to an audience.

Editing

It isn't always necessary to edit taped material, but without selective editing, you may very quickly bore your audience.

Less is more! The pros pull out the most important, salient material for viewing and leave the rest on the cutting room floor. Your material should follow a logical progression. Don't only show the talking head(s), but put them into context—in what environment is your material being recorded? Is there any accompanying action? Try to reveal the relationship between people in the room. It is possible to help explain some of what is happening through the judicious use of voiceover, or graphics—there are no hard and fast rules; be creative.

Etiquette

The relationship between videographer and interviewee is often key to success. Being aware of being recorded can be very disconcerting for a subject—put subjects at ease first. Just as the microphone is the surrogate for the viewers' ears, the camera lens takes the place of their eyes. In effect, the camera is a stand-in for the audience—one that can be oppressive and overbearing, or if handled well, a kind friend or confidant.

Most television documentary recorders do not ask interview subjects to speak directly to the lens . . . this journalistic style allows the interview subjects to make eye contact with the interviewer and forget about the machine that is in the room. More experienced television personalities can be trained to peer naturally into a lens, ignoring the people around it. This is a skill that takes training and practice. Often the greatest challenge for many nonactors is speaking directly to the camera. Remembering lines while speaking into the lens can be especially frustrating. If you are creating this kind of segment, leave lots of extra time for retakes. Although sometimes having the presenter's script on poster boards can help, it's easier to use a teleprompter that projects the script on the front surface of a half-silvered mirror mounted directly in front of the camera. This kind of equipment may be available in your media departments. Another solution is to plan to have only a few sentences while the speaker is on camera, then read the rest from a script. In editing, the sections that are read from the script can be covered with other pictures.

It's best not to do covert taping unless you like trouble! If you are able to incorporate comedy into your video it can help to produce more effective, attention-grabbing materials—but only use a *little* bit of humor. A small amount of light relief goes a long way in the right place, *but* what is humorous to you may not be to someone else! For example, see John Cleese's *Videos for Business Training.*

GENTLE WARNINGS

Receipt of written consent should be sought from subjects recorded outside the classroom setting—providing your classmates don't mind being videotaped. Many medical professionals are used to obtaining informed written consent; various institutions have their own formalities for acquiring this consent. We would strongly urge you to consider obtaining written consent, most especially if your material may be viewed by a number of people, or potentially in a number of different settings. It is *very* important to receive (and file) *written*, informed consent from the parents or guardians of minors. When dealing with this legal paperwork, it can be daunting for the signer.

Words of caution also apply to copyright. Please be aware that the majority of music, video, and photographic material found on the web, in libraries, or on disk that seem to be free is copyrighted. This means that legal protection has been assigned to authors and photographers protecting them against unauthorized copying of their work. The good news is that you can find noncopyright, public domain media in many places, but it is your responsibility to confirm its public domain status.

Exhibit 16-1 is an example of a release form. You can use it as a guide in creating your own release form. The wording can be adapted for adults only. Please be aware that because this is a legal document, it should be approved by your institution before use.

CONCLUSION

We live in an environment ripe with moving images. Visual and oral media can be powerful tools for education. Video materials can be simple or complex and may be used on their own or in tandem with other technologies, and they may also be used to supplement more traditional materials.

It should be challenging to stretch your intellectual and technical abilities, but any serious amateur can make a video worth watching. The onus to understand or to interpret a piece of video should not be left to the viewer. Your work may make complete sense to you, but the audience does not necessarily know or care about how you made it. Stand back, put yourself in the shoes of someone viewing it cold, and try it out on your friends or colleagues. Is it really accomplishing what you intended it to?

We hope that the process of making a video will open up new avenues of creativity and imagination for you. Good luck!

EXHIBIT 16-1

Acknowledgment, Consent, and Assignment

I, _____, acknowledge (as the parent/guardian of my child, _____ [Insert child's name] _____) that [*insert institution's name*] is producing video.

I acknowledge that this video is being produced for the purpose of furthering the educational goals of [*insert your institution*]. Any profits from the sale or commercial use of this material will be applied to the educational work of [*insert your institution*].

I hereby grant and release to [*insert your institution*] the right to film, tape, and photograph my child and record his/her voice in connection with the materials and hereby assign all of his/her rights, title, and interest in the materials, and their footage, including his/her copyright interests therein, to [*insert your institution*].

I acknowledge that [*dept. of institution*] will be the sole owner throughout the world of the copyright and all other rights in this material, as well as in any photographic materials, written works, bibliographies, syllabi, or other materials based upon the programs (related works).

The [*dept. of institution*] and its respective licensees and others acting with their permission have my consent to use my child's name, likeness, picture, and appearance in the materials and associated projects. I also grant my consent to use the above, as well as any biographical materials I have provided or may in the future provide, to advertise and publicize the material and related works.

The rights and releases granted herein apply to all formats in which the material may be marketed or presented, including, but not limited to television, the web, cable casting, written works, and educational and home video use.

This acknowledgement, consent, and assignment has been signed as a contract under seal on this:

_____ day of _____, 200[?]

Name: _____
Signed: _____
Home address: _____
_____
_____
Home telephone number: _____
E-mail address: _____

EXAMPLE

Thomas Allardi—Physical Therapist, Massachusetts General Hospital, Boston

We frequently videotape our patients for a number of reasons. A common one is to complete a basic gait analysis. In order to accomplish this, a patient's step must be broken into its component elements. Video helps us to observe each component many times over.

Videotaping can help us work with children with cerebral palsy who are often diagnosed with muscular imbalance. In order to offer treatment, we carefully analyze interrelated movement between knees, hips, and toes. A recording allows us to efficiently evaluate this and to communicate to colleagues and our patient's parents the specific nature of the case.

Videotaping is an important tool used after an examination in order to consult with colleagues without need to use the physical therapist's unique language. As you can imagine, as with most medical specialties, when a puzzling case comes to our attention, it is far more effective for us to consult our colleagues with a review of video.

Parents are often reluctant to see their child wearing an assistive device, but we have been able to show before and after examples of recommended appliances that would be in the best interest of their child. Video evidence often reassures these parents.

A bonus of using video recording is that because most of our child patients do not stand still long enough to repeat their movement, we can use video for immediate review!

REFERENCE

Annenberg Media. (2006). [Online Simulcasts]. Retrieved July 8, 2006, from http://www.learner.org

RECOMMENDED READING / RESOURCES

Anderson, M. Brownell (Ed.). (2003). Really good stuff: Reports of new ideas in medical education. *Medical Education, 37,* 1025–1049.

Brigham and Women's Hospital. (2006). *Surgery webcasts.* Available at http://www.brighamand womens.org/surgerywebcast

Cleese, J. [Video series]. *Videos for business training.* Retrieved July 8, 2006, from http://www. rctm.com/Products/celebritiesgurus/johncleese.htm

Curran, V. R., & Fleet, L. (2005). A review of evaluation outcomes of web-based continuing medical education. *Medical Education, 39*(6), 561–567.

Curran, V. R., Kirby, F., Allen, M., & Sargeant, J. (2003). A mixed learning technology approach for continuing medical education. *Medical Education Online, 8*(5). Retrieved July 10, 2006, from http://www.med-ed-online.org/pdf/t0000036.pdf

Holloway, S., Lee, L., & McConkey, R. (1999). Meeting the training needs of community-based service personnel in Africa through video-based training courses. *Disability and Rehabilitation, 21*(9), 448–454.

Howe, M. J. A. (Ed.). (1983). *Learning from television: Psychological and educational research.* London: Academic Press, Inc. Ltd.

Lewis, M. L., & Kaas, M. J. (1998, August). Challenges of teaching graduate psychiatric-mental health nursing with distance education technologies. *Archives of Psychiatric Nursing, 12*(4), 227–233.

Makoul, G. (2001, April). Essential elements of communication in medical encounters: The Kalamazoo consensus statement. *Academic Medicine, 76*(4), 390–393.

McCombs, R. (2005). Shooting web video: How to put your readers at the scene. *USC Annenberg Online Journalism Review.* Retrieved July 8, 2006, from http://www.ojr.org/ojr/stories/050303mc combs/index.cfm

Rose, J. (2002). *Producing great sound for digital video* (2nd ed.). Gilroy, CA: CMP Books.

Schneps, M. H., & Sadler, P. (1985). *A private universe* [Teacher workshop guide and video series]. Cambridge, MA: Harvard-Smithsonian Center for Astrophysics, Department of Science Education.

Science Education Department, Harvard-Smithsonian Center for Astrophysics. (2006). *Factors influencing college success in science.* Available at http://www.ficss.org

Utz, P. (n.d.). How-to info and books for videographers: Learn video equipment, setup, operation, and production. Retrieved August 29, 2006, from http://videoexpert.home.att.net

Utz, P. (2005). *Today's Video* (4th ed.). Jefferson, NC: McFarland Publishing.

CHAPTER 17

Multimedia in the Classroom: Creating Learning Experiences with Technology

Karen H. Teeley

INTRODUCTION

Health professions educators have new roles to fill in an era of increasing technology. Multimedia has grown from simple A-V (audio-visual) to a never-ending, ever-growing list of technological opportunities. The challenge for the instructor is not just to master new, complicated technology, but also to find more meaningful ways to engage the students. Expectations are higher with each succeeding generation as students are exposed to technology at earlier ages. Today's students have grown up with technology; they have been raised on the Internet, they Google for information and have thrived in the online communities of instant messages, chat rooms, electronic mailing lists and e-mail. Students expect educators to be adept with the current technology and its applications (Prensky, 2001).

With increasing student enrollments in the health professions, the additional challenge is to be able to reach more students with more content, yet maintain that all-important student-teacher relationship so vital in educating health professionals.

Aside from technological sophistication, today's students are skilled in the art of multitasking or parallel processing (Prensky, 2001) and lose interest quickly if the learning environment is not dynamic or interesting or both. How can instructors use technology to reach and engage the students and create opportunities for the students to apply what they learn? This chapter will look at multimedia and multidelivery formats including web-based course tools, the Internet, and other learning activities designed to create meaningful learning experiences.

DEFINITION AND PURPOSE

There are numerous definitions of multimedia, but for purposes of this chapter, multimedia simply means using more than one type of media and integrating the use of text, graphics, sound and/or video. Barr and Tagg (1995) describe paradigm shifts taking place in higher education from teacher-centered to learner-centered education.

Educators are no longer the experts; teachers have become persons with expertise (Wilson, 2004). Since students have access to volumes of information via the Internet, the instructor can no longer possibly keep ahead of the abundance of information, but instead must guide the student into making the information meaningful. Students struggle with prioritizing information and organizing it in meaningful ways. The instructor's role changes from the traditional sage on the stage to the role of the guide on the side (Collison, Elbaum, Haavind, & Tinker, 2000).

Educators must be knowledgeable in new and emerging multimedia technology to be able to reach and engage students in ways the students are willing to learn. With increased competition for students, institutions must reach more students more effectively. Multimedia technology and a variety of delivery methods provide the flexibility for faculty and institutions to engage both classroom and distance learners.

THEORETICAL FOUNDATIONS

Background Information and Research Leading to Development and Use of Strategy

Creating learning environments through multimedia technology has roots in our knowledge of adult learning. Components of adult learning are described by Knowles (1990) and emphasize that adults are self-directed, are interested in topics that are relevant to their lives, like to be actively involved in the learning process, and have control over where and how they learn so they can learn at their own pace. Knowles's theory of andragogy makes the following assumptions about the design of learning: (1) adults need to know why they need to learn something; (2) adults need to learn experientially; (3) adults approach learning as problem solving; and (4) adults learn best when the topic is of immediate value (Knowles, 1990).

It is important that the instructor know the learners' needs and design learning activities that are relevant to those needs. The students should be actively involved in learning, with the instructor acting as a facilitator or guide. The instructor who recognizes that adults have different learning needs can tailor instruction design to the characteristic ways adults prefer to learn. Adult learning theory is important in multimedia instructional design for several reasons: (1) it is important to tailor the content specifically to the learner's level or it will not be effective (Lee & Owens, 2000); (2) learner goals and objectives must utilize a variety of learning activities if adults are to be engaged in the learning (Fink, 2003); and (3) by engaging in meaningful activity, students feel like they are making significant, sustainable contributions (Teeley, Lowe, Beal, & Knapp, 2006).

Educators are familiar with Benjamin Bloom's taxonomy of educational objectives, as they have been a standard framework since the 1950s (Bloom, 1956). Educators generally refer to the cognitive domain most frequently. They include, from the lowest to the highest:

- Knowledge
- Comprehension
- Application
- Analysis
- Synthesis
- Evaluation

Fink (2003) responds to the changing needs of students and educators by introducing a new taxonomy, called a *taxonomy of significant learning* in his 2003 publication, *Creating Significant Learning Experiences*. He addresses needs that are not easily met by Bloom's taxonomy, such as learning how to learn, leadership and interpersonal skills, ethics, communication skills, character, tolerance, and the ability to adapt to change (see **Figure 17-1**). Fink defines learning in terms of change, stating that, "For learning to occur, there has to be some kind of change in the learner. No change, no learner. And significant learning requires that there be some kind of lasting change in the learner" (p. 30).

Foundational Knowledge. At the base of most other kinds of learning is the need for students to know something. Knowing, as used here, refers to students' ability to understand and remember specific information and ideas. It is important for people today to have some valid basic knowledge, for example, about science, history, literature, geography, etc. They also need to understand major ideas or perspectives, for example, what evolution is (and what it is not), what capitalism is (and is not), and so forth. **Special Value:** Foundational knowledge provides the basic understanding that is necessary for other kinds of learning.

Application. This familiar kind of learning occurs when students learn how to engage in some new kind of action, which may be intellectual, physical, social, etc. Learning how to engage in various kinds of thinking (critical, creative, practical) is an important form of application learning. But this category of significant learning also includes developing certain skills (e.g., communication, playing the piano) or learning how to manage complex projects. **Special Value:** Application learning allows other kinds of learning to become useful.

Figure 17-1   The taxonomy of significant learning.

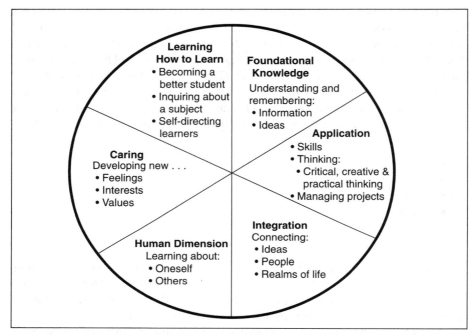

From Fink, L. D. (Ed.). (2003). *Creating significant learning experiences*. San Francisco: Jossey-Bass, pp. 31. Used with permission.

Integration. When students are able to see and understand the connections between different things, an important kind of learning has occurred. Sometimes they make connections between specific ideas, between whole realms of ideas, between people, and/or between different realms of life (e.g., between school and work or between school and leisure life). **Special Value:** The act of making new connections gives learners a new form of power, especially intellectual power.

Human Dimension. When students learn something important about their own self and/or about others, it enables them to interact more effectively with themselves or with others. They discover the personal and/or social implications of what they have learned. What they learn or the way in which they learn sometimes gives students a new understanding of themselves (self-image) or a new vision of what they want to become (self-ideal). At other times, they acquire a better understanding of others—how and why others act the way they do or how the learner can interact more effectively with others. **Special Value:** This kind of learning informs students about the human significance of what they are learning.

Caring. Sometimes a learning experience changes the degree to which students care about something. This may be reflected in the form of new feelings, interests, and/or values. Any of these changes means students care about something to a greater degree or in a way other than they did before. **Special Value:** When students care about something, they then have the energy they need for learning more about it and making it a part of their lives. Without the energy for learning, nothing significant happens.

Learning How to Learn. This occurs when students learn something about the process of learning itself. They may be learning how to be a better student, how to engage in a particular kind of inquiry (e.g., the scientific method), or how to become self-directing learners. All of these constitute important forms of learning how to learn. **Special Value:** This kind of learning enables students to continue learning in the future and to do so with greater effectiveness.

TYPES OF LEARNERS

Students enter the health professions in different stages in their lives. While some are traditional college students, most students have very busy lives with jobs and children and other additional family obligations. With the added expense of college tuition, it is a rare student who does not have to work in addition to attending school and fulfilling clinical placements. This changing profile of the learner suggests that most students fulfill the pedagogical requirements of the adult learner (Jairath and Stair, 2004). The more flexible and self-paced the course delivery is, the more likely the students will be able to fit it into their schedule and be successful. Traditional students in higher education in the first decade of the 21st century include the generation called, "millennials" (Howe & Strauss, 2000). These are students born between the years of 1982 and 2002. They are global, connected, and interactive. Although they grew up in a media age, they will undoubtedly have varying levels of proficiency that will require access to support functions.

Web-based courses using a platform such as Blackboard or WebCt require a comprehensive orientation to the format. Students must become quickly proficient in navigating the tools and how to troubleshoot common problems such as disabling pop-up blockers and mastery of e-mail and attachment functions. Most importantly, students need to know how to access help.

Prensky (2001) differentiates *digital natives* from *digital immigrants*. He describes digital natives as the students who are *native speakers* to the digital language of computers, video games, and the Internet; those who are not native to the digital language (most instructors) are said to be *immigrants*. Immigrants have to learn a new language and adapt to a new environment. "Digital natives are used to receiving information really fast, they like to parallel process and multi-task and they function best when networked" (p. 2). He suggests that it is unlikely that digital natives are going to learn the immigrant's language, so in order to reach these students, immigrant instructors must learn to communicate in the language style of the student.

Conditions for Learning—Hybrid Design

A web-based, or hybrid design course requires that the students are self-directed and are accustomed to working independently. Although beginning college students may do well with the technology, the discipline and organization required means that the more mature student will be better prepared and ultimately more successful. The course must be well planned in advance since the students will have access to the entire course once they are registered and enrolled. Clear instructions and troubleshooting guides should be readily available and included in a course orientation or overview.

Hybrid design is the best of both worlds; it allows for the development of independent study style and self-discovery in the online portion, yet the classroom component provides the intimacy found in the face-to-face classroom environments. The design promotes community building both online and in the classroom, once the students have been assigned to their groups.

Multimedia delivery formats have the potential to better engage the students by creating self-directed, lifelong learners. Goals for multimedia-multidelivery format include:

- Create a positive learning environment
- Effect greater interactivity and increased engagement in the course
- Address different learning styles
- Retain information after the course
- Develop an ability to transfer knowledge
- Make information meaningful
- Develop self-directed learners
- Develop a love of knowledge and lifelong learners
- Create collaborative learners
- Promote community building

RESOURCES

Personnel

The most essential resource for a hybrid or web-based design is the availability of faculty facilitators to manage the smaller discussion groups of 6–12 students. A group that is too small does not have the diversity of input and opinions to make it interesting, and a group that is too large becomes unwieldy for both the students and the facilitator especially if there are multiple postings and responses required within a short time.

Technology

Students and faculty need access to home computers with access to the Internet and e-mail accounts. Classrooms must also have computer and Internet access, plus projection equipment for CDs, tapes, videos and PowerPoint presentations. Faculty must be proficient in the use of the classroom technology. If the educational setting offers training for faculty, it is advised to take advantage of new and emerging technology. Nothing seems to diminish the important role of the faculty quicker than stumbling through technological setup in front of a class.

Faculty Development

Faculty development for online course development is essential in addition to ongoing design support and technology support.

USING THE METHOD

There are numerous how-to texts available for web design courses, and many of these resources are listed in the *Recommended Reading* section at the end of this chapter. This section will look specifically at developing a hybrid (or blended) course and incorporating within the course design multiple media types aimed at engaging the student in the learning experience. The key to successful implementation of a hybrid course is allowing sufficient time for planning the course itself as well as allowing time to train faculty facilitators. See **Table 17-1**.

Planning

Taking an existing course and adapting it for use online requires *reconceptualizing* the learning material (O'Neil, Fisher, & Newbold, 2004). Each module or learning section needs to be reassessed in light of new available options. How are the module's objectives best met given the skill level of the faculty and the available technology? Can the content be packaged and available online for viewing at the students' own pace? Does the content lend itself to small group

Table 17-1 Taxonomy Design Worksheet

Goals	Fink's taxonomy	Learning activities—in class	Learning activities—outside class	Types of media/delivery	Feedback and assessment
1. Describe basic elements of the financing of health-care delivery including Medicaid, Medicare, and managed care options.	Foundational knowledge	Lecture Textbook CD Interactive game	Online vignettes Self-paced PowerPoint Clinical setting	Instructor-led lecture CD-ROM Interactive game PowerPoint WebCt	Preclass online quiz Midterm or final exam 1-minute papers
2. Evaluate opportunities for disparities in present-day system.	Application Integration Caring Human dimension	Discussion Debate Case studies	Clinical setting Online discussion question Online reflection Literature/stories	WebCt Text-based case studies Discussion board Internet audio Internet video	Discussion of grade Weekly reflection Project presentations
3. Investigate resources for eliminating disparities.	Integration Caring Learning how to learn	Discussion Debate	Clinical setting Links to web sites	Self-directed Internet exploration	Project presentations

discussions that can be facilitated on a discussion board? If the students read the material online in preparation for the next face-to-face class, then can class time be better spent in classroom activities and discussions instead of simply imparting content? What activities, case studies, and discussions are better suited for an online discussion or a face-to-face class?

For integrated planning, use a course design worksheet based on goals and learning objectives. See Table 17-1, which is based on Fink's taxonomies (Fink 2003).

Feedback and Assessment

How will the students receive feedback? How will they be assessed and graded? Discussion questions need to be carefully constructed to elicit thoughtfully researched responses. Clearly defined rubrics are helpful for the students as well as the faculty facilitators to assure uniform grading criteria.

Expectations

In addition to the traditional course content with objectives and outcomes, the online and hybrid faculty need to clearly set the tone and the expectations. The students will most likely have access to the online component of the course before they meet face to face (of course this is optional). What the students see on their first visit will most likely determine their first impressions of the class. Will it be visually appealing and friendly or chaotic and hard to navigate? A friendly welcome from the professor with the hybrid course expectations clearly explained will allay fears and set the tone for a positive learning experience.

Dispel the myth that less class time means less work. Clearly define the students' expectations for workload plus the expectations of the new role for the faculty facilitators. When can the students expect responses from the faculty and how will their grades be communicated? Develop a list of course frequently asked questions and add to it as the course evolves.

Training and Orientation

New roles and expectations for faculty facilitators must be clearly defined, as this is most likely a brand new role. Time involved should not be underestimated and should be agreed upon at the start of the course to prevent any unwelcome surprises. Rubrics for grading are helpful for new faculty as well as timelines and sample responses to the students' discussion postings. How to resources for moderating online discussions will help support the faculty as they grow in this new role.

Group faculty training with hands-on Internet and web course access is ideal for introducing the faculty facilitators to the course design and to hear concerns and questions before the class begins. Practice discussion questions help the faculty work together to anticipate student issues. Once the training period is over, it is helpful to establish a private discussion area on the course's web site just for faculty to communicate with each other; they will undoubtedly have common questions from students and it will be helpful to have a *community* as a resource.

Student orientation to the hybrid design needs to be just as thorough as the faculty orientation, especially if this is a new way of learning. In addition to on-line resources, the first face-to-face class meeting should be spent going over required computer skills, course layout and navigation tips, expectations for timely assignment submissions, organization tips, appropriate communication strategies (netiquette), and most importantly, how much time will be allowed to complete the assignments.

POTENTIAL PROBLEMS

For Students

The most challenging problem is for the students to embrace a new way of learning. Although the students may be accustomed to the technological features, this course requires a lot of independence and self direction, and the student who is not ready for this different way of learning can feel lost and resentful. Poor organizational skills and impaired time-management can also derail a student if they get behind. Students who are not web savvy need to get up to speed quickly. Varying computer skills and access to high speed internet can also be problematic in this course style. On-line quizzes are a particular challenge for varying internet speeds, and students can experience a high degree of frustration on top of the quiz anxiety when the internet is inaccessible.

For Faculty

Course development takes a considerable time commitment just in the planning stages, and once the course is implemented. The first few "editions" need continued tweaking and modifying to work out the bugs. Because of the nature of technology, plus the addition of new areas of content, the course will never be finished, but will always be evolving.

EXHIBIT 17-1

Course Development Workflow Checklist

1. Outline the course into teaching modules.
2. ID online and face-to-face segments.
3. Define learning objectives for each module.
4. Outline module content.
5. Define feedback and assessment strategies.
6. Identify integration link each week between online and classroom.
7. Identify resources for content support.
   a. Web sites, books, articles
8. Determine teaching/learning activities to address course content and objectives.
9. Determine assessment tasks.
   a. Quizzes/tests
      i. Develop test questions based on objectives.
      ii. Provide rationale for answers.
   b. Discussion board questions/case studies
      i. Develop questions based on module objectives.
      ii. Clearly define instructions for posting and responding including length and deadlines (create a visual chart).
      iii. Provide rubric for correct answers.
      iv. Communicate rubric to other course faculty.
      v. Design method for weekly faculty communication with course coordinator.
   c. Other written assignments
10. Develop grade plan based on above assessment tasks.
11. Communicate all the above in the course syllabus.
    a. Include time management expectation for students (3 hrs prep per each hour of class).
    b. Include help desk resources and academic technology support.
12. Communicate all of the above to clinical faculty in a faculty orientation/ training session.
    a. Develop clinical faculty training materials.

Source: Fink, 2003.

CONCLUSION

Students entering the health professions in the 21st century are different learners than their instructors. Internet access to new information and the convergence of technology is a way of life and must be an integral part of the classroom if the goal is to be meaningful engagement and lifelong learning. Instructors need to learn to reach students so that they will use the material and foster a love of learning. A successful student is one who knows that learning will not end with graduation but will graduate with the necessary tools and skills to make lifelong contributions to their profession.

APPLIED EXAMPLE

Community Health Nursing—A Hybrid Course

The decision to use a hybrid model emerged from growing class sizes and increased need to deliver more content in less time. A creative way was needed to better engage the students in learning and increase the connectivity between the students and the faculty in light of the larger class sizes. The course coordinator/designer met with instructional designers and web course experts from the college's academic technology department. Goals and timelines were established with an 8-month planning time frame. In addition, the first hybrid model was scheduled to run as a pilot project with only three modules online. Once some of the bugs were worked out of the pilot, the full hybrid course had five modules online with seven face-to-face classes.

The community health nursing class content was already in modules and online in a web-enhanced format. Most of the documents, such as the syllabus, handouts, and forms, were already online, as was the test question database. This reduced some of the redesign time. The course modules were reevaluated, taking into consideration the best way to engage the students with the material. Online and web-based activities were selected with multiple learning styles in mind. The class was scheduled to meet every other week online, followed by a face-to-face class the next week.

One of the major hurdles in the online course management is the increased faculty time required for the reading and responding to multiple discussion posts. With a class size of 70 students and two to three posts per week, it would quickly become unmanageable to respond to more than 200 posts each week. Since the course already employed clinical faculty for a student/faculty ratio of six to seven students per faculty, it seemed logical to include the clinical faculty in the course design as *faculty facilitators*. As the students were assigned to their clinical groups, the same groups were carried over into the classroom and the clinical/faculty facilitator was responsible for managing the discussion posts for their group. This worked out especially well by engaging the clinical faculty in the classroom portion, and it provided much needed continuity for the students, thereby connecting the classroom and the clinical settings.

For the on-line component, the students had assigned readings and activities followed by discussion questions and responses due on specific dates. The responses were important as they were designed to engage the students in an online community and promote a back-and-forth discussion, as opposed to just posts. Faculty facilitators were guided in their role as facilitators and were discouraged from jumping into the discussion, but rather were encouraged to let the discussion flow among the students. The facilitators graded the students' postings using a private mailbox but responded to the groups' postings as a whole once all the postings were complete. Once the faculty facilitators posted their response to the student group, they were encouraged to share their response with other faculty members on a private (faculty only) faculty forum message board. The faculty forum was also available to faculty to share ideas and concerns throughout the class.

In order to keep the classroom times interesting by leaving time for activities and discussions, the students were required to read the assignments *before* class and complete an online quiz based on the material. Because this was structured as a learning experience rather than a test, the students could take the test up to two times and only their highest score was recorded. This worked well because the students came to class with questions and were already engaged in the material. The students also liked this because they received immediate feedback from the online test.

Academic misconduct was minimized as much as possible by stating up front that the quizzes and tests were *open book*. The questions were designed to be higher level, i.e., *application* and *integration* rather than simply *knowledge based* (Fink, 2003) and required fuller comprehension of the material. Midterms and final exams, while also online, were built on a WebCt feature of a computerized random selection of questions so that no two tests were alike. Misconduct is always a concern with online tests, but by enabling the students to take the quizzes more than once and enabling the random selection feature, the opportunities were minimized.

One of the most successful features of the course was the presentation project students made based on reading current literature about a selected vulnerable population group (Leffers & Martin, 2004). The learning goal was to evoke a caring response by immersing the reader into the personal struggles of the population. This goal is consistent with Fink's taxonomies of significant learning (Fink, 2003) of both the caring and human dimension taxonomies.

The students presented their project as a group to the class utilizing creative multimedia methodologies. A selection of their presentations included formats such as video production, radio show simulation, a Jeopardy game, and others that engaged the rest of the class and communicated the message of heartfelt vulnerability. The best way to keep up with new and meaningful delivery methods is to take notes from the students; they will let instructors know how they like to learn.

Feedback for the hybrid delivery method was elicited from both students and the clinical faculty facilitators. The responses were organized into four themes, time management, participation, learning opportunities, and technology. The results were favorable for the hybrid style in general, as most students like the flexibility and opportunities to participate. Some students still would prefer to sit in class and *be taught*, but for the most part, the students enjoyed the learning experience, and students and faculty alike benefited from the increased engagement in the discussions. See survey results in **Table 17-2.**

Table 17-2   Survey Results

	Student—advantages of hybrid model	Student—disadvantages of hybrid model	Faculty facilitator—advantages of hybrid model	Faculty facilitator—disadvantages of hybrid model
Time/schedule	• Fits schedule better. • More flexible; less stressful. • Quizzes can be taken in a relaxed environment. • More time for readings. • Less commuting time. • Lets me organize my time better.	• Writing out the discussions is time consuming. • Seems to be more work involved, too much time researching answers to discussions. • Hard to keep organized; the time management is difficult. • Very time consuming, makes you prefer classroom lectures.	• The students seem to manage their time better.	
Participation	• More engaged with material. • Really enjoy learning others' opinions. • More communication with classmates. • Students who don't speak easily in class speak up online. • More time for a better prepared response.	• Don't like sharing with other students. • Feel disconnected from the classroom professor. • Miss the classroom interaction with other students. • Online discussions feel like busy work.	• Very interesting discussions, I love reading them! • Allows the students to clearly express their thoughts. • I learn a lot about the students from their postings; I would never get that otherwise.	• The students don't like reading all the discussions and responses. • I worry that the students view the online sessions as an "off" week.

	• More feedback from peers. • Smaller groups, more attention. • Good for someone like me who does not speak up in class, yet has a lot to say.	• Online doesn't feel "real"; hard to take it seriously. • I would rather sit in class for 2 hours and listen to the professor than to read on my own and share my thoughts on the Internet. • Too much computer screen time; would rather have more face-to-face time. • Others' discussions are too long to read.	• Would love to see more of the course online!	• Hard to give feedback—at this level, students still need feedback on basic grammar and APA format; I find it hard to use this format to make comments.
Learning opportunities	• Forces you to look things up and learn more. • Like the independent learning—I learn more on my own. • Enables students to learn in different ways. • Need to really read to participate in class. • I am learning more through the discussions and quizzes than I am in the classroom.	• Feel different instructors grade discussions differently; it's not fair. • Find the different assignments confusing. • We have to learn quite a bit on our own.	• The students did great research in preparation for the discussion questions. • The discussion questions seem to cover a great deal of material. • The students seem to learn more from the assignments. • The students seem to be able to organize their thoughts better by putting them in writing.	

continued

Table 17-2 Survey Results—continued

	Student—advantages of hybrid model	Student—disadvantages of hybrid model	Faculty facilitator—advantages of hybrid model	Faculty facilitator—disadvantages of hybrid model
	• The discussions allow us to think about what we read. • The Internet connectivity leads us to different web sites with a lot of new information. • The discussions make you really think about the readings instead of just memorizing. • Ties in the clinical practice with class. • The discussions revealed whole new areas of interest for me.		• The students seem better at tying together the classroom and the clinical.	
Technology	• Improves my technology skills by forcing me to use the WebCt features.	• If the Internet is down, participation is difficult. • The technology is confusion. • Frustrating to work on an old PC. • Culture shock compared to other nursing classes.		• I don't like correcting online; I would rather have a Word document I can print out and make comments on.

REFERENCES

Barr, R. B., & Tagg, J. (1995). From teaching to learning—a new paradigm for undergraduate education. *Change, 27*(6), 12.

Bloom, B. S. (Ed.). (1956). *Taxonomy of educational objectives; the classification of educational goals handbook I: Cognitive domain.* New York: McKay.

Collison, G., Elbaum, B., Haavind, S., & Tinker, R. (2000). *Facilitating online learning: Effective strategies for moderators.* Madison, WI: Atwood Publishing.

Fink, L. D. (Ed.). (2003). *Creating significant learning experiences.* San Francisco: Jossey-Bass.

Howe, N., & Strauss, W. (2000). *Millennials rising: The next greatest generation.* New York: Vintage Press.

Jairath, N., & Stair, N. (2004). A development and implementation framework for web-based nursing courses. *Nursing Education Perspectives, 25*(2), 67.

Knowles, M. (1990). *The adult learner: A neglected species* (4th ed.). Houston: Gulf Pub. Co.

Lee, W. W., & Owens, D. L. (2000). *Multimedia-based instructional design.* San Francisco: Jossey-Bass.

Leffers, J., & Martin, D. C. (2004). Journey to compassion: Meeting vulnerable populations in community health nursing through literature. *International Journal of Human Caring, 8*(1), 20.

O'Neil, C. A., Fisher, C. A., & Newbold, S. K. (Eds.). (2004). *Developing an online course: Best practices for nurse educators.* New York: Springer.

Prensky, M. (2001, October). Digital natives, digital immigrants. *On the Horizon, 9*(5), 1–2.

Teeley, K., Lowe, J., Beal, J., & Knapp, M. (2006). Incorporating quality improvement concepts and practice into a community health nursing course. *Journal of Nursing Education, 45*(2), 65–71.

Wilson, L. O. (2004). *Teaching millennial students.* Retrieved August 6, 2005, from, http://www.uwsp.edu/education/facets/links_resources/Millennial%20Specifics.pdf

RECOMMENDED READING

Brookfield, S. (2003). Adult cognition as a dimension of lifelong learning. In J. Field and M. Leicester (Eds.), *Lifelong learning: Education across the lifespan.* New York: Routledge Falmer. Retrieved January 8, 2006, from http://www.open.ac.uk/lifelong-learning/papers/393CD0DF-000B-67DB 0000015700000157_StephenBrookfieldpaper.doc

Brookfield, S. (1986). *Understanding and facilitating adult learning.* San Francisco: Jossey-Bass.

Collison, G., Elbaum, B., Haavind, S., & Tinker, R. (2000). *Facilitating online learning: Effective strategies for moderators.* Madison, WI: Atwood Publishing.

Conrad, R., & Donaldson, J. (2004). *Engaging the online learner.* San Francisco: Jossey-Bass.

Fink, L. D. (Ed.). (2003). *Creating significant learning experiences.* San Francisco: Jossey-Bass.

Fink, L. D. (2005). *A self directed guide to designing courses for significant learning.* Retrieved July 8, 2006, from http://www.ou.edu/idp/significant/Self-DirectedGuidetoCourseDesign1.doc

Howe, N., & Strauss, W. (2000). *Millennials rising: The next greatest generation.* New York: Vintage Press.

Matthews-Denatale, G., & Cotler, D. (2005). *Faculty as authors of online courses: Support and mentoring.* Retrieved December 30, 2005, from http://www.academiccommons.org/commons/essay/matthews-denatale-and-cotler

Novotny, J. M., & Davis, R. (Eds.). (2006). *Distance education in nursing.* New York: Springer.

O'Neil, C. A., Fisher, C. A., & Newbold, S. K. (Eds.). (2004). *Developing an online course: Best practices for nurse educators.* New York: Springer.

Palloff, R. M., & Pratt, K. (2001). *Lessons from the cyberspace classroom.* San Francisco: Jossey-Bass.

Palloff, R. M., & Pratt, K. (2003). *The virtual student.* San Francisco: Jossey-Bass.

Prensky, M. (2001, October). Digital natives, digital immigrants. *On the Horizon, 9*(5), 1–6.

CHAPTER 18

Electronic Communication Strategies

Arlene J. Lowenstein

DEFINITION AND PURPOSES

Educational institutions are increasingly moving toward a computer-enriched environment (Mitra & Steffensmeier, 2000). The use of computers for electronic communication takes many forms, including, but not limited to, bulletin boards; chat rooms; e-mail; forums and threaded discussions around specific topics; electronic libraries; use of the Internet, which is worldwide; and intranets, which are established within one school or organization; the Nightingale Tracker used for communication in the clinical arena; and even iPods (Effink et al., 2000; Kimeldorf, 1995; Read, 2005). E-mail use has been growing significantly in educational settings and has brought about dramatic changes in communication between students, faculty, and staff (Gatz & Hirt, 2000).

Enrichment is the key phrase. Computer technology is a valuable teaching tool, but it must never replace the teacher. Faculty members can use computers as one strategy to enhance the teaching-learning process, but the need for human contact should also be considered. Effective use of this technology depends on the learning objectives (Little, Hannum, & Stack, 1996). E-mail journaling may be appropriate for learning objectives that are geared toward the individual, whereas threaded discussions or group e-mail discussion may be more appropriate for objectives that include learning to work with group processes.

Computers can be used to stimulate students to become actively involved in the teaching-learning process by giving them tools they can manipulate to control their learning environment (Morgan, 1995). Computer use can be asynchronous, which does not require that both parties communicate at the same time. Students and faculty can read and answer messages at their convenience. E-mail messages can be longer and more detailed than traditional voice mail messages. The instructor is responsible for introducing students to the resources available, providing guidelines for use, and troubleshooting with the student when technical problems occur.

THEORETICAL RATIONALE

Mitra and Steffensmeier (2000) carried out a longitudinal study of students following a university decision to provide a computer network, create an intranet for student use, and provide students with laptop computers. The computer-enriched environment was positively correlated with students' ability to facilitate communication and positive student attitudes toward computers in general. Ease of access was a major influence in fostering those positive attitudes in the teaching and learning process.

Levin (1999) studied the use of electronic communication in teacher training. Four types of communication were explored: (1) student-to-peer e-mail journal entries, (2) student-to-keypal e-mail exchanges with teachers in another state, (3) e-mail exchanges between students and instructor, and (4) a threaded discussion using student-to-group messages. Although there were many personal and supportive messages, the most frequent purpose of the student-to-peer e-mail exchanges were messages that provided an opportunity to reflect on their growth as teachers and to discuss teaching resources and planning instruction. Reflective comments were also found in student-to-keypal exchanges, but not as often as in student-to-peer messages. Student-to-keypal messages tended to use more descriptions and comparisons of programs, although supportive feedback and reflection were also found.

Student-to-instructor exchanges were often found in addition to journal assignments. The exchanges provided a mechanism for students to have a running discussion with the instructor that lasted for several weeks. These messages tended to revolve around the topic of student development as teachers and included planning lessons and curriculum discussions. Personal issues and technical problems were also discussed. The main purpose of the student-to-group discussions was reflection, which was the content of many of the messages. The discussions also provided a forum for feedback and moral support. Reflective, self-analytical thinking was fostered the most by the student-to-group discussions. Student-to-peer discussions included more than personal and supportive messages; they also shared issues and problems (Levin, 1999).

Most faculty members are routinely faced with two issues in class. The first issue is that of encouraging students to become more active in preparation for class, including reading assigned material and reflecting on it prior to class. A second issue is to encourage students who are silent during class discussions and who do not offer ideas or opinions. By using technology to serve pedagogy and facilitate learning, Parkyn (1999) addressed those issues by developing a discourse community of students who were assigned to use a collaborative electronic journal. Students were assigned to small groups, with no more than 10 to 12 students per group. Each group was responsible for writing a collective, weekly journal. The journal provided an opportunity for students to discuss ideas about the reading assignment, respond to comments of other students, and become aware of how other students responded to the entry. Students were found to be better prepared for class discussions, and peer-mediated learning was higher than that found in the traditional classroom. Some students found the journal to be a safer environment in which to discuss ideas than the open classroom. This safe environment was fostered through the use of a pseudonym or journal name used by each student, known only by the individual student and instructor (Parkyn, 1999). Overall, students were able to share with one another in a way that transformed individual learning into collaborative and effective learning.

CONDITIONS

Access to the technology and technology support services, along with faculty comfort with computers, are the most important conditions for utilizing this teaching strategy. Students who are not familiar with the equipment or computers can be given a period of time to learn and practice if support is available. Faculty members also need time and support to develop expertise in using e-mail or other computer-assisted strategies. Students should be able to access computers at home or at school. If passwords are necessary, then a process needs to be defined to ensure student access to the needed material.

TYPES OF LEARNERS

Electronic communication can be used by all levels of students. Electronic communication strategies work well in both graduate and undergraduate educational settings. Computers are rapidly becoming part of the educational landscape. Students are increasingly being exposed to computers well before entering postsecondary education; however, many nursing students seek to enter the profession or graduate school at a later age than the traditional postsecondary student. Although some of these students will be computer savvy, many have not been exposed to computer usage. It is important to determine the students' level of computer comfort when making assignments, and to be supportive as the students work their way through the computer learning curve.

RESOURCES

Although many faculty members have been exposed to and use computers, others have not and do not, and the same is true for students. Regardless of faculty expertise level, training with technical support follow-up must be made available (Bates & Poole, 2003). Knowledgeable and friendly technical support is very important. Working with computers can be extremely frustrating and stressful for novices unless an adequate support system to troubleshoot problems and encourage the users is in place. Learning to work with computers takes practice and persistence, but the process can be well worth the time and energy. Technical support personnel can alert faculty members to new programs that are available. For example, Oosterhof (2000) described a process that can be used by faculty with large classes to individualize e-mail through the use of macros and worksheets. Universities and colleges are becoming increasingly wired for computer usage, with fiber optic or other cabling systems. They are developing intranet systems as well as Internet links that faculty members are able to access and use for instructional purposes. Coordination between the information systems department and faculty is needed to avoid problems caused by underestimating the use and need for assistance.

USING THE METHOD

The choice of which technology is to be used depends on the learning objectives, the need for asynchronous processes, and the resources available. The Internet may be assigned for finding references and in-depth research. However, students must understand the need to validate the data found, since many web pages are not peer reviewed, and the accuracy of the material cannot be guaranteed unless it is an electronic version of a journal article. A bulletin board, chat room, or threaded discussion can be developed for use by a specific class. Mobile technology including handheld personal digital assistants (PDAs), cell phones, and laptop computers can be used in the clinical area to maintain contact with the faculty member (Effink et al., 2000). IPods can be used for more than music, and students can store and transmit data (Read, 2005). Choice of communication method also depends on the need for group interaction, peer-to-peer-interaction, or student-to-instructor interaction. Passwords may be necessary to gain access for some venues.

Technology changes and evolves rapidly. Cell phones take pictures; iPods collect data. It is important for faculty to be aware of new methodologies as they develop (Bates & Poole, 2003; Morersund, 1997). Faculty should also be aware of potential financial issues involved for students interested in purchasing or required to purchase their own equipment.

Instructions for use must be clear. It is important to assess students' comfort level with computers and to provide resources to assist them. The process for finding help for technological problems should be developed and communicated to students. E-mail messages can be more informal than student papers or written journals. Typos, spelling, and grammar may not need correction in e-mail messages, as long as students understand that good grammar, spelling, and proofreading are required for paper assignments. Many schools have ethical policies for computer usage and e-mail. Students should be informed of those policies and be expected to adhere to them.

POTENTIAL PROBLEMS

Faculty and student comfort with the systems is the first major problem that needs to be considered. Many individuals are technologically challenged and avoid using computers, especially if they have had bad experiences in beginning attempts. Technological problems often occur, from full computer crashes to loss of messages that have not been saved or were overwritten. Knowing where to go for help becomes very important in these instances. Remembering passwords when they have not been used frequently can be difficult, and a system needs to be available to retrieve a password without compromising security. Misspelled addresses can be frustrating and time consuming when a minor error, such as an extra dot, causes the message to go astray. Finding the error in an address or message can be difficult because of the tendency to read the word as the reader thinks it should be, thereby reading over the error. Computers are famous for carrying out commands literally. What the user wrote in the command may not have been what the user intended, but computers do not recognize intentions. Small errors can cause major problems and are often difficult to discover. At the same time, however, with the proper support, computers can enhance learning and be fun and enjoyable to use.

Privacy and avoiding embarrassment can be important issues. E-mail messages are not private, even though they feel as if they are. Both students and faculty need to be made aware of that fact. In chat rooms, bulletin boards, and other group venues, it is possible for students to use an alias or pseudonym, as Parkyn (1999) had students do in the discourse communities he developed. He found that students expressed more opinions when they were free of personal harassment or disparaging remarks directed at their true self.

Time for e-mail is an important issue for the instructor, especially if the selected method involves one-to-one student-instructor conversations. Class size is an important parameter in deciding if the instructor has the time to respond effectively to students. There are other methods to work with larger classes. Oosterhof's (2000) method of individualizing e-mail allowed for consolidating messages and providing some automatic answering options. His method was used successfully with large classes. Replies to students can be brief but need to be meaningful. Both large and small classes can benefit from the use of electronic communication when the technology is geared to meet specific teaching-learning objectives.

EXAMPLE

Electronic Journaling

The history of nursing ideas course was developed to enable graduate students to view nursing theory in the context of nursing history and growth of the profession. The course description and objectives are shown in **Exhibit 18-1**. A major mission of the nursing program and the school is to prepare students for leadership within the profession. Understanding dynamics of change and recognizing decision makers is important to the development of leadership skills necessary to carry out that mission. The critical-thinking objective is used to prepare students to recognize decision makers and those dynamics of change within the nursing profession and in the provision of health care.

EXHIBIT 18-1

History of Nursing Ideas Course Syllabus

Course Description

This course focuses on the contributions of nursing history, nursing theory, and contemporary issues in the social evolution of nursing as a profession. The nature of nursing theory and the relationship between philosophy, theory, and science are explored. The evolution of nursing knowledge within the social context of history is emphasized.

Objectives

Upon completion of the course, the student should be able to:
1. Identify major issues associated with the development of nursing as a profession.
2. Examine the influences of hospitals and the rise of medicine in the development of nursing.
3. Utilize critical thinking to analyze the components of theories and the history of development in nursing.
4. Examine the relationship between historical development in nursing, nursing theory, and nursing science.
5. Apply theory in domains of practice. Analyze contemporary nursing within the framework of its historical development.

The nursing program offers a generic master's program for students who have no nursing background but hold a baccalaureate in another field. This course is taught to those students in the first semester of their first year in the program. This course is also required for all registered nurses (RNs) who enter the graduate program, although they have the option to take the course at any point in their program plan of study. For entry-level students, the course attempts to establish an understanding of the profession in which the students will be entering, and specifically the importance of theory-based practice. This course also emphasizes the use of theory-based practice for the RN student. For both groups, the course sets the groundwork for the development of leadership skills and understanding the expectations of scholarly work in graduate study. Other courses in the curriculum build on the leadership and theory framework of this course, and a scholarly project that requires self-directed scholarly work is the culmination of the program.

These students bring a variety of backgrounds to the course. Entry-level students have included students with a previous master's degree in public health or another field, a heavy science background, or a doctorate in another field; professional musicians; emergency medical technicians; peace corps volunteers; or, at the other extreme, students fresh out of college with a liberal arts or science degree. Some have had experiences with the healthcare system or cared for an ill friend or relative, and that experience influenced the decision to enter nursing, whereas others have different reasons for their decision. The RNs also have varied backgrounds and enter the program with clinical expertise that they can share with the entry-level students. All of these students have something special to offer their fellow students and the instructor. They range in age from 21 to well over 50, all bringing life experiences with them. It is a wonderful group to work with, but it is challenging because of the students' expertise and status as adult learners. Principles of adult learning must be considered in the design of teaching strategies for this course.

The course is presented along a timeline, looking at past to present to future. Influences on the development of the profession are explored over that timeline. Students look at such issues as the impact over time of sociocultural influences and changes, war, religion, economics, immigration, new diseases, new technologies, the development of medicine and health care, nursing practice, and nursing education. The era of the late 1960s and 1970s brings in the impact of the civil rights, women's rights, and consumer rights movements and the reaction of nurse leaders in recognizing the need for a stronger professional view of nursing and the development of nursing science. The development of a nursing body of knowledge becomes a major focus of the course for many weeks. Students conduct group presentations for their colleagues, explaining a specific nursing theory, including appropriate research, critiques, and applicability to practice.

No single reference book can be used for the content of this course. In order to effectively contribute to class discussions, students must read various articles and book chapters and become familiar with other sources, which may include the Internet. Students must be actively involved in the learning process to benefit from this course. Students must carry out a certain amount of discovery on their own, with instructor assistance in finding appropriate resources.

In designing the course for my first time teaching, I followed the format that other instructors had used—the development of weekly topics with reading assignments for each. A book of readings, developed for purchase and adhering to copyright laws, was made available to provide students with easy access to the articles. Special attention was given to the reading selections to be sure they would provide different perspectives for discussion and new information applicable to course objectives. In addition, students formed groups in which they were responsible for a nursing theory presentation. They were expected to conduct a literature review for the particular theory and present a bibliography to the class. A term paper was also required, which presented another aspect of the students' theories or discussed the historical issues that were presented in class.

The group presentation and paper assignments required students to seek out literature and be able to discuss it orally or in their term paper. Preparing for class discussions was problematic, however. Some students took advantage of the reading collection and contributed well to the class discussion, whereas others were quiet or contributed general knowledge that did not relate to readings. These students were missing out on the richness that the readings provided. Another problem was finding ways for the instructor to assist students in preparing their presentations and papers. Although regular office hours were available, many students used the time just before or after class to talk with me. The time was rushed, and, although I was aware of some resources that could help, I did not have time to explore additional resources that would have been helpful to them.

All students in the school had access to an e-mail account that could be used within the learning resources center, but it was a new experience for many of them. I had become quite comfortable in using e-mail and found it to be a valuable form of communication. The next time the course was offered, I decided to require an electronic journal that would allow students to discuss readings with me prior to class and to turn in their term paper outlines and/or project for feedback and assistance (see **Exhibit 18-2**). My objectives were to encourage students to read before class, to encourage students who found it difficult to speak in class to discuss what they had read, and to be available for questions about assignments. In addition, papers from the previous class had shown that students were not comfortable with the format for citing references and needed feedback prior to turning in the final paper. I added an annotated bibliography to the assignment to help them understand citation formats and to gain skill in abstracting information from a journal article.

This was only one of four courses that the entry-level students took as part of their program. They were beginning basic nursing, with clinical experience that took time and was their primary interest. It was important to keep the assignments at a manageable level and to keep their interest in the topic. The basic nursing course was designed so students would begin to recognize and use a theory base in their practice. For that class, they were able to use the information they worked with in history of nursing ideas class, which helped them to see the relevance of what we were doing.

EXHIBIT 18-2

E-mail Journal Examples

Student No. 1

In Carper's article, "Fundamental Patterns of Knowing in Nursing," the author states the importance of wholeness and incorporating all of the patterns of knowing in nursing. The American Nurses Association policy statement states that, "Nursing is a scientific discipline as well as a profession" (ANA Policy Statement, p. 7). I concur that all of the components stated [earlier in this e-mail] explain the profession of nursing well; however, I do not believe the theorists have put enough emphasis on the synergistic effect of the different components that constitute the profession of nursing. Although placing the branches of nursing together is great, one needs to look beyond that and see what happens when they work together and create this new dimension of nursing. The sum of these components truly makes the nursing profession unique. I believe it is important for nurses to be aware of the synergistic effect of the wholeness of nursing.

Student No. 2

Hello, Dr. Lowenstein, this is [name omitted] from your Nursing History class. I'm e-mailing this from my house, but if you need to reply to anything, I use my [e-mail address omitted] e-mail address more.

Well, I'm not sure if anyone had picked this one either, but I read "The Seeing Self: Photography and Storytelling as a Health Promotion Methodology," by Mary Koithan. I enjoyed how this article addressed the issue of our world being too fast paced and impersonal these days because I believe this is very true. It also cited that more and more diseases today are related to stress, which is obviously detrimental to our well-being. The author stresses the importance of finding other ways to block out the confusion and busyness of everyday life and to center ourselves and concentrate on our wellness. She referred to these methods as aesthetic modalities that would promote health, empower the person, and make them aware of the connection between mind, body, and spirit. Such aesthetic modalities must work wonders for some people who are skeptical about modern medicine. It is good that we have these additional ways of healing because it is very individual and self-promoting. I found this article very interesting and hope to read more on similar subjects. I will see you in class on the 18th!

Student No. 3

The article I found dealt with the use of drawing to gain information about children and their experiences and feelings. The article "Children's Drawings: A Different Window," by Judy Malkiewicz and Marilyn L. Stember discussed that children will offer more of their feelings and experiences through drawings than through conversation with a healthcare provider. It is thus very useful for nurses to use this artistic technique to help them understand their younger patients and know how to address their needs, especially since younger children cannot express themselves well through verbal communication. The only obstacles that the authors presented were those involved with the interpretations of such artwork. Many times healthcare providers overanalyze these pieces, as well as underestimate their significance.

The article also discussed several different types of drawing exercises that can be used. Draw-a-Person, Kinetic Family Drawing, House-Person-Tree, Draw-a-Situation, and others provide the means to enter the child's world in various situations and roles that the child encounters. Each specific type of drawing serves a unique and specific purpose.

On a personal note, I worked at [employer omitted] for three years as a Child Life Assistant. In this position, I worked with the kids to keep them occupied with arts and crafts, tutor them on schoolwork, help them understand procedures using medical play, and educate them and their families on the things that were happening during their hospital stays. Most of the children on the unit were experiencing chronic illnesses such as cystic fibrosis, cancer, AIDS, spina bifida, and others. Thus we saw the children repeatedly and for long durations of time. Among our many activities and tools was the use of drawing. It provided a great release for the kids, and it told us a lot about how they were feeling about their care. It tuned us in to their fears, how we could reduce them, and how we could prevent them. I thought it was a wonderful thing. Also, the drawings were a source of pride for the kids. We displayed them all over the units and entered them into national competitions with the hospitals of the Children's Miracle Network. That was why my interest was struck by this particular article, but I can attest to the fact that these drawing exercises are valuable for both caregiver and patient. The article was from the book *Art & Aesthetics in Nursing*.

The use of theory-based practice was not as clear for the RN group, which was a factor that I needed to acknowledge in my responses to their e-mails. The RNs were encouraged to read articles relating theory to practice and to comment on how they viewed using the theory in their own nursing practice.

Instruction to students included the following:

A journal and annotated bibliography are responsible for 20% of the course grade. A weekly journal discussing your reactions to the readings and class discussion should be submitted by e-mail. For the weekly journal, pick out the major points within the reading and comment on them. This can be somewhat informal, I do not need the whole citation for that reading, and try to keep your comments to two or three paragraphs in length. Of course, if you feel that a reading deserves more depth, I will gladly look forward to reading your comments. I will respond to each message, to acknowledge receipt or to discuss some of your points. I may also ask you to bring up the point you are making in the class discussion, so the rest of the class can benefit from your thoughts. I understand that you may not be able to read every article every week in advance of class, but that should be the exception, not the rule. If that happens, please read the article after class and comment on your reactions to the article in light of the class discussion.

An annotated bibliography, consisting of a minimum of four articles over the course of the semester, should also be submitted by e-mail, in addition to the weekly journals. The annotated bibliography should follow the following guidelines:

- The content of the article should be relevant to the course objectives; include one article from the journal *Advances in Nursing Science*; and include the article citation in APA format, an abstract of the article including major issues and findings, and a brief critique and reaction to the article. The selection of articles is in addition to the assigned readings but may include articles to be used in the presentation or final paper.
- You are also encouraged to use e-mail to correspond with me regarding any questions you may have about your presentation, paper, or any other issue you feel the need to discuss. I will be pleased to give you feedback in these areas. Of course you may schedule an appointment if you wish further assistance with these projects.

I have been very pleased with the response from the journals and annotated bibliographies. Students who were not familiar with e-mail found it to be very helpful by the end of the semester and were often proud of their new skill. They usually became comfortable after a few tries, although it may have been stressful at first. Although technical problems did arise periodically, most students were successful in using the system. Technical problems included difficulty getting an e-mail address and being unable to open attachments, especially when different operating systems were being used. To address that problem, I suggested that students not use the attachment feature, but rather paste the text directly into the e-mail message, which was usually successful. Computer crashes and lost messages occurred sporadically, but most students were able to cope. To avoid complaints about needing to be on campus to use e-mail, I accepted e-mails from school or home addresses.

The responses added much to the class discussions. Students did contribute experiences or ideas that they had expressed in the e-mails and that I felt would benefit the class discussion. Students demonstrated a deeper understanding of issues and content. I did not penalize students for missing a week or two, but instead worked with them to be sure they had met the course objectives.

An added advantage to using e-mail was the ability to discuss e-mail and other computer applications during the technology topic discussion. Class discussion included looking at the present and future, identifying the technology issues and how they have and potentially will influence both nursing practice and nursing education.

The amount of e-mails can be difficult to manage for the instructor. With a class of 35, I needed to set aside time to read and respond to e-mails in a timely fashion. In some cases, no long response was necessary; I was able to acknowledge the e-mail with few words. For others, a longer conversation was in order. I have learned to pay attention to each e-mail as soon as I receive it and to respond immediately and not allow them to pile up. I was able to move the e-mails into a permanent file, sorted by student, with a separate permanent file for my responses. This allowed me to return to the messages if questions arose and to be sure students had met course objectives.

Although some students do read early, most of them wait until it is close to class. There were times when I was unable to read all of the messages before the class discussion, but these instances were usually spread out enough to allow me to at least acknowledge and possibly bring something up in the class discussion that I was not able to reply to in the message. Overall course and professor evaluations have improved with use of the e-mail journals (see Exhibit 18-3). Students have felt a closer relationship with me, and I have been able to assist students with problems or issues that would not have surfaced in other formats. Students have demonstrated improved skills and benefits from the course content. I will continue to use journals to achieve those learning objectives.

EXHIBIT 18-3

Evaluation Comments

1. "I liked the structure of the course in regards to the group project on theorists rather than doing a lot of heavy reading. I also liked the seminar/discussion style of the course. The reading was intensive, though, but the e-mail system was *great!*"
2. "I really enjoyed the readings and found the journal keeping and e-mailing very rewarding. I felt I definitely learned a lot about nursing that I didn't know about. Acceptance of my comments and experiences made the work very unthreatening."
3. "Enjoyed use of e-mail, very effective, allow for better student/teacher interaction. Thank you."

REFERENCES

Bates, A. W., & Poole, G. (2003). *Effective teaching with technology in higher education.* San Francisco: Jossey-Bass.

Effink, V. L., Davis, L. S., Fitzwater, E., Castleman, J., Burley, J., Gorney-Moreno, M. J., et al. The Nightingale Tracker Clinical Field Test Nurse Team. (2000). A comparison of teaching strategies for integrating information technology into clinical nursing education. *Nurse Educator, 25*(3), 136–144.

Gatz, L. B., & Hirt, J. B. (2000). Academic and social integration in cyberspace: Students and e-mail. *The Review of Higher Education, 23*(3), 299–318.

Kimeldorf, M. (1995). Teaching online—techniques and methods. *Learning and Leading With Technology, 25*(2), 26–31.

Levin, B. B. (1999). Analysis of the content and purpose of four different kinds of electronic communications among preservice teachers. *Journal of Research on Computing in Education, 32*(1), 139–155.

Little, D. L., Hannum, W. H., & Stack, G. B. (1996). *Computers and effective instruction: Using computers and software in the classroom.* New York: Longman.

Mitra, A., & Steffensmeier, T. (2000). Changes in student attitudes and student computer use in a computer-enriched environment. *Journal of Research on Computing in Education, 32*(3), 417–435.

Morgan, T. (1995). Using technology to enhance learning: Changing the chunks. *Learning and Leading With Technology, 25*(2), 50–55.

Oosterhof, A. (2000). Efficiently creating individualized e-mail to students. *Journal of Computing in Higher Education, 11*(2), 75–90.

Parkyn, D. L. (1999). Learning in the company of others: Fostering a discourse community with a collaborative electronic journal. *College Teaching, 47*(3), 88–90.

Read, B. (2005). Duke U. assesses iPod experiment and finds it worked—in some courses. *Chronicle of Higher Education, 51*(43), A26.

RECOMMENDED READING

Bachman, J. A., & Panzarine, S. (1998). Enabling student nurses to use the information superhighway. *Journal of Nursing Education, 377*(4), 155–161.

Barber, K., Wyatt, K., & Gerbasi, F. (1999). On-line interactive evaluation in course and clinical instruction. *Nurse Educator, 24*(2), 37–40.

Bates, A. W., & Poole, G. (2003). *Effective teaching with technology in higher education.* San Francisco: Jossey-Bass.

Bonnel, W., Wambach, K., & Connors, H. (2005). A nurse educator teaching with technologies course: More than teaching on the web. *Journal of Professional Nursing, 21*(1), 59–65.

Britt, P. (2004). Mobile elearning takes hold. *Intranets, 7*(6), 1–3.

Conrad, R., & Donaldson, J. A. (2004). *Engaging the online learner: Activities and resources for creative instruction.* San Francisco: Jossey-Bass.

Korn, K. (1999). Nutrition information on the Internet. *Journal of the American Academy of Nurse Practitioners, 11*(8), 355–356.

Nidiwane, A. (2005). Teaching with the Nightingale Tracker technology in community-based nursing education: A pilot study. *Journal of Nursing Education, 44*(1), 40–42.

Oosterhof, A. (2000). Efficiently creating individualized e-mail to students. *Journal of Computing in Higher Education, 11*(2), 75–90.

Parkyn, D. L. (1999). Learning in the company of others: Fostering a discourse community with a collaborative electronic journal. *College Teaching, 47*(3), 88–90.

Smith, R. (2004). Personal digital assistants: Expanding uses in the academic and clinical setting. *Journal of Hospital Librarianship, 4*(3), 89–94.

Zwim, E. E. (1998). Media, multimedia, and computer-mediated learning. In D. M. Billings & J. A. Halstead (Eds.), *Teaching in nursing: A guide for faculty* (pp. 315–329). Philadelphia: W. B. Saunders.

CHAPTER 19

Teaching by Distance Education

Kathy P. Bradley and Mariana D'Amico

DEFINITIONS AND PURPOSE

The trended use of a variety of technologies and instructional systems has brought about a change in education and instructional delivery. Distance education is described as an instructional delivery method occurring when learners and educators are separated by time and/or distance during the teaching-learning process. The use of accelerated learning technologies has created dramatic changes in how health professions students learn. Distance education represents the convergence of a host of opportunities and challenges (Keller, 2005). Greene and Meek (1998) described distance education as a quasi separation of the educator and learner requiring central involvement in the planning, development, and delivery of instruction. The use of distance education has provided alternative educational opportunities that may not otherwise be available due to learners' constraints, such as family, work, geographic, or social commitments.

INTRODUCTION

Today distance education is offered using a variety of media-based technology. The technology allows instructors to deliver content in live and delayed-time formats. The use of technology allows teacher-learner interaction in two ways: synchronous and asynchronous. Synchronous interaction involves real time, live, and conversational methods during the instructional delivery. Asynchronous is described as delayed, either occurring before or after the instructional setting or delivery (Miller & King-Webster, 1997).

The purpose of this chapter is to describe the use of synchronous distance education learning methods used in teaching in the healthcare professions. These two interactive videoconferencing systems allow for synchronous videoconferencing technologies for students at remote sites. Students enrolled in healthcare professions courses require the maximum level of interaction in order to help them master the complex knowledge, skills, and behaviors required by the profession (Gallagher, Dobrosielski-Vergona, Wingard, & Williams, 2005). Healthcare professions are increasingly challenged to meet the needs of learners and provide care in rural areas. The use of new synchronous instructional trends is available for providing needed health-related professional education. The educational trend for the 21st century continues to include the use of synchronous technologies to offer effective and innovative healthcare education. Examples of a planning process, possible pitfalls, and strategies for success will be shared from the literature and from experiences (Tucker, 2001).

THEORETICAL FOUNDATIONS

Educational technological theories are also referred to as techno-systemic or systemic theories. They are generally focused on the improvement of the instructional message through the use of appropriate technologies. Historically, research efforts in distance education have focused primarily on the capacity of computers to process information and explore ways to improve the quality of interaction between the learner and the content. The technological upsurge in the last 20 years has had a significant influence on educational institutions in terms of the use of technological development and the evolving concept of curriculum development and instructional delivery methods (Anderson, Beavers, VanDeGrift, & Videon, 2003).

In the 1960s, technology was viewed as the pioneering methodology of education. In 1968, the United States established the Commission on Instructional Technology to analyze the benefits of technology for educational purposes. The commission's report identified the use of technology as a contributing force to an educational revolution. The report called for studies to examine methodologies that effectively improved the acceptance and progression of the use of distance education (Bertrand, 1995). The report highlighted future studies resulting in the National Education Association (NEA) establishing research-driven quality benchmarks for distance learning in higher education. These benchmarks were formulated from practical strategies in use by leading U.S. universities. The categories of quality measures included institutional support, course development, teaching/learning, course structure, student support, faculty support, and evaluation and assessment (National Education Association, 2000). These benchmarks are used to establish standards for distance education courses.

The term *technology* is broadly used in the literature to describe all technology, including computers, videoconferencing, Internet, and resources to provide instruction from the systematic application of scientific knowledge to solving practical problems. The main focus of a synchronous educational technology theory is to propose an organization for the use of instructional methods that could be used to effectively transmit learning content to individuals at another site. The use of learning or instructional technology is an approach that involves a process that places emphasis on components of communication and the selected learning methodologies. Instructional technology is a method to systematize learning in a general applied method (Ely, 2000). Prégent (1994) described distance education as a meta approach to the relationship between theory and practice. Instructional technology is an interdisciplinary process and applicable in all fields of study. Instructional technology involves the process of organizing the learning environment with the selected instructional methods and means. It involves a systemic conception of instruction (Ely).

There are two main educational trends within the technological movement; system theory and hypermedia theory. The system theory approach offers numerous models that have been applied in secondary and postsecondary institutions. Von Bertalanffy (1998) expanded system theory's scientific roots to include an analysis of the parts and processes associated with a life form. Romiszowski (1986) outlined stages of the systems approach and instructional systems. The principal implementation methods included organizing the instructional process into a flowchart of performance objectives and then sorting the identified objectives into appropriate learning taxonomies for usage. **Figure 19-1** highlights this process. The process then allows the instructor to select the necessary elements, including groups, texts, audio-scripto-visual devices, videoconferences, computers, etc. Information is gathered on the learners' characteristics and needs, and the learning objectives are modified accordingly. Then operational plans for teaching and learning are developed. This method takes into account the learners' characteristics, the performance needs, organization, use of systems theory, and the needed learning conditions.

External learning conditions include the technology. Internal learning conditions involve the cognitive processing required by the individual learner to master the performance or knowledge expectations (Anderson, Beavers, Van-DeGrift, & Videon, 2003). Prégent (1994) described the applicability of the systems approach as appropriate for all disciplines. He described the instructor as the stage director or informational engineer who determines what is to be learned. The instructor also develops the plans needed for learning to occur and assesses the activities and means necessary to promote accomplishing the specific learning outcome. The instructor provides feedback and corrects any inadequate performance or learning. The instructor assumes the role of motivator (Bertrand, 1995).

Hypermedia educational theories originate with the selection of the use of the technology or cybernetics. Hypermedia theory is based on behavioral and communication learning approaches. The potential use of technology in healthcare

Figure 19-1   Outline of effective distance education learning process.

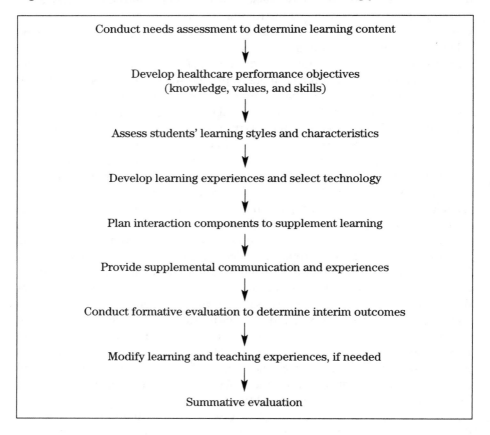

Conduct needs assessment to determine learning content

Develop healthcare performance objectives
(knowledge, values, and skills)

Assess students' learning styles and characteristics

Develop learning experiences and select technology

Plan interaction components to supplement learning

Provide supplemental communication and experiences

Conduct formative evaluation to determine interim outcomes

Modify learning and teaching experiences, if needed

Summative evaluation

education has become commonplace. Hypermedia theories originate with the use of media in education or cybernetics. This approach is based on behavioral and communication theories. The focus in the hypermedia approach is to model the informational processing by using the selected media. Early foundations of this approach were used in mathematical fields. Computers, discs, videoconferencing, and Internet-based instruction are examples of selected media. Five fundamental organizational principles of a hypermedia environment include a variety of interactions, open modeling, domain independence, cooperative instruction, and multimediatization of the presented information (Anderson et al., 2003). The use of multimediatization allows for learning using various forms of media in numerous ways. The most important learning phenomenon is the evolution of the learning principles used in educational technology requiring experimentation of the content and interactivity. Interaction exploration and discovery of the needed content using technology allows greater student access to the learning process.

Learning theories related to distance education and the use of instructional technology research provides a foundational viewpoint for an interactive healthcare curriculum and the appropriate use of selected instructional technologies. The selected learning theories and technologies are used to enhance the learners' outcomes. Universities worldwide offer distance learning strategies. Implementation requires an acceptance of the learning technology, the use of innovative teaching methods, and interactive implementation methods as a required learning process (Keller, 2005). The primary instructional focus continues to be on the interactive process designed to obtain the targeted learning outcomes and performances, not the selected technology (Tucker, 2001).

TYPES OF LEARNERS

Distance education is becoming a routine part of higher education. Most universities offer distance education courses. Universities that use distance education allow for a broader, more diverse student audience. Distance learning is appropriate for a variety of educational programs and learners. This chapter addresses the use of distance education in preparing healthcare professionals, who are generally upper division or graduate-level students. Rapid advances in the health professions and the related technology have fostered innovative teaching and learning methodologies. Healthcare students expect to be adequately prepared to practice as professional care providers. Consumers expect competent, knowledgeable practitioners. Studies involving a variety of health professionals have examined learning outcomes and the pros and cons of educating future health professions using distance education methodology. The literature regarding the effectiveness among healthcare professions continues to be limited in scope; however, numerous studies have described successful learning outcomes (Anderson et al., 2003).

Studies examining the success of distance education and student profiles indicate learner and instructor familiarity with technology was beneficial to the overall learning outcomes. Also, learner motivation and a sense of interactivity were highly predictable of learner success (Gallagher et al., 2005). Older adults tend to select distance education courses due to conflicting life priorities. Distance education programs allow these individuals more opportunities to pursue a healthcare career. The level of motivation to succeed among these learners is helpful for successful learning outcomes. Larger sample sizes and an examination of learning outcomes for the health professions are needed for more reliable and sophisticated statistical analysis. An important touchstone of distant education has been the ability to contribute to the development of individual learners regardless of life circumstances. Synchronous distance education is appropriate for all types of healthcare learners if attention is paid to the learners' access to education, adjustment to the new learning environment, individual development, knowledge and awareness of learners in context, and the importance of understanding the learners' perspective of distance education (White, 2005).

CONDITIONS FOR LEARNING

The literature for distance education has provided various suggestions for implementation. Successful distance education methods allow for attention provided to the development of individual learners. This process requires an understanding of the learning needs of the distance learners and their individual learning contexts. Studies examining learner characteristics have identified a positive relationship between self-motivation and distance learning success. Five central distance education themes have been described: (1) the learner's access to education is the first critical component of the teaching learning process; (2) the learner should have easy access to the learning materials and an understanding of the technology; (3) instructions should be given as to the best way to negotiate content mastery within the technological environment; (4) it should be expected that there will be an adjustment to the new learning environment; and (5) it is recommended that the instructor spend time identifying the learner's needs and characteristics, individual development needs, knowledge and awareness of learners in context, and the importance of understanding the learner's perspective of distance education (Sherry, 1996).

Two crucial conditions for effective distance education are the quality of the instructional process and the technology. As an example, a telemedicine project was conducted to prepare a patient education program for childbirth preparation classes. The instruction originated from a large regional hospital and was projected to a remote site at a small rural hospital. Over six months, three classes were administered. Formative learning outcomes were examined and the identified advantages included the availability of the learning programs, improved program attendance, and the convenience to the rural participants. The primary disadvantages of the project were the technical problems that occurred, particularly audio quality. This study supported the importance of quality technology systems and support services to the learning process (Byers, Hilgenberg, & Rhodes, 2003).

The available studies examining distance education using videoconferencing or other synchronous teaching methods all indicated the quality of the instruction, the interaction of the learning, and attention to the learners' needs and characteristics are critical to the learning outcomes. These data are similar to traditional learning outcomes studies. When all of the aforementioned variables are controlled, the critical condition for success is the quality of the technology and immediate technical support (Hilgenberg & Tolone, 2000). With few exceptions, students learning in distance education programs have similar learning outcomes when compared to traditional teaching methods (Fitzpatrick, 2001; McKissack, 1997). Studies have supported the need for student learning preferences to be honored, the provision of experiential educational experiences, and supportive learning conditions. It should be expected that technological problems must be immediately addressed in order to allow for learning to occur. University support for quality technology and technical support is critical for obtaining the required educational outcomes needed by healthcare professionals. Examples of a quality planning process, possible pitfalls, and strategies for success will be shared from the literature and from experiences of one allied health program with a distant satellite site.

RESOURCES

Identifying the needed resources for successful synchronous learning requires knowledge about how effective instruction is provided. Supportive learning aids need to be developed and the technology support must be seamless. Although the learners are participating in the learning process from an electronic classroom, the need for interaction with the content and the professor is critical to the learning process. Learners on the distant site may become co-dependent on written instructions. Professors need to be aware of the intended objective of written assignments and ensure the directions are clear. Learning outcomes are accomplished if the learning experiences are interactive. Also, handouts and readings supplement the presented content if the sound and video transmission are of a good quality. Poor learning outcomes have been noted with poor sound and video transmission (Mills, Bates, Pendleton, Lese, and Tatarko, 2001; Saba, 2005). When these resources are secured, distance education teaching and learning methods are appropriate for healthcare professionals.

Synchronous distance learning technology must support the learning ideas. New system technology includes Internet-based videoconferencing or the video over Internet protocol (VOIP). The distance learning course allows two or more sites to deliver and receive lectures. Communication is interactive between the sites. Each site is equipped with dedicated videoconferencing equipment, cameras, and microphones. Instructors may need a personal wireless microphone. Televisions allow the instructor to view students on both sites. The remote site views a video image of the instructor and other students at the transmission site. The instructor may use PowerPoint slides, SmartBoard, or Tegrity software to supplement the projected learning content. A document camera may be used to project documents or demonstrations of techniques for management of a hand contracture. Various other technology allow for interaction, demonstrations, games, and other experiential learning activities. The existing technology is only effective with fostered interaction and supportive experiential and flexible presentations (Anderson et al., 2003).

USING THE METHOD

The presented model has been applied by an occupational therapy program at the Medical College of Georgia. The literature describes the elements used in this model as supportive of effective learning outcomes. A model for distance education is proposed to guide other healthcare programs considering the use of asynchronous distance technology or the virtual classroom. The model may be applied to traditional classroom content as well as practice application teaching-learning experiences. The model continues to advocate for the critical element of instructor-learner and learner-to-learner interaction using a variety of experiential teaching methods. The decision to consider the use of distance education centers on matching the appropriate technology to the appropriate learning need. The technology choice is always secondary to the learners' needs and the programs' required knowledge, values, and skills competencies. The importance of the instructor-learner interaction is critical to the success of any professional educational program implementing instructional technology methods. The learner must also have experiential learning activities to support the retention of knowledge (Grimes, 2002).

Administrative and Financial Support

Within the proposed distance education model is the required prerequisite administrative commitment and support. The administrative support will require a financial commitment from the institution for upgraded technology. University administration and the healthcare education program should create a financial pro forma to project the start-up costs of offering a synchronous educational program. The financial foundation should include: (1) the cost of the selected instructional technology; (2) a determination of the number of enrolled students needed to justify the financial expenditures; (3) the cost of faculty development for learning how to appropriately use the technology with selected appropriate instructional design strategies; (4) the cost of the selected technology and technical support expenses; and (5) ongoing upgrades or operational expenses.

Faculty and Student Support and Commitment

Faculty support and commitment, as well as student support and commitment, are collateral development areas needed to enhance the knowledge, skills, and buy-in for learning within a technological learning environment. Initial faculty skills in using the selected technology will be varied. Planning for faculty and student professional development skills will result in significantly improved skills within a short time period. Students' exposure to the distance videoconferencing includes an orientation to guide the learners' acceptance of the technology and for the appropriate learning style. Students must be cautioned that their every move or comment may be broadcast to more than one location at any given moment.

Program Competencies

The next steps of this strategy involve thorough planning of the learning needs and competencies. The educational program should continue to remain the key focus of the designed distance educational experience. Targeted learning competencies are based on professional standards and the learning styles of the learners. The importance of determining the learning needs continues to be the primary focus. The targeted learning outcomes of any healthcare profession should remain the same regardless of the selected instructional methods or the selected technology. Instructional and technological teaching methods are selected to accomplish the required learning outcomes and meet the needs of the learners. It is important to assess the learning style characteristics of the students. Learning outcomes are not selected to accommodate the available technologies. For an example, what would a client education program for clients with cancer require? The learning needs are identified first, and then the instructor can design methods that would provide the required information to the learners and the future clients.

Curriculum Design

The selected curriculum design will remain constant for the required educational experiences for a curriculum taught by using technology or traditional curriculum design methods. Both areas require organized and planned educational experiences that are guided to promote lifelong learning, as well as individually motivational and experiential learning activities that involve a variety of experiential teaching methods.

Selected Technology

The selected technology is identified to best meet the learners' needs. Too often instructors are pressured to use technology that is more cost-effective or available. It is inappropriate to select technology based on availability or the bells and whistles the selection offers. The technology selection should be guided by sound instructional design choices that optimally facilitate the desired knowledge, skills, values, and interaction needed for competency and lifelong learning needs. The model proposed in this chapter requires an interactive relationship between curriculum design, instructional design, technology selection, and the financial implications (Boettcher, 2000).

Commitment

Many institutions embark on distance education without first analyzing the impact on the teaching, the faculty, and the learners. The financial impact of the administration and the control of intellectual property are also serious synchronous learning issues. The eagerness to join the technology marketplace has resulted in distance education disasters (Oblinger & Kidwell, 2000). A need for new higher learning administrative strategies and polices that embrace change but also creates an organizational plan that anticipates consequences is needed. The level of faculty, student, and administrative commitment is a good predictor of distance education success. Guidelines are available to assist the instructor in making the decision whether to enter into the distance education arena. Educators need to respond to several issues before getting started in distance education, including the following:

1. How does one get started? For example, clarify the needed infrastructure of support and needed financial resources. Conduct a needs assessment to determine the number of potential learners. Determine what type of distance program is needed. Determine if the need is for entry healthcare professions, postprofessional education, or client and family centered care. Determine the available technology and the learning needs of the faculty and learners. Critically analyze university support of the quality of the offered technology and support systems. Determine if the fac-

ulty and adjunct healthcare providers would accept the distance learning concept and be prepared for technology mastery.

2. Assume the role of devil's advocate and identify any potential barriers to successful implementation. For an example, technological errors or down time interfere with the teaching-learning flow. Determine how faculty would assist learners to recapture the lost teaching-learning interaction for the needed learning competencies. Identify workload issues when teaching using distance methods. Published opinions vary on the amount of extra time required for teaching using distance methods, but there is consistency in that distance teaching requires more instructor time. Critically analyze if the faculty want to participate in distant teaching. Faculty views could influence the learning process and the potential outcomes. Recognize that some faculty may experience degrees of technology discomfort. Discontentment with actual face-to-face student interaction also may be a concern. Faculty and administrators need to address these perceptions or concerns before starting a distance education program. Opponents of distance education question the loss of valuing the traditional teaching process. Many earlier publications revealed that educators feared the use of distance education as a job threat. Once the instructors engage in distance education, they are comforted that the role of the instructor is paramount to distance education success (Hilgenberg & Tolone, 2000). It is important to identify the potential barriers or threats to success and work with faculty to jointly pose effective strategies to resolve the potential barriers to success.

3. Preparation of successful distance education strategies requires the faculty and administration to jointly identify the strengths and weaknesses of initiating distance education. Action plans should be developed to jointly plan for success. Identification of the needed development and resources should be planned for with targeted timelines. The faculty will need to develop a level of expertise in instructional technology and implementation strategies. Faculty will require more time to design these needed experiential learning materials and activities. Faculty will need support to stay abreast of frequent technology advances (Martin, 2005).

Healthcare educators must carefully address the aforementioned identified needs and suggested strategies. Valuing the use of technology and synchronous distance education will be essential to successful application. Faculty should identify potential barriers and plan professional development and alternative solutions to resolve potential issues (Boaz, Foshee, Hardy, Jarmon, & Olcott, 1999; Dupin-Bryant, 2004).

POTENTIAL PROBLEMS

There are negative impacts on learning outcomes when the audio or video transmission is poor. The potential disruption needs to be anticipated with backup instructional plans to ensure student learning. Clear interaction and communication is required for effective professional learning. The literature clearly states technology problems directly contribute to poor learning outcomes (Hilgenberg & Tolone, 2000). Interruptions in audio and video have severe consequences for the learning environment for the transmission and remote learning sites (Anderson et al., 2003).

Experiential learning and interactivity are basic distance education requirements. If these events do not occur, the students at the remote site often disengage as they feel they are watching television. The lack of interaction results in poorer learning outcomes. The instructor must make assertive efforts to keep the students at the remote site engaged and promote active participation with meaningful learning activities. Initial assessment of the learning styles of the students is helpful in planning meaningful learning experiences.

The interaction between campuses should be positive and interactive. Faculty should role model the needed level of support and connection between the various learning sites. Students should be aware that casual conversations during class or break will be broadcast. It is important that the faculty member present equal interaction for all learning sites. Student expectations and faculty support should be equal. It is important to avoid any tendency to respond to questions that are not open to all learners and all campuses. All learners should be included and feel valued.

Faculty need to be proficient with the technology and to be aware of projection expectations such as the size of the font used in PowerPoint presentations or the use of demonstrations that may be easily viewed by all students. Avoid the use of projected web sites that are not easily viewed by all students.

New faculty will need to be coached in the most effective methods for distance teaching and for the most effective use of the technology. Knowledge of potential pitfalls help new faculty members to minimize the negative impact of these issues.

CONCLUSION

A profusion of studies provide arguments both for and against distance education. The dichotomy of opinions is due to the complexity of variables that contribute to a successful distance education experience. Earlier studies focused on learner outcomes and satisfaction rates. Numerous studies indicated the overall outcomes were comparable to traditional educational methods if the instruction considers learning style, interactivity, and the quality of communication and experiences. Student learning styles and motivation do have an effect on overall success. If learning preferences are effectively considered, the learning outcomes have been comparable to traditional education methods. Factors contributing to failures are the quality of the technology and the support personnel. Most studies have examined if distance education is as effective as traditional education. If the instructor meets the expected learning considerations such as organization, interactivity, effective communication, and experiential learning, the outcomes are comparable. Distance students prefer organization, experiential learning, and interaction with the instructor. Selection of the appropriate technology methods should consider the needed program competencies and learner characteristics. Technology should be suitable for the learning needs of health profession students. The quality of the technology support is critical to the students' learning and the overall success of the distance education program (Anderson et al., 2003).

APPLIED EXAMPLE

The Medical College of Georgia's department of occupational therapy offers a distance education program that includes two campuses. The model of implementation for using video over Internet protocol included a meeting of academic, technology, and operational personnel to identify the needs for transitioning and implementation. Key issues were identified to ensure seamless teaching-learning outcomes prior to implementation of the new technology. The technology will be used to project learning to 108 occupational therapy (OT) students. The institution and university system has made financial commitments to upgrade the technology prior to implementation (thus meeting the administrative and financial support prerequisite discussed earlier). Faculty have all attended a professional development seminar related to the new technology and brainstormed the developmental skills needed to use the technology appropriately. The faculty team leader designed some teaching vignettes to illustrate how the technology could be used. The faculty held an orientation for enrolled students to cover the changes and guidelines for success once the new technology would be demonstrated. The new Internet protocol was implemented gradually so that all glitches could be worked out before the older technology was phased out (it had faculty and student support and commitment).

A special academic affairs committee critically analyzed the implementation of the new technology and examined the program competencies to ensure the teaching-learning process remained the focal point of teaching. The profession's standards were reviewed, and the competencies and targeted outcomes were updated to ensure accreditation standards. Benchmarks for technology, learning, and faculty and student outcomes were developed to ensure success from student, faculty, and administrative perspectives (program competencies were reinforced).

The curriculum design remained constant for the required teaching-learning experiences as the educational experiences were the most important outcomes. Faculty mentors were assigned to faculty with less than optimal results to enhance the teaching-learning outcomes. It was noted that faculty who were structured and organized and proficient in the technology received the best student ratings for teaching-learning effectiveness. Faculty mentorships help all new faculty be successful in teaching using the technology. Mentorships and faculty development were also provided related to the planning of the educational experiences. Efforts are made to make the students be active and self-motivated to engage in the learning activities. Experiential teaching methods, such as case-based learning, video analysis of real clients and their families, and client simulations are implemented and used (curriculum design takes place).

Faculty felt pressured to move to the new technology, so a team of participants from academia, administration, and the technological departments were formed to troubleshoot any potential problems. A collaborative team effort was adopted by all groups in order to provide proactive communication, troubleshooting, and sound interaction between the curriculum design, instructional implementation, and the selected technology. The collaborative team interaction is a process, not an event, so the communication is ongoing strategy (selected technology is identified).

As a part of the distance education process, all parties (students, faculty, administrators, and technicians) need to remain committed to the process. Benchmarks are established to critically analyze the impact on the teaching, the faculty, and the learners. The financial impact of the administration and the control of intellectual property is examined each semester. Administrative decision-making policies are to be established to critically examine the distance education success. Annually, the team conducts a strengths, weaknesses, opportunities and threats (SWOT) analysis to determine future distance education needs. The team develops an annual strategic plan to ensure distance education success. The process requires the faculty and administration to jointly identify methods to implement a successful distance education process (they have made a commitment).

REFERENCES

Anderson, R., Beavers, J., VanDeGrift, T., & Videon, F. (2003, November 5–8). *Videoconferencing and presentation support for synchronous distance learning.* 33rd ASEE/IEEE Frontiers in Education Conference. Boulder, CO, pp. 1–6.

Bertrand, Y. (1995). *Contemporary theories and practice in education.* Madison, WI: Atwood Publishing.

Boaz, M., Foshee, B., Hardy, D., Jarmon, C., & Olcott, D., Jr. (1999). *Teaching at a distance: A handbook for instructors.* Monterey, CA: Archipelago Productions.

Boettcher, J. V. (2000). The state of distance education in the United States: Surprising realities. *Syllabus: New Directions in Educational Technology, 13*(7), 36–40.

Byers, D. L., Jr., Hilgenberg, C., & Rhodes, D. M. (2003). Telemedicine for patient education. In M. Moore & J. J. Savrock (Eds.), *Distance Education in the Health Sciences, 8,* 135–147.

Dupin-Bryant, P. A. (2004, March). Teaching styles of interactive television instructors: A descriptive study. *American Journal of Distance Education, 18*(1), 39–50.

Ely, D. (2000). Looking before we leap—Prior questions for distance education planners. *Syllabus: New Directions in Educational Technology, 13*(10), 26–28.

Fitzpatrick, R. (2001). *Is distance education better than traditional classroom?* Retrieved February 28, 2006, from http://www.clearpnt.com/accelepoint/articles/r_fitzpatrick_060101.html

Gallagher, J. E., Dobrosielski-Vergona, K. A., Wingard, R. G., & Williams, T. M. (2005). Web-based vs. traditional classroom instruction in gerontology: A pilot study. *Journal of Dental Hygiene, 79*(3), 1–10.

Greene, B., & Meek, A. (1998). Distance education in higher education institutions: Incidence, audiences, and plans to expand. *Issue Brief. National Center for Education Statistics* (Report No. NCES-98-132). Washington, DC: National Center for Education.

Grimes, E. B. (2002). Use of distance education in dental hygiene. *Journal of Dental Education, 66,* 1136–1145.

Hilgenberg, C., & Tolone, W. (2000). Student perceptions of satisfaction and opportunities for critical thinking in distance education by interactive video. *American Journal of Distance Education, 14*(3), 59–73.

Keller, C. (2005). Virtual learning environments: Three implementation perspectives. *Learning, Media, & Technology, 30*(3), 299–311.

Martin, M. (2005). Seeing is believing: The role of videoconferencing in distance learning. *British Journal of Education Technology, 36*(3), 39–50.

McKissack, C. E. (1997). *A comparative study of grade point average (GPA) between the students in traditional classroom setting and the distance learning classroom setting in selected colleges and universities.* Unpublished doctoral dissertation, Tennessee State University.

Miller, W., & King-Webster, Jill. (1997). *A comparison of interactive needs and performance of distance learners in synchronous and asynchronous classes.* Las Vegas, NV: American Vocational Association.

Mills, O. F., Bates, J. F., Pendleton, V., Lese, K., & Tatarko, M. (2001). Distance education by interactive videoconferencing in a family practice residency center. *Distance Education Online Symposium News, 11.* Retrieved August 12, 2006, from http://www.ed.psu.edu/acsde/deos/deosnews/deosnews11_7.asp

National Education Association. (2000, June 13). Quality online: Maintaining standards in the distance education course. In *Syllabus: New Directions in Education Technology,* (10), 10.

Oblinger, D., & Kidwell, J. (2000). Distance learning: Are we being realistic? *Syllabus, 13*(7), 31–38.

Prégent, R. (1994). *Charting your course: How to prepare to teach more effectively* (M. Parker, Trans.). Madison, WI: Magna Publications.

Romiszowski, A. J. (1986). *Developing auto-instructional materials: From programmed texts to CAL and interactive video.* London, New York: Nickols Publishing.

Saba, F. (2005, October). *Critical issues in distance education: A report from the United States Department of Education, 26*(2), 255–272.

Sherry, L. (1996). Issues in distance learning. *International Journal of Educational Telecommunications, 1*(4), 337–365.

Tucker, S. (2001). Distance education: Better, worse, or as good as traditional education? *Online Journal of Distance Education Administration, 4*(4), pp. 1–13. Retrieved February 26, 2006, from http://www.westga.edu/~distance/ojda/winter44/tucker44.html

Von Bertalanffy, L. (1998). *General system theory: Foundations, development, applications.* New York: Braziller.

White, C. (2005, October). Contribution of distance education to the development of individual learners. *Distance Education, 26*(2), 165–181.

CHAPTER 20

Web-Based Instruction

Judith Schurr Salzer

INTRODUCTION

Rapidly evolving technology, in combination with the explosion in medical information and knowledge, has increased the use of web-based teaching and learning during the past decade. Today's students in healthcare professions require fast access to the most current information on which to base their critical thinking and to apply evidence-based practice. Web-based instruction provides a variety of educational tools to broaden the scope of learning experiences and prepare students to function optimally in a technologically rich healthcare environment.

DEFINITION AND PURPOSE

As transition from the Industrial Age to the Information Age continues, the Internet offers educators an increasing range of teaching options. Courses may be developed that are totally web-based asynchronous (no face-to-face or real-time interaction), totally web-based synchronous (no face-to-face interaction with class meetings online in real time), partially web-based with some face-to-face meetings either in a single classroom or multiple classrooms using distance technology (with asynchronous or synchronous online interaction), or traditional with supplemental web-based components (e-mail, forums, chat rooms, class content). During the 2001 to 2002 academic year, 55% of all 2- and 4-year institutions offered credit-granting distance education with 90% of these offering asynchronous computer-based courses. Eighty-eight percent of institutions offering or planning to offer distance education planned to begin using or increase use of asynchronous computer-based Internet instruction as the main means of delivering distance education courses (Waits & Lewis, 2003). Although virtual colleges, which exist only in cyberspace, are increasing in number and gaining acceptance as a credible means of obtaining a degree, research indicates that employers continue to prefer applicants with traditional degrees (Adams & DeFleur, 2005). Online degrees from traditional colleges and universities are less controversial, perhaps because it is often difficult to ascertain whether a program was attended on-campus or online.

Rather than being used as an all or none strategy, the Internet is often integrated into courses as one of many teaching strategies as educators transition pedagogy from face-to-face to online delivery. Research and documented experience are providing increasing evidence that web-based instruction is applicable to a wide variety of students and subject matter including courses with clinical components or skill acquisition. As the rapid evolution of technological innovations continues, educators will be challenged to incorporate ever-new technologies into their instruction while developing pedagogically sound instructional strategies.

THEORETICAL FOUNDATIONS

Web-based instruction is the newest addition to a variety of distance education tools. Distance education began with correspondence courses and video tapes, then CD-ROM, and evolved to include two-way video with two-way audio and asynchronous or synchronous computer-based Internet instruction. Today, many courses and programs use multiple delivery systems such as combining asynchronous computer-based Internet instruction for delivery of didactic content with two-way video/audio for seminar discussions. Although technology has advanced to the point where personal computers support web-based education to most individuals with computer and Internet access, the pace of technological advancement requires frequent updating of equipment, and individuals limited to dial-up Internet access currently experience serious disadvantages.

As with any innovation, use of the Internet for educational instruction has had early adopters, late adopters, proponents, and detractors. Teaching online is different from traditional teaching and requires a paradigm shift. In online teaching, a shift occurs from instructor-focused to student-focused (Chaffin & Maddux, 2004), in which the authority figure instructor becomes instead a facilitator of student learning (Ryan, Hodson-Carlton, & Ali, 2005). This shift requires motivated instructors who are innovative, creative, and willing to learn new teaching methods by trial and error.

Published research is increasingly available to document faculty and student perceptions of online learning and effectiveness of online teaching. Ali, Hodson-Carlton, and Ryan (2004) investigated graduate students' perceptions of learning online. Students found online learning convenient and asynchronous discussions an effective means of communication. Timely faculty feedback was considered crucial. However, undergraduate and graduate students' perceptions may differ. Although undergraduate and graduate students were equally satisfied with online learning and equally willing to assume responsibility for their learning, undergraduate students felt more connected to instructors and classmates (Billings, Skiba, & Connors, 2005). Students' native language, gender, and prior computer experience do not appear to have an effect on their academic achievement or course satisfaction in an online setting (Barakzai & Fraser, 2005). Similarly, faculty find web-based courses to be equal to or better than traditional courses in flexibility and student participation (Johnson, Posey, & Simmens, 2005). Anecdotal descriptions of successful web-based courses range in content from critical care (Jeffries, 2005), health assessment (Lashley, 2005), and epidemiology (Suen, 2005) to methods of validating critical thinking skills (Ali, Bantz, & Siktberg, 2005).

Although the use of web-based education will continue to expand in the future, a number of pragmatic issues have yet to be resolved. Online course development and teaching are more time-consuming than traditional instruction. Many institutions fail to provide faculty with adequate time to learn the required technology and develop courses for online delivery, resulting in workloads that do not accurately reflect the time commitment required. As a result, significant disincentives currently exist for many faculty members to teach web-based courses.

Some educators continue to be intimidated by rapid technologic advances in web-based educational applications. However, the impact of the Internet on all courses and health professionals cannot be ignored. Students have quick and ready access to the most current information on the Internet and are increasingly expecting instructors and courses to be dynamic and interactive. In addition, computer literacy and Internet skills are now essential for survival in today's workplace and a vehicle to lifelong learning. As a result, educators are recognizing that the traditional delivery system is only one of many varied ways of learning (Draves, 2000).

TYPES OF LEARNERS

Student age, gender, or computer skills should not be deciding factors in determining whether web-based courses are appropriate for an individual (Barakzai & Fraser, 2005). Instead, an individual's cognitive style is key to predicting successful academic achievement in an online environment. Individuals categorize and manage information in varying ways. Those with a field-dependent learning style who prefer a more social learning environment in which they are taught content are likely to do less well in a web-based environment than those with a field-independent learning style who enjoy conceptual challenges and are less dependent on face-to-face social interaction (see Chapter 1, "Effective Learning: What Teachers Need to Know"). Classes may also be composed of a mix of non-traditional adult and traditional young adult learners who have differing motivations, purposes, and intellectual skills (Neal, 1999). Participation in web-based learning requires students to be self-directed and able to function in an environment with limited or no face-to-face faculty and peer interaction. Students must also possess basic computer skills and have some degree of comfort operating in a computer-based environment (Murphree, 1999).

Before electing to pursue web-based courses, students should assess whether their readiness and learning style are compatible with an online environment. Many self-assessment tools are now available through online organizations and schools offering web-based educational options. After completing the questionnaire, students receive feedback with an assessment of their probability of success in a web-based course. A sample of self-assessment tool web sites is provided at the end of this chapter.

When students register for a web-based or enhanced course, their technology skills and knowledge of Internet navigation should be assessed before class begins. A short preparatory class for those lacking required skills is needed, as well as a class for all students on navigating the institution's online library resources. The lack of adequate knowledge and skills in online navigation can prevent even the most motivated student from taking control of his or her own learning.

CONDITIONS FOR LEARNING

Variations of web-based instruction integration into courses continue to evolve and gain in popularity. Although fundamental principles of good teaching and learning are applied in web-based courses, a paradigm shift is required. Teaching online is simply not the same as teaching in person. The instructor is no longer the authority figure providing new information in a passive setting, but rather is a facilitator of learning in a dynamic, interactive environment (Chaffin & Maddux, 2004). This paradigm shift involves faculty learning new pedagogies and adjusting their roles to ones that require "high energy levels and creativity" (Ryan et al., 2005, p. 361). Further, faculty members often need to develop new skill sets, including the use of new technology and incorporating it into teaching.

Specific elements of web-based instruction may be integrated into courses to enhance the learning process depending on the level of the course, course content, and instructor's experience with technology and web-based instruction. Commonly, courses transition to a web-based format over time as instructor comfort and experience increases. A traditional course may begin its transformation to becoming web-based through the addition of an online syllabus, content outlines, and communication tools such as a bulletin board for posting announcements. Over time, content may be delivered online, replacing some face-to-face classes, and asynchronous and/or synchronous communication tools may be used for class discussions and answering content questions. Instructors may transition their courses to be completely web-based or may find some combination that works best for them such as maintaining face-to-face interaction through monthly seminar discussions.

At the other end of the spectrum, entire programs and schools exist only on the Internet with faculty located all over the country or globe. Some schools are actually virtual, with no brick and mortar existence. Web-based degree-granting programs span the range from offering little interaction with faculty, a do-it-yourself type of program, to frequent faculty communication and specific, concentrated on-campus requirements.

It is impossible to say with certainty where the trend toward web-based instruction will lead with the rapid development of new technology, but using the Internet to teach and learn is clearly here to stay. Although some may continue to prefer traditional teaching methods, it appears likely that this mode of instruction may soon become outdated. As instructors become increasingly creative in their online teaching, incorporating new technologies as they develop, there appear to be few limitations to the development of web-based global education.

RESOURCES

Any instructor with a computer and Internet access is able to add several helpful online components to courses. Instructor web pages with links to course-related material may be created by novice computer users with specialized software. Free software is available for download to provide chat rooms for synchronous student discussions, and new applications are under continuous development. More commonly, institutions provide a platform for online courses, which is often maintained on a server separate from the institution's main server. The platform provides course components that each instructor selects to include in a course template. Course content, links, communication tools, articles, videos, or other features may be loaded directly into the course template.

Courses that are developed and managed online require institutional support in the form of equipment (hardware and software), services, and faculty time and recognition. The infrastructure is expensive to establish and maintain. Faculty members require up-to-date computers, supporting software, and Internet access. A server and educational platform must be purchased and regularly updated with security maintained. An expert staff specializing in using and maintaining the environment must be trained, updated, and available to students and faculty at all times. Faculty training on course development incorporating various teaching strategies in the online environment is essential. In addition, best practices and innovations in technology and the online environment must be communicated to faculty through periodic professional development.

Because not all faculty members adapt to the technical environment at the same pace, support and mentoring groups help those who may be overwhelmed or intimidated by the technology. Support groups also provide a forum for sharing implementation experiences and problem-solving strategies.

Institutional administrative support is required for faculty release time to develop online courses. Administrators must understand that an online course with faculty-student interaction requires a lower student-to-faculty ratio than a traditional course. Monitoring and guiding online communication among class members, in addition to direct faculty-to-student communication, requires a significant faculty time commitment. Institutions that commit resources to support online course delivery will likely require faculty to effectively use the resources provided. However, administrative policies for merit and tenure need to be adjusted to recognize the knowledge, skills, and time required to develop and teach courses in an online environment.

In addition to student course evaluations, a process for peer review of web-based courses assists faculty to continuously improve their online courses. Excellent evaluation tools for web-based courses are available online. Increasingly, institutions are developing their own evaluation criteria for online courses based on national criteria. A variety of free online newsletters is also available to inform instructors of best practices, new innovations, and methods of problem solving. Local, regional, and national conferences on web-based teaching and learning enable faculty to network with others teaching online, share best practices, and evaluate new innovations.

USING THE METHOD

This discussion focuses on the practical integration of web-based instruction into traditional courses, one of the most common applications of online instruction and often the first phase of transitioning courses to fully web-based instruction. Regardless of the format, any course must be carefully planned, including identifying which online components will enhance the teaching and learning environment and considering students' varying learning styles. During course development, instructors must keep in mind that online tools themselves do not improve teaching or learning. A tool's effectiveness is determined by the manner in which it is integrated to support course objectives and learning outcomes and to create a community of learners (Funaro & Montell, 1999).

Web-based tools generally impact communication through the transmission of information or by enabling two-way communication. Information may be transmitted to students by posting the syllabus, class outlines, or other resource information to be electronically accessed by the student at a convenient time. Chat rooms, e-mail, electronic bulletin boards, forums, and quizzes provide means for two-way electronic "talking" between instructor and students and/or among classmates. Faculty members should become comfortable with using new tools prior to their implementation and should provide students with an orientation to the technology, new tools, and expectations for their use.

Although basic information transmission may be accomplished through instructors' personal web pages created on the world wide web, tools available in commercial structured learning environments provide a standardized system for transmission of specific types of information. Information paths and pages enable instructors to provide the full syllabus, class content outlines, Power-Point presentations with audio voiceover or video lectures, and link directly to online content, web sites or virtual demonstrations (e.g., heart sounds).

In courses delivering content online, course material should be divided by topic into 5 to 10 modules, with each module being a separate component of the course. Objectives, competencies, and outcomes are developed for each module (Draves, 2000). Module content is divided into lessons which are chunks of information of less than 10 minutes in length (slide shows, videos, online lectures). Content outlines to guide study may be printed by students. Self-quizzes and other learning exercises provide students with activities to reinforce learning and meet the needs of students with varying learning styles. Free, downloadable software is available to easily create crossword puzzles, matching, and multiple choice activities.

Pages created for faculty and student profiles help class members get to know each other and course faculty in courses that are completely web based or with limited face-to-face contact. Management tools enable instructors to track students' hits and identify students who may be falling behind. Students may track their grades and view statistics on each test or assignment, such as the class grade range, median, and mode. A calendar tool may be used by both instructors and students. Information about class schedules or content may be posted by instructors. Students may post clinical activities for instructor review or personal schedules that can be made visible only to the posting student. Posting and viewing slide shows and videos are generally supported by current technology except in areas with dial-up-only Internet access. New user-friendly tools that are continuously under development are incorporated into frequent updates of commercial structured learning environments.

Online interactivity is essential for a web-based course to promote student achievement and satisfaction. Two-way synchronous or asynchronous communication is facilitated by e-mail, bulletin boards, forums, chat rooms, and quizzes. Because student access to the tools is available 24 hours a day, 7 days a week, faculty members must inform students of the limits established for faculty input.

Some faculty members prefer to use the tools only during the traditional work week, whereas others also check in during evenings and weekends. The more often faculty communicate with students, the more often students will take advantage of the communication tool. Fast response and feedback from instructors is commonly cited by students as an advantage of web-based courses. Slow response and limited interaction from faculty results in low satisfaction and poor course evaluations. Some faculty hold office hours in chat rooms on a regular basis, enabling students to "drop in" to discuss content, ask questions, or "talk" about the course in a synchronous online environment. Although a high level of interaction is essential in an online environment, it requires a greater than usual faculty time commitment.

E-mail is familiar to most faculty and students. Either personal e-mail accounts or e-mail embedded in commercial structured learning environments may be used for asynchronous one-to-one communication. E-mail embedded in commercial structured learning environments may be used to communicate only with course faculty and those students who are registered in the course. Faculty members may send the same message to all class members or communicate with individual students. Students may provide information, clarify content, or ask questions directly of the instructor. Successful use of e-mail requires an agreement among users on the frequency of checking for messages. More frequent checking results in greater interaction.

Electronic bulletin boards are used by instructors and students to post messages to the entire class. Similar to a bulletin board, a forum provides for asynchronous communication among members of a designated group. In large classes, forums provide for more productive conversation among students in smaller groups. Forums may be used by students to work through an assigned discussion question between scheduled classes. Forum discussions may be monitored by instructors for both content and student participation. Instructor comments provide positive feedback to the group, redirect the discussion, or suggest resources. Students have the opportunity to think about their answers or to do some reading prior to posting comments. **Figures 20-1** and **20-2** demonstrate a student-initiated, faculty-monitored forum discussion. Again, expectations and rules must be communicated to students to avoid rambling pages that lack substance. The expected content and minimum number of postings per student need to be clearly stated and understood by students. Postings may be graded using a grading rubric, counted as class participation, or used as a critical-thinking exercise.

Real-time synchronous conversations can be conducted in chat rooms that are commercially available for free download or within a commercial structured learning environment. Use of a chat room requires setting a date and time to "meet" in a designated room. Student groups may use chat rooms to discuss projects or class content. Instructors may meet with small groups of students for topical discussions, to discuss problems, or to clarify content between scheduled

Figure 20-1   Forum listing on bulletin board.

Interesting case [Forum: Group 1]
- ☐   144. Kathy Benton (Thu, Mar. 2, 2000, 16:40)
  - ☐   145. Instructor (Thu, Mar. 2, 2000, 20:40)
  - ☐   146. Annie Freund (Sat, Mar. 4, 2000, 15:24)
    - ☐   147. Instructor (Sun, Mar. 5, 2000, 12:32)
      - ☐   148. Donna Rider (Sun, Mar. 5, 2000, 13:38)
      - ☐   149. Annie Freund (Sun, Mar. 5, 2000, 14:03)
  - ☐   150. Kathy Benton (Sun, Mar. 5, 2000, 16:18)
    - ☐   151. Instructor (Mon, Mar. 6, 2000, 08:45)

Figure 20-2   Forum dialog under Figure 20-1 forum listing.

Subject: Interesting Case
[Prev Thread] [Next Thread]

[Prev Thread] [Next Thread]
Article No. 144: posted by Kathy Benton on Thu, Mar. 2, 2000, 16:40

I saw something this week that I haven't seen before and wanted to ask you guys about it. I saw a 3-year-old who we diagnosed with a right otitis media. She presented with serosanguineous drainage from the ear, but she did not have myringotomy tubes. She did have a perforated ear drum. We treated her with Floxin 6 drops twice a day and amoxicillin by mouth. I have not looked at the literature yet, but I wanted to know if you guys have seen this presentation of otitis media and how you treated it. Kathy

[Prev Thread] [Next Thread]
Article No. 145: [Branch from no. 144] posted by Instructor on Thu, Mar. 2, 2000, 20:40

What was the history on this child? Did she have upper respiratory infection symptoms, ear pain, fever? What dose of amoxicillin did you use? Prof. Sanders

[Prev Thread] [Next Thread]
Article No. 146: [Branch from no. 144] posted by Annie Freund on Sat, Mar. 4, 2000, 15:24

I saw a similar case this week. The child presented with bloody ear drainage and was diagnosed with acute otitis media with perforation. We treated the child with amoxicillin and Floxin. I haven't had a chance to look at the literature yet, but will let you know if I find anything. Annie

(continues)

Figure 20-2   Forum dialog under Figure 20-1 forum listing (*continued*).

[Prev Thread] [Next Thread]
Article No. 147: [Branch from no. 146] posted by Instructor on Sun, Mar. 5, 2000, 12:32

It's interesting that each of you have seen this since it is not that common. Makes me wonder if there is an unusual underlying cause like a virus. What was the age of your patient, Annie? What other symptoms did she have? Prof. Sanders

[Prev Thread] [Next Thread]
Article No. 148: [Branch from no. 147] posted by Donna Rider on Sun, Mar. 5, 2000, 13:38

Dr. Patton saw a child this week whose mother reported seeing bloody drainage on the sheet when they got up in the morning. The mom described the drainage as a quarter-sized amount or slightly more, and she said she thought it came from his ear. On exam there was no evidence of ruptured ear drum. One tympanic membrane was slightly hazy, but the other was normal appearing. We did not find any evidence of bleeding from the nose, mouth, etc. We did not diagnose as a ruptured tympanic membrane. Kathy, what did the tympanic membranes look like on exam? Donna

[Prev Thread] [Next Thread]
Article No. 149: [Branch from no. 147] posted by Annie Freund on Sun, Mar. 5, 2000, 14:03

The child was 20 months and has had 2 previous episodes of otitis media this winter. She also attends daycare. She is the first case like this I have seen and I thought it was unusual. Annie

[Prev Thread] [Next Thread]
Article No. 150: [Branch from no. 144] posted by Kathy Benton on Sun, Mar. 5, 2000, 16:18

I found a good article online in Contemporary Pediatrics, May 1999. You can access it from www.contpeds.com and go to past issues. Kathy

[Prev Thread] [Next Thread]
Article No. 151: [Branch from no. 150] posted by Instructor on Mon, Mar. 6, 2000, 08:45

Good. Sounds like we need to discuss this further this week. Please see what else you can find in the current literature and bring the references to seminar. Also, make sure you have the relevant history and physical findings of children you have seen with ear drainage. See you Wednesday. Prof. Sanders class meetings. Some chat rooms permit the instructor or all participants to print conversations out at the completion of the chat session. A printed record of the discussion and action agreed upon is helpful to both instructors and students.

Online testing is widely available, often with immediate grading and student feedback. Although essay questions generally require hand-grading at this time, programs for computer grading are under development. Quiz-type tools in commercial structured learning environments have several uses. Self-administered quizzes with immediate feedback aid students' study of online content. Graded tests assess students' knowledge throughout the course. In addition, a quiz tool may be used as another form of asynchronous communication. Open-ended questions provide a framework for students' clinical journal entries or notes and provide for timely instructor-to-student feedback. At the same time, students' clinical progress may be closely monitored to identify student problems and provide for early intervention (see **Figure 20-3** and **Figure 20-4**).

Figure 20-3   Sample SOAP note using quiz tool construction.

Question 1: Enter complete, concise subjective information.

Student Response:

A 21-month-old female comes to clinic today for a sick visit accompanied by her mother. Child has had a fever, runny nose, and cough. The fever has been for 2 days up to 102 axillary. She has had a cough that sounds "hacky" for about 3 days, and she has had a runny nose for about 1 week. Her appetite has been decreased, but she is drinking okay. She has had 6 oz. of juice and 6 oz. of milk today. Her elimination pattern is normal. She has had 3 wet diapers already today. Her activity level has been decreased, and mom thinks that she is sleeping more than usual. Her cough is waking her up some at night, but then she goes right back to sleep. She has not had any vomiting or diarrhea. She is in a small daycare with 4 other kids, and mom does not think that she has had any illness exposures. She has not been to daycare in 2 days. The only medicine she has had is acetaminophen for the fever, and it has brought the temperature down, but after it wears off it goes back up. The last dose of acetaminophen was 3 hours ago. Dad smokes in the house.

Comments:

Allergies? Acetaminophen dose? The progression of this illness would be easier to follow if you begin at the beginning: child was well until 1 week ago when she began having a runny nose. Hacky cough began 3 days ago and fever up to 102 axillary began 2 days ago. Add in when her decreased eating, decreased activity level, and increased sleeping began. Work on being more concise.

(continues)

Figure 20-3   Sample SOAP note using quiz tool construction (*continued*).

Question 2: Enter pertinent objective information.

Student Response:

Weight—29 lbs. Temperature—100.8 tympanic
General—ill appearing but in no acute distress; quiet and cooperative for exam
HEENT—normocephalic; sclera clear, conjunctiva pink, right tympanic membrane slightly injected with good light reflex, clear landmarks, good mobility; left
tympanic membrane slightly injected with good light reflex, sharp landmarks,
good mobility; nares patent, turbinates erythematous with purulent white
drainage; pharynx clear, tonsils +2 with no erythema or edema; mucoid post
nasal discharge
Mouth—mucous membranes pink and moist, lips dry
Cardiovascular—clear S1, S2, without murmur; capillary refill brisk, peripheral
pulses strong and equal
Lungs—coarse breath sounds bilateral; crackles in lower lobes bilateral, posterior >
anterior; no wheezing or retracting; respirations even, unlabored, rate 28; no grunting
Abdomen—soft, nontender, no masses or hepatosplenomegaly
Genital—normal external female genitalia without discharge or rash
Skin—warm, dry, without rash, good turgor
Lymphs—shotty, nontender, posterior cervical nodes bilateral

Comments:

Was the white nasal discharge really purulent? Was it thick or thin?

Question 3: Enter your assessment with rationale.

Student Response:

Pneumonia—bilateral, likely viral
Rationale: According to the articles by Schidlow & Callahan and Churgay, crackles
and wheezes are sounds that indicate compromise of the lower respiratory tract.
Churgay's article pointed out that most pediatric pneumonias are viral in origin,
but a bacterial source should be considered because antibiotics would then be
crucial to the treatment plan. The articles I reviewed all indicated that children
with a bacterial pneumonia are usually sicker, in more respiratory distress, and
with higher fevers than those with viral pneumonia. After my reading, I have a
much better understanding of how to diagnose and differentiate pneumonia.

Comments:

Good job.

Question 4: Enter your plan with rationale.

Student Response:

My preceptor obtained a chest X-ray that showed patches of consolidation and
admitted the child for treatment of pneumonia. After my reading, I would not

Figure 20-3   Sample SOAP note using quiz tool construction (*continued*).

have done this. Because the child was in no distress and appeared mildly ill, I'm not sure I would have obtained an X-ray. The articles indicated that pneumonia in young child is a clinical diagnosis because X-rays may be unreliable. In addition, obtaining an X-ray would not have changed my treatment for this child. My plan would have been:

1. Amoxicillin 400 mg/5 ml, 1 teaspoon by mouth twice a day (60 mg/kg/day)
2. Push oral fluids—juices, Gatorade
3. Cool air humidifier at night for the coughing—instruct mom on use and cleaning
4. Instruct mom on what signs to look for that would indicate the child was working hard to breathe—mom to call or go to emergency department if they occur
5. Discuss dangers of passive smoke exposure
6. Return in 48 hours if child is still running a fever > 101
7. Return in 3 days for follow-up

Rationale: Although 90 percent of childhood community-acquired pneumonias are viral, it is very difficult to distinguish them from the bacterial causes. Because of this, antibiotic therapy is usually given (James, 1999). Aside from viruses, streptococcus pneumoniae, staphylococcus aureus, H-flu, and group A strep are the main pathogens causing pneumonia. Streptococcus pneumoniae is by far the most common cause and can be treated with penicillin or erythromycin in those allergic to penicillin (James, 1999). I used amoxicillin because it can be given twice daily at 60–80 mg/kg/day, and it is generally well tolerated by children and is inexpensive.

Comments:

Good. Be specific when you ask parents to "push fluids." How much, how often? I would also have arranged to call the family the next day to see how the child has been doing since the visit. To implement your plan, you need to feel comfortable that the parents are capable of assessing the child accurately at home. In this case, it certainly sounds reasonable. I am not familiar with amoxicillin that comes 400 mg/5 ml. Please let me know what your reference is for this.

Question 5: What references did you use?

Student Response:

Churgay, C. (1996). The diagnosis and management of bacterial pneumonias in infants and children. *Primary Care: Clinics in Office Practices,* 23: 821–835.
Lassieur, S. M. & Jacobs, R. F. (1999). Pediatric pneumonia: Recognizing usual and unusual causes. *The Journal of Respiratory Diseases for Pediatricians,* 1: 42–50.
Latham-Sadler, B. & Morell, V. (1996). Pneumonia. *Pediatrics in Review,* 17: 300–310.

Comments:

You refer to an article by James (1999), but it is not listed in references. Please provide this reference. Nice job. I see much progress in your critical thinking on these cases.

Figure 20-4   Sample student weekly self-assessment using quiz tool construction.

Question 1: What are your strengths, weaknesses, and areas you need more experience in during your remaining clinical time?

Student Response:

I feel comfortable talking with parents and younger children. Parents seem to be responding to me by asking questions about their children and listening to what I have to say. I'm finally feeling like I know how to answer some of the questions. I'm not as comfortable with adolescents and have had limited experience dealing with them. Because we see few adolescents in this practice, is there somewhere I could get more experience with them?

Comments:

It is good when you start to feel like you know what you're doing! There is a teen clinic not far from you that we have used for students in the past. Let me see if they would be able to have you work with them for some of your clinical training. You can also ask around to see if there are other appropriate sites. Let me know if you find anything and I'll look into it.

Question 2: What problems have you encountered in the clinical setting that are obstacles to your learning? What can you do about them?

Student Response:

The only problem is that Dr. Towner is so busy at times that I don't get to ask him his rationale for a diagnosis or treatment. I don't feel that I can try to slow him down because there are so many patients to be seen. I'm not sure what to do.

Comments:

Have you thought about arranging for a routine, 15-minute meeting with Dr. Towner to ask your questions? Take a look at your day and see when 15 minutes might be convenient for him. Write your questions down and be very concise. Make sure you do not take more than the prearranged time. Keep me posted on what you decide to do.

Increasingly web-based courses are being developed for interdisciplinary use. Interdisciplinary online discussions of clinical or ethical case studies and virtual patient scenarios enable students to view issues from the perspectives of different professions. Students gain a greater appreciation for varying approaches and teamwork in problem solving.

POTENTIAL PROBLEMS

Although innovative and state-of-the-art, web-based instruction is not without problems and disadvantages for administrators, faculty, and students. Both faculty and students may be surprised by the increased time required in web-based courses. Students may not understand the increased responsibility for their own learning that is required in online courses and may believe that expectations are the same as in a traditional classroom (Ryan et al., 2005). As students assume more responsibility for their learning, faculty must relinquish some control of the learning process that they had in traditional courses and instead become facilitators of student learning. Since online course development is time consuming, faculty may be unpleasantly surprised to find that online courses need frequent updating, not only of content, but to incorporate new technology. Dynamic, ongoing interaction in an online environment is an advantage, but misunderstandings may easily occur when the written comments are interpreted differently than if the comments were spoken. Body language and voice inflections that contribute to interpretation are absent in the online environment.

The electronic environment poses several threats to courses dependent on web-based instruction. Electrical outages eliminate the ability of individuals in affected areas to participate in web-based courses, sometimes for extended periods. Users depend on ISPs for connection to the Internet, but ISPs vary in efficiency, reliability, and quality. As Internet users increase, access problems will increase as ISPs become overloaded. Users also depend on the efficient functioning of an institution's server for the commercial structured learning environment. When the server goes down or is undergoing maintenance, all coursework ceases. Security breaches through the invasion of courses by hackers could compromise student confidentiality or result in the modification or theft of course materials. Institutional firewalls must be continually updated and tested, and students should be advised to install a firewall on personal computers.

Administrators are faced with the expense of continuous maintenance and upgrading of servers, hardware, and software. Far from being a lucrative means of providing education, most institutions are finding that online courses are more expensive than traditional courses to develop and implement. Administrators initially anticipated that online instruction would enable faculty to teach larger classes and to positively impact the bottom line. The increased demand on faculty time arising from the ease of student-faculty online communication is beginning to be realized. Although web-based instruction provides many advantages and is able to reach students who would not otherwise be able to continue their education, administrators no longer consider web-based courses to be an extremely profitable venture in the short run.

Faculty members need to learn new technology skills and how to apply appropriate teaching strategies. High motivation and a willingness to invest time in the learning curve are required, but without the expectation of recognition or early reward. Developing online courses is teaching innovation that should be expected, respected, and rewarded, but in most institutions it is ignored as an important scholarly activity. Similarly, current intellectual policies for web-based materials are inconsistent and often do not allow for faculty ownership of online courseware (University of Illinois, 1999).

Courses with limited or no face-to-face meeting may lead some students to feel isolated and prevent them from developing the identity, cohesion, and rapport usually found in face-to-face classes (Funaro & Montell, 1999; Neal, 1999). Student isolation may also interfere with learning. Computer access is becoming less of a problem since many institutions now require students to have updated or new personal computers; however, high-speed DSL or cable Internet access might not be available to students in remote areas. Students limited to dial-up access may be prevented from full participation in a web-based course. The additional expense of a computer and Internet access may create an additional financial burden for students.

CONCLUSION

Adventurous educators are increasingly venturing into the realm of web-based instruction. Although clearly a trend that will continue into the future, the parameters and limits of web-based instruction are currently untested and unknown. Innovative educators must continue to document and share their experiences as they employ creative uses of the Internet in teaching and learning.

APPLIED EXAMPLE

Hybrid Teaching and Learning: Combining the Best of Both Worlds

Elizabeth Friedlander

The educator's challenge to help learners develop problem-solving and critical-thinking skills has never been greater. Changing societal expectations for educational preparedness, the increased pace of knowledge development and the subsequent need to stay abreast of new information, and the dynamic technological culture pose tremendous challenges and opportunities for today's educators, learners, and educational institutions (Morton, 1999). Educators must remain focused on the task of designing and evaluating learning environments that support the development of skills for lifelong learning (Driscoll,

2000). This involves a reexamination of all components of the traditional pedagogy, including curricular design, the role of the instructor and learner, and content delivery methods (Knowles, Holton, & Swanson, 1998).

Asynchronous online learning environments have the potential to support learning that is collaborative, problem based, and facilitates the development of lifelong learning skills (Palloff & Pratt, 1999). However, many faculty and learners continue to prefer traditional classroom learning to online learning. The most frequently cited reason is a strong preference for face-to-face learning (Charles & Mamary, 2002). In a recent study, nurses expressed a strong need for personal interaction with faculty and other learners in a learning environment (Friedlander, 2006). One solution is to consider a hybrid approach that combines the online benefits of enhanced access, convenience, and innovative teaching and learning strategies with classroom opportunities for personal interaction, networking, and socializing.

Advanced Assessment and Diagnostic Reasoning of the Adult is a five-credit course designed to facilitate the development of comprehensive health history, physical examination, and diagnostic reasoning skills in nursing students enrolled in the acute care, adult, gerontology, women's health, and psychiatric nurse practitioner tracks of a graduate nursing program. The course description and objectives are shown in **Figure 20-5**. The course is taught in the fall semester of the second year of a 3-year curriculum for entry-level students. The course is also required for RN and post-master's students as it lays the foundation for the assessment and critical thinking skills required of nurse practitioners. The course

---

Figure 20-5   Course description and objectives.

Course Description: This course focuses on the performance of comprehensive wellness-oriented screening and symptom-driven exams with appreciation of normal adult life-cycle variations. Emphasis is placed on mastery of interviewing and psychomotor assessment skills, diagnosis of common problems, and exploration of the health promotion and treatment plan.

Objectives: *Upon completion of this course, the student will be able to:*

1. Incorporate medical diagnoses and nursing diagnoses in the assessment and diagnostic reasoning of adult patient problems.
2. Perform a comprehensive and sensitive health history and physical assessment that reflects life-cycle variations and cultural diversity.
3. Utilize diagnostic reasoning skills in the assessment and differential diagnosis, of patient symptoms and physical examination findings.
4. Establish interpersonal skills during interviews with patients.
5. Communicate the health history, physical assessment, differential diagnosis, and health promotion plan verbally and in writing using appropriate format and terminology.

consists of three credits of classroom theory and two credits of clinical practicum in the nursing laboratory and patient care setting. In response to a need for enhanced course access, improved class schedules, and classroom space, the theory component of the course was revised and placed online in the fall of 2005 using an online course platform designed by the institution. The courseware is user friendly and hosts asynchronous course room discussions along with DL-101, an introductory course to online learning for new users, and access to electronic library resources, technical support, and e-mail for course instructor(s) and peer learners.

The 14-week course is divided into 15 online learning units. The learning units are shown in **Figure 20-6.** Students progress through the units at a pace of one unit per week. With the exception of the introductory unit, the instructional design of each subsequent online unit is identical to minimize learner frustration, facilitate mastery of the technology, and keep the focus on the learning. The introductory unit contains a link to DL-101 and several web sites offering information and tips on netiquette and a copy of the course syllabus. Students are asked to post a personal introduction along with individual learning goals for the semester. Each subsequent unit begins with a list of required readings from the course textbooks, online articles, and web sites. Course textbooks consist of a selection of health assessment, differential diagnosis, and health promotion texts. Articles are exclusively full-text downloads available electronically through the institution's library. Web sites are accessed through clicking active links on the reading list. Required reading materials are thereby readily available to students through remote access.

Following completion of required readings, students view a PowerPoint presentation outlining the essential learning for the unit. Students are encouraged to print a copy of the presentation to use as a guide during the laboratory practicum. Once the readings and PowerPoint presentation have been completed, students progress to the course room discussions. Each unit hosts one to four asynchronous discussions that surround the analysis of case studies designed to explore the differential diagnosis of common complaints pertinent to the unit's topic. For example, case studies for the unit on neurological assessment addressed the differential diagnoses of headache and confusion, while the musculoskeletal unit case studies assessed back pain and joint pain. Students are taken through the differential diagnosis process by a series of questions that prompt students to develop a list of potential differentials, elicit additional history, conduct a symptom-driven physical exam, order diagnostic tests, and consider health promotion education and screening. A sample case study is shown in **Figure 20-7.**

Students are required to post a response to each of the unit's case study discussions. For large case studies, students either work electronically in groups to produce a group posting to the case study, or students are assigned to analyze a specific portion of the case study. Postings must be well developed, thoughtful, informative, and must demonstrate critical thinking. Students are also required to respond to at least one other student's posting each week. Postings must consist of more than an "I agree" type response. Questions, comments, and related learning that students would like to share with the group are posted to an asynchronous discussion thread titled "Questions/Comments." This helps to keep case study discussions on task and free of unrelated communication. Each unit ends with a 10-question online quiz designed to evaluate student learning of content presented in the unit.

Figure 20-6   Online learning units.

Online Learning Units

Unit 1: Introduction

Unit 2: Health History and Differential Diagnosis

Unit 3: Assessment of the Skin

Unit 4: Head and Eye Assessment

Unit 5: ENT Assessment

Unit 6: Respiratory Assessment

Unit 7: Cardiovascular Assessment

Unit 8: Assessment of the Abdomen and Rectum

Unit 9: Musculoskeletal Assessment

Unit 10: Neurological Assessment

Unit 11: Health Promotion

Unit 12: Assessment of Elders

Unit 13: Women's Health Assessment

Unit 14: Men's Health Assessment

Unit 15: Adolescent Health Assessment

The practicum for each unit takes place the following week in the nursing laboratory. The session begins with a review of the online quiz and is followed by a question-and-answer period to clarify points of learning. Once students are clear on the concepts, an instructor-produced video of the physical examination pertaining to the system is shown. Instructor demonstration using student volunteers is discouraged to prevent embarrassment and protect student privacy. Following the video, students work with laboratory partners to practice a system-specific history and physical examination. The practicum is

Figure 20-7   Sample case study.

Unit 7 Case Study Discussion: Mrs. Brown is a 73-year-old female with a history of DM, HTN, dyslipidemia, atrial fibrillation, CHF, and is s/p an inferior wall MI 3 years ago. She presents for routine follow-up. This morning you received a phone call from her daughter who is her health proxy, stating that her mom has been more short of breath than usual, not sleeping well at night, and has developed swelling of her ankles and a weepy ulcer on the lateral aspect of her left ankle. The daughter is quite concerned about the possibility of an infection because that leg seems more red and swollen than the other leg. The daughter also asks you if you can refill her mother's acarbose, metformin, losartan, furosemide, verapamil, simvastatin, and warfarin. She also thinks her mother has run out of sublingual NTG tablets.

Please post a reply to one of the following questions:

Question 1:
What are the differentials for Mrs. Brown's symptoms, and what are your priorities as you approach the assessment of Mrs. Brown?

Question 2:
What else do you need to know for health history, and what information do you need to gather on physical examination?

Question 3:
What labs and diagnostic tests do you consider ordering, and what consults would you obtain?

Question 4:
You decide to assess how Mrs. Brown is managing her care at home. What data do you gather in order to make the assessment?

---

driven by a related chief complaint. Each student has an opportunity to role-play the nurse practitioner and elicit a symptom analysis and history of present illness and conduct an appropriate physical examination. The history and physical is written up, submitted, and critiqued. Students are encouraged to write up the "visit" on the spot to simulate an actual clinical encounter. Subsequently, student written communication skills improve dramatically over the course of the semester.

The nursing laboratory is equipped with state-of-the-art simulation technology and students gain experience in assessing abnormal lung and heart sounds through the use of clinical case-based scenarios. Synthetic models are available for demonstrating and practicing breast, rectal, and prostate examinations. Live, professional models are used for the gynecologic exam practicum. The capstone experience of the course occurs in the final 3 weeks, when students have the opportunity to perform complete histories and physical examinations on patients in a tertiary care setting. Students submit write-ups of their assessments, which include a complete history, physical exam, assessment (which often includes a discussion of differential diagnoses), and a problem list. Students consistently report the clinical experience helps to pull the learning from the semester together.

NS 760 Advanced Assessment and Diagnostic Reasoning ran for the first time as a hybrid course in the fall of 2005 with 19 students. Sixteen of the 19 students completed evaluations of the hybrid design. Fifteen of the 16 students had never taken a hybrid course before. All sixteen students felt the hybrid instructional design was better than an all-online or all-classroom design. One student commented,

> It was better than both the traditional and online courses. I learned much more from reading and writing posts related to case studies than I would have learned from a 3-hour lecture. The lab time gave us plenty of time to answer questions that were too difficult to ask online. (December 5, 2005, anonymous course evaluation.)

Another student commented, "It allowed for lab time and face to face interaction but also made you take responsibility for your own work" (December 5, 2005, anonymous course evaluation). Many students liked the convenience and independence and felt the course provided a greater opportunity for input and learning from every student. "I think online case discussion actually increased my class participation compared to other classes because it was less intimidating!" (December 5, 2005, anonymous course evaluation).

Students liked the online case studies and lab time best. They also liked the organization of the course and the freedom of doing work on their own time. They least liked the occasional problem with the technology and posting online late or last as the case studies seemed completely discussed and they felt they had nothing to add. All students felt the course met their individual learning goals and that they would take the course again and recommend the course to other students. Only one student felt she did not have enough contact with fellow students and the instructors. All students reported feeling satisfied with the course and the majority felt very satisfied. Several students commented that the course exceeded their expectations, including one who said, "The course was more beneficial than I had expected."

Another student commented, "I was really nervous as I had never taken an online course, but it worked out really well."

Yet another student noted, "The course exceeded my expectations. I am now an advocate of online learning!" (December 5, 2005, anonymous course evaluation).

Students identified organization, instructor presence in the course room, and instructor enthusiasm for and comfort with the method as the keys to successful online learning. As with all learning situations, understanding, patience, and a sense of humor go a long way toward supporting students and minimizing frustrating learning experiences. As one student noted, "The instructor made it both interesting and fun and was very understanding about time constraints and working out the 'kinks' of an online format" (December 5, 2005, anonymous course evaluation).

REFERENCES

Adams, J., & DeFleur, M. H. (2005). The acceptability of a doctoral degree earned online as a credential for obtaining a faculty position. *American Journal of Distance Education, 19*(2), 71–85.

Ali, N. S., Bantz, D., & Siktberg, L. (2005). Validation of critical thinking skills in online responses. *Journal of Nursing Education, 44*(2), 90–94.

Ali, N. S., Hodson-Carlton, K., & Ryan, M. (2004). Students' perceptions of online learning—implications for teaching. *Nurse Educator, 29*(3), 111–115.

Barakzai, M. D., & Fraser, D. (2005). The effect of demographic variables on achievement in and satisfaction with online coursework. *Journal of Nursing Education, 44*(8), 373–380.

Billings, D. M., Skiba, D. J., & Connors, H. R. (2005). Best practices in web-based courses: Generational differences across undergraduate and graduate nursing students. *Journal of Professional Nursing, 21*(2), 126–133.

Chaffin, A. J., & Maddux, C. D. (2004). Internet teaching methods for use in baccalaureate nursing education. *CIN: Computers, Informatics, Nursing, 22*(3), 132–142.

Charles, P. A., & Mamary, E. M. (2002). New choices for continuing education: A statewide survey of the practice and preferences of nurse practitioners. *The Journal of Continuing Education in Nursing, 33*(2), 88–91.

Draves, W. A. (2000). *Teaching online.* River Falls, WI: Learning Resources Network.

Driscoll, M. P. (2000). Constructivism. In *Psychology of learning for instruction* (2nd ed., pp. 373–396). Boston: Allyn and Bacon.

Friedlander, E. A. (2006). *Online continuing nursing education: A study of factors related to nurse practitioner participation.* Unpublished doctoral dissertation. Capella University, Minneapolis, MN.

Funaro, G. M., & Montell, F. (1999, December). Pedagogical roles and implementation guidelines for online communication tools. *Asynchronous Learning Networks Magazine, 3*, Article 5. Retrieved April 5, 2006, from http://www.sloan-c.org/publications/magazine/v3n2/funaro.asp

Jeffries, P. R. (2005). Development and testing of a hyperlearning model for design of an online critical care course. *Journal of Nursing Education, 44*(8), 366–372.

Johnson, J., Posey, L., & Simmens, S. J. (2005). Faculty and student perceptions of web-based learning. *The American Journal for Nurse Practitioners, 9*(4), 9–18.

Knowles, M. S., Holton, E. F., & Swanson, R. A. (1998). *The adult learner* (5th ed.). Houston, TX: Gulf Publishing Company.

Lashley, M. (2005). Teaching health assessment in the virtual classroom. *Journal of Nursing Education, 44*(8), 348–350.

Morton, E. (1999). Transforming education: Don't reengineer the existing system. *Vital Speeches of the Day, 65*(16), 487–491.

Murphree, V. (1999). Using the virtual classroom. *Occupational Health & Safety, 68*(9), 28–29.

Neal, E. (1999). Distance education. *National Forum, 79*(1), 40.

Palloff, R. M., & Pratt, K. (1999). *Building learning communities in cyberspace: Effective strategies for the online classroom.* San Francisco: Jossey-Bass Publishers.

Ryan, M., Hodson-Carlton, K., & Ali, N. S. (2005). A model for faculty teaching online: Confirmation of a dimensional matrix. *Journal of Nursing Education, 44*(8), 357–365.

Suen, L. (2005). Teaching epidemiology using WebCT: Application of the seven principles of good practice. *Journal of Nursing Education, 44*(3), 143–146.

University of Illinois. (1999). Teaching at an Internet distance: The pedagogy of online teaching and learning. Retrieved April 7, 2006, from http://www.vpaa.uillinois.edu/reports_retreats/tid_final-12-5.pdf

Waits, T., & Lewis, L. (2003). *Distance education at degree-granting postsecondary institutions: 2000–2001*. Retrieved April 7, 2006, from http://nces.ed.gov/surveys/peqis/publications/2003017

RECOMMENDED READING

White, K. W., & Weight, B. H. (Eds.). (1999). *The online teaching guide: A handbook of attitudes, strategies and techniques for the virtual classroom.* Boston: Allyn and Bacon.

INTERNET RESOURCES

Student Self-Assessment Tools

Center for Independent Learning

http://www.cod.edu/dept/CIL/CIL_Surv.htm

Community College of Philadelphia

http://faculty.ccp.edu/dept/ccpde/self_asmt.html

OnlineLearning.net

http://www.onlinelearning.net/ole/holwselfassess.html?s=522.30606163q.074d 302c50

Peterson's Distance Learning Assessment

http://www.petersons.com/dlwizard/code/default.asp

Educational Platforms—Commercial Structured Learning Environments

Blackboard

http://www.blackboard.com/us/index.aspx

e-College

http://www.ecollege.com/indexflash.learn

WebCT

http://www.webct.com/

Online Course Evaluation

Guiding Principles for Faculty in Distance Learning

http://www.ihets.org/progserv/education/distance/guiding_principles

The Online Course Evaluation Project

http://www.montereyinstitute.org/ocep.html

Quality on the Line—Benchmarks for Success in Internet-Based Distance Education

http://www.ihep.com/Pubs/PDF/Quality.pdf

Virtual Clinical Sites

The Auscultation Assistant

http://www.med.ucla.edu/wilkes/intro.html

Epidemiologic Case Studies

http://www2a.cdc.gov/epicasestudies

Eye Simulator/Virtual Patient

http://cim.ucdavis.edu/EyeRelease/Interface/TopFrame.htm

Lung Sounds

http://www.rale.ca

Multimedia Educational Resource for Learning and Online Teaching (MERLOT)—course content for sharing

http://www.merlot.org/Home.po

Normal and Abnormal EKGs and Heart Sounds

http://www.bioscience.org/atlases/heart

Virtual Hospital

http://www.vh.org

Virtual Patient Reference Library

http://research.bidmc.harvard.edu/VPTutorials

Software for Learning Exercises

Half-Baked Software

http://www.halfbakedsoftware.com

Hot Potatoes crossword, matching, multiple choice

Quandary—create an interactive case study

CHAPTER 21

Philosophical Approaches to Clinical Instruction

Martha J. Bradshaw

INTRODUCTION

The purpose of clinical instruction is to give the student opportunities to bridge didactic information with the realities of nursing practice. In guided situations, students blend theoretical knowledge with experiential learning, in order to effect a synthesis and understanding of those endeavors known collectively as *nursing*. Clinical learning is directed by a nurse educator who operationalizes his or her practical knowledge about teaching. Through use of this practical knowledge, the instructor translates a formal curriculum into active engagement with students (Johnson, 1984). Clinical instruction has become more challenging because of changes in the healthcare environment and the need for health professionals to fulfill increasingly diverse roles. Instructors need to examine their personal philosophies (underlying beliefs) about teaching, especially considering the changes in traditional models of clinical learning. The need for clinical judgment, especially in complex patient settings, calls for both content-specific knowledge and an ability to use the information for decision making (Botti & Reeve, 2003). Students need directed guidance from a practice-oriented instructor in applying knowledge to specific care situations.

ROLE OF THE CLINICAL INSTRUCTOR

In the clinical setting, planning and selection of clinical learning activities tends to be instructor-driven. Depending upon the amount of experience and sense of self-efficacy held by the instructor, the nature of clinical learning may become more student centered. In either case, the teacher guides the students in applying theory to patient care. The faculty role in clinical instruction is as diverse and demanding as are the settings. The instructor is expected to be competent, experienced, knowledgeable, flexible, patient, and energetic. The instructor should be capable of balancing structure with spontaneity. Clinical learning is aimed at knowledge application, skill acquisition, and professional role development. The instructor must be aware of didactic information the students are studying, in order to provide parallel opportunities for application. Students are led in practicing and improving nursing care skills, and need guidance in valuing the skills (Clark, Owen, & Tholcken, 2004). By recognizing the importance of a skill and performing it safely and efficiently, students will increase confidence in their abilities to provide direct patient care. Clinical instructors also help students understand and respect the uniqueness of each client and family in order to individualize holistic nursing care (Northington, Wilkerson, Fisher, & Schenk, 2005).

Paterson (1994) describes two approaches to clinical instruction: *task mastery* and *professional-identity mentoring*. Task mastery instruction is based on the instructor's decisions about what behaviors and ways of thinking are important for nurses and, therefore, need to be reproduced in students. In essence, nursing instructors are gatekeepers, allowing students to enter the profession once they have demonstrated their abilities. With the professional-identity approach, the instructor serves as a mentor, guiding students in decision making and inculcation of hallmarks of professional practice. Task mastery may be suitable with novice students, but the professional-identity approach has a more far-reaching effect on students as they progress in their nursing programs.

The successful student clinical experience—measured in terms of learning outcomes and an internalized sense of fulfillment—is largely influenced by the planning and selection of learning activities available to the students. Selection of activities, as well as actual teaching, is value-laden and reflects the faculty member's philosophical approach to clinical learning and the role or roles the instructor chooses to fulfill. The roles in which individual instructors see themselves may include interaction with students, serving as a role model, or functioning as an expert reference. Roles that students see as important for clinical instructors to hold have been identified as resource, evaluator, encourager, promoter of patient care, and benevolent presence (Flagler, Loper-Powers, & Spitzer, 1988). Once this self-image is determined, teachers consciously or subconsciously shape situations that enable them to enact their various roles. This action enhances teacher effectiveness because the instructor is most comfortable in fulfilling preselected roles.

In addition to self-image, other personal attributes influence the instructor's thinking regarding student assignments. There is some indication that background knowledge and preferences for orientation to practice strongly influence planning and decision making by teachers (Yaakobi & Sharan, 1985). Therefore, an instructor with a concrete, structured practice background (such as surgical nursing) may select or plan patient assignments that are more structured than those selected by an instructor from a less structured background (such as psychiatric nursing). The potential conflict exists between teacher and student regarding learning and practice preferences. With careful planning and collaboration with the students, the clinical instructor can best shape the learning situations to meet students' needs (Sutcliffe, 1983).

FOUNDATIONS FOR SELECTION OF CLINICAL ACTIVITIES

Another philosophical perspective that governs clinical learning is the instructor's view of the *purpose* of the clinical learning experience. The three most common purposes are for students to (1) apply theoretical concepts, (2) experience actual patient situations, and (3) see and implement professional roles. Based on the chosen perspective, the instructor selects the agency or unit and plans the type of clinical assignment that is best suited for the identified purpose. The realism of clinical activities brings added benefit to any of the three types of experiences.

The planning and supervising of clinical learning call for the instructor's own philosophical stance to be blended with the selected goal(s) of the clinical experience. Student assignments may have one of the following goals:

- Learn the **patient**: provide one-to-one total care
- Learn the **content area**: practice a variety of care activities in one setting
- Learn **role(s)**: function as a staff or team member, as a practitioner, administrator, or other selected roles

Assignments can be based on theories of action:

- **People-centered**: interpersonal interaction systems
- **Health**: promotion, maintenance, functioning
- **Nature of practice milieu**: decision making, leadership, collaboration (Reilly & Oermann, 1985)

The instructor who selects a student focus for clinical assignments may value empowerment as part of his or her philosophical approach to teaching. The aims of this approach are the cultivation of responsibility, authority, and accountability in novice practitioners (Manthey, 1992). Selected clinical activities directed toward empowerment could include:

- **Analytic nursing**: use of actual experiences (instructor or student based) to define and solve problems
- **Change activities**: develop planned change and identify resources to effect this change

- **Collegiality**: professional interactions (instructor-student, student-student, student-staff) to solve problems and promote optimal care
- **Sponsorship**: Collaboration and interaction with preceptors, administration; analysis of bureaucratic system (Carlson-Catalano, 1992)

Within the framework of the assignment, the instructor then makes decisions about which activities will enhance learning outcomes. This process again reflects the teacher's values, beliefs about how learning should take place, and how teacher role fulfillment will influence this learning. For example, the instructor who values participatory learning and role modeling will be actively involved in many aspects of the student's activities, and his or her presence will be felt by the student—at the bedside or interacting with staff members. Purdon (1992) points out that such role-modeling has positive benefits for students, such as reducing fears and seeing effective communications. The instructor who wishes to foster independence in students may take on the role of resource person and become centrally available to students as needed. The instructor who places emphasis on organization and task accomplishment will oversee numerous student activities and facilitate completion of the assignments within a designated period. Many instructors value all of these activities as a part of student learning. To accomplish all of these activities calls for a great deal of diversity and planning by the teacher. There are clear advantages for students to be engaged in more than one type of learning experience from one clinical day or week to the next. This broadens the possibilities for learning plus strengthens understanding of multiple roles and diversity of settings. Students who experienced multiple clinical placements described themselves as more adaptable in new environments (Adams, 2002).

Some philosophical approaches to teaching and role assumption by educators are more subtle, yet promote more complex, higher order learning. More specifically, the teacher who values empowerment and accountability in students will take on a less directive role and assume one that is more enabling. The instructor who wishes to promote independence in students must be willing to release a certain amount of control, in order to give freedom for students to learn and grow.

Periodic, timely feedback is essential. Students can only recognize strengths and areas for improvement when they are given objective, constructive feedback. Feedback should be not only evaluative but also encouraging to bolster confidence and independence. Augustine (1992) investigated feedback by clinical instructors and discovered that, in addition to group feedback, such as in conferences or orientation, students felt the need for personal feedback from the instructor until they were certain of what the instructor wanted from them. This need indicates not only the value of the instructor as a guide but also the emphasis students place on feedback for clinical success or failure.

Dimensions of feedback given by instructors reflect the instructor's philosophy and teaching style. Augustine (1992) found that instructors are less likely to give positive feedback in the patient's room than elsewhere, and instructors give a high amount of cautionary or negative feedback during procedures. These findings exemplify the gatekeeping role of the instructor, with a more negative quality to feedback.

CLINICAL ACTIVITIES AND PROBLEM SOLVING

The instructor who promotes problem-solving abilities in students fashions clinical activities to meet this goal. Discovery learning is one way in which student autonomy and problem solving can be enhanced. Students can have experiences where they can realize, or discover, patient responses to certain aspects of care, or how structuring an activity differently is more time saving. These discoveries boost self-esteem when students see what they have learned on their own, or that they have the ability to resolve certain problematic situations. Discovery learning also has been found to increase student motivation, interest, and retention of learned material (DeYoung, 1990). The instructor then is rewarded by seeing growth take place in the students.

Another approach to promoting problem-solving abilities is by placing emphasis on the clinical, or patient, problem, rather than on the clinical setting. Student assignments that take place in familiar, repetitive settings enable students to deal with patients *in that setting*. As Gaberson and Oermann (1999) point out, practice settings for clinical learning are moving away from acute care environments, and students should be equipped to work with clinical problems in diverse settings. In addition to learning how to deal with clinical problems, students also experience professional socialization through role discontinuity. In making the transition from instructor-directed, structured, familiar assignments to empowering, unstructured, undefined patient problems, students experience new ways of defining their own roles and responsibilities as practitioners.

STUDENT-CENTERED LEARNING

The strategy of reciprocal learning not only meets clinical learning needs but promotes collegiality as well. Reciprocal learning usually takes the form of peer teaching, or student-to-student instruction. This learning informally occurs within most clinical groups and can become more purposeful and goal-directed through instructor planning. By pairing students for specific learning activities, the student learner gains information, experience, and insight in new ways. Learners receive individualized, empathetic instruction and may feel more relaxed with a peer than with a faculty teacher. The student teacher also learns about instruction, helping, and working with others. Student teachers also assume the responsibility of role models and collaborators (Goldenberg & Iwasiw, 1992).

From the viewpoint of the instructor, student-centered learning increases student accountability and independence. This is especially beneficial for students who are closer to graduation and need to break ties to the instructor. As students increase independence, the instructor can receive satisfaction from this new level of student performance. Students appreciate the trust that the instructor conveys to them. In fact, the promotion of cooperative learning, active involvement, and the recognition of diverse ways of learning are attributes that students rank highly in effective teachers (Wolf, Bender, Beitz, Wieland, & Vito, 2004).)

FACULTY DEVELOPMENT

The powerful influence of the instructor as a person should not be overlooked. Development of an effective clinical instructor and the evolution of a meaningful, positive clinical learning experience are based on insight, planning, and implementation by the faculty member. Therefore, individual teachers need to cultivate an appropriate self-image as a teacher. In addition, the clinical instructor should indulge in periodic self-reflection: Is my own clinical competence being maintained? Are my own views on nursing and the teaching–learning process congruent with student perspectives and needs? Should teaching strategies, types of assignments, or communication skills be revised? The effective faculty member may need to reshape his or her own teaching perspectives to better blend with those perspectives held by the clinical students.

CONCLUSION

The philosophical approach to teaching is the foundation by which the instructor operationalizes his or her own practical knowledge. The responsibilities for the instructor are great, calling for clinical expertise, role modeling, and understanding of teaching and learning principles for a variety of students, settings, and clinical experiences.

Carlson-Catalano (1992) pointed out that much of the instruction that takes place is related to how the instructor has internalized professional values and developed a self-image as a practitioner and role model. The clinical instructor is a pivotal person for developing positive or negative self-concepts in students (Kelly, 1992). The instructor who wishes to promote empowerment in students must see himself or herself as empowered to do so. Only then can needed socialization and empowerment take place. The empowered instructor is able to visualize the potential learning opportunities in the clinical environment (Chally, 1992). The nature of clinical practice has been redefined, and so must the nature of clinical learning experiences.

Faculty members need to adapt to these changes and be willing to give up their comfort zone of familiar, yet limited, clinical settings and methods of instruction (Mundt, 1997). Effective clinical instruction emerges from conscious efforts by the instructor. These efforts should be based on background knowledge, strongly formed values, and a well-defined self-image as a nurse teacher. Applying these personal resources enables the teacher to bring about effective clinical instruction. Formal and personal learning outcomes then are achieved.

REFERENCES

Adams, V. (2002). Consistent clinical assignment for nursing students compared to multiple placements. *Journal of Nursing Education, 41*, 80–82.

Augustine, C. J. (1992). Dimensions of feedback in clinical nursing education. *Dissertation Abstracts International,* 54-02A (1992):0433.

Botti, M., & Reeve, R. (2003). Role of knowledge and ability in student nurses' clinical decision-making. *Nursing and Health Sciences, 5*, 39–49.

Carlson-Catalano, J. (1992). Empowering nurses for professional practice. *Nursing Outlook, 40*, 139–142.

Chally, P. S. (1992). Empowerment through teaching. *Journal of Nursing Education, 31*, 117–120.

Clark, M. C., Owen, S. V., & Tholcken, M. A. (2004). Measuring student perceptions of clinical competence. *Journal of Nursing Education, 43*, 548–554.

DeYoung, S. (1990). *Teaching nursing.* Redwood City, CA: Addison-Wesley.

Flagler, S., Loper-Powers, S., & Spitzer, A. (1988). Clinical teaching is more than evaluation alone! *Journal of Nursing Education, 27*, 342–348.

Gaberson, K. B., & Oermann, M. H. (1999). *Clinical teaching strategies in nursing.* New York: Springer.

Goldenberg, D., & Iwasiw, C. (1992). Reciprocal learning among students in the clinical area. *Nursing Outlook, 17*, 27–29.

Johnson, M. (1984). Review of teacher thinking: A study of practical knowledge. *Curriculum Inquiry, 14*, 465–468.

Kelly, B. (1992). The professional self-concepts of nursing undergraduates and their perceptions of influential forces. *Journal of Nursing Education, 31*, 121–125.

Manthey, M. (1992). Empowerment for teachers and students. *Nurse Educator, 17*, 6–7.

Mundt, M. H. (1997). A model for clinical learning experiences in integrated health care networks. *Journal of Nursing Education, 36*, 309–316.

Northington, L., Wilkerson, R., Fisher, W., & Schenk, W. (2005). Enhancing nursing students' clinical experience using aesthetics. *Journal of Professional Nursing, 21*, 66–71.

Paterson, B. (1994). The view from within: Perspectives of clinical teaching. *International Journal of Nursing Studies, 31*, 349–360.

Purdon, J. E. (1992). Fear of persons with HIV infection: Teaching strategies for helping students cope. *Journal of Nursing Education, 31*, 138–139.

Reilly, D. E., & Oermann, M. H. (1985). *The clinical field: Its use in nursing education*. Norwalk, CT: Appleton-Century-Crofts.

Sutcliffe, L. (1993). An investigation into whether nurses change their learning style according to subject area studied. *Journal of Advanced Nursing, 18*, 647–658.

Wolf, Z. R., Bender, P. J., Beitz, J. M., Wieland, D. M., & Vito, K. O. (2004). Strengths and weaknesses of faculty teaching performance reported by undergraduate and graduate nursing students: A descriptive study. *Journal of Professional Nursing, 20*, 118–128.

Yaakobi, D., & Sharan, S. (1985). Teacher beliefs and practices: The discipline carries the message. *Journal of Education for Teaching, 11*, 187–199.

SECTION V

CLINICAL TEACHING

Clinical teaching is one of the most significant features of health professions education. The transition from academia to the real world of practice and its challenges is made easier. Chapters in Section V are introduced by philosophical underpinnings that should guide each instructor when planning and carrying out clinical instruction, and then are concluded by issues and cautionary suggestions for faculty. The clinical teaching chapters evolve from introductory skills lab to addressing complex situations such as student preceptor issues and service-learning. Critical thinking and the development of higher-order thinking are key components of the chapter on concept mapping.

Student learning by giving care to patients combines academic knowledge and clinical skills. Since external placements are becoming more difficult to obtain, one method to address this has been the use of faculty-based clinics. Issues involved in working with students in this environment are presented. This type of clinic benefits faculty, students, and patients. Faculty maintain their clinical skills through dual roles as teachers and practicing clinicians, while faculty supervision provides a safe environment for both students and their patients. The clinic provides a service for patients, and students can achieve a higher degree of self-awareness of personal strengths and weaknesses and enhanced critical thinking skills.

CHAPTER 22

The New Skills Laboratory: Application of Theory, Teaching, and Technology

Deborah Tapler and Judy Johnson-Russell

INTRODUCTION

Creation of an effective skills laboratory can energize learning by students and facilitate the transition from practice of required skills to direct care delivery to clients. The skills laboratory provides an atmosphere for students to experience the acquisition of new skill knowledge and implementation using multiple modes of teaching and learning. With emerging restrictions of clinical placement of health-related students, the skills lab can be used as a learning environment without the presence of clients (Duffin, 2004). Nursing programs are debating proposals to allow students to spend much more clinical time in practice labs instead of actual hospital units. With unlimited hours of operation, the lab can provide needed opportunities to practice procedures, evaluate learning outcomes, and reinforce critical thinking objectives. As technology increases in complexity through the use of advanced human-patient simulators, the skills laboratory can now provide almost true-to-life clinical situations.

DEFINITIONS AND PURPOSES

Acquisition of new knowledge and skills are an important component of the educational curriculum for healthcare professionals. Nurses must be able to perform procedures such as wound care, intravenous therapy, and endotracheal suctioning. Through the use of a skills laboratory, these and other integral patient care skills are learned and practiced before implementation on patients. The instructor educating students about skills uses several sources for instruction.

Theory-based practice guides the educator when preparing to teach new nursing skills. Theory has a direct link to practice. Educational theories relate

313

the instructor to students through the development of effective learning strategies appropriate for selected students. Theory also influences practice through
theory-driven research that impacts patient care. For example, germ theory dictates the procedure of successful handwashing, which is a skill that every nursing student must master to prevent infection. When learning in the skills lab,
the student must progress beyond the how of a procedure to the more complex
level of thinking to ask, "why?"

Evidence-based practice must also be used in the skills laboratory. Evidence-
based practice is a systematic approach to problem solving that can be applied
to nursing care delivery as well as education (Pravikoff, Tanner, & Pierce, 2005).
Teaching skills that are based on valid research provides students with state-of-
the-art information for safe implementation of skills in actual clinical experiences. Research must be applied to practice through the use of the best evidence
currently available for clinical decision making in order to ensure the delivery
of the most effective care possible. It is imperative to educate students about the
process of accessing research evidence as part of a lifelong learning goal. Elements of procedures and relevancy of skills change as knowledge and technology grow. The skills laboratory must reflect the most current information when
educating nurses for the future.

The purpose of this chapter is to explore the purposes, diverse uses, and effectiveness of a skills laboratory. Based on current theory, valuable teaching
modalities, and advanced technology, the skills laboratory can be an effective
tool of education for a wide range of health-related disciplines.

THEORETICAL RATIONALE

Knowles's theory of adult learning has shaped the way that educators present
information to adult learners (Knowles, 1989). Adults approach a learning situation differently than children. With life experiences to color the acquisition of
new knowledge and skills, adults thrive in a learning environment that is open
to creativity, values personal knowledge, and is relevant to immediate learning
goals. Adult learners desire to make individual choices and decisions. Education
in the skills laboratory is hands on and relevant to direct patient care. Students
are allowed and encouraged to self-evaluate their competence prior to clinical
placement (Clarke, Davies, & McNee, 2002). They develop self-confidence in
the use of psychomotor skills without fear of failure. After the students attend
traditional learning presentations such as lecture, the adult learners are motivated to learn those things in the skills lab that they know will be necessary to
accomplish course objectives. Practice in the skills lab allows the students to
cope effectively with future patient interactions. The skills lab can also provide

academic assistance when a student has difficulty integrating knowledge regarding a psychomotor skill.

Benner's theory of skill acquisition plays an important part in the nursing education curriculum (Benner, 2001). Benner proposed a model for the nursing profession, based on the Dreyfus Model, explaining that nurses function at various levels of skill from novice to expert. The novice level is characterized by a lack of experience of the situations in which the person is involved and is expected to perform. The beginning nursing student functions at the novice level. The nursing curriculum gives students entry to nursing situations and allows them to gain the experience through skills development. The skills lab acts as an instrument to transfer knowledge and skills to novice nursing students so that they may progress to increasingly more complex levels of understanding. The skills lab can be used to teach about situations in terms of "objective attributes" such as intake and output, blood pressure, and temperature (Benner, 2001, p. 20). These features of the task world of nursing have to be learned before actual situational experiences with patients. The behavior of the novice is rule governed and very limited and inflexible. Faculty members impart rules to guide performance before the information makes sense to students. Practice and rehearsal of new behaviors allows the students to gain confidence in their abilities despite little understanding of the contextual meanings of recently learned nursing concepts. Thus, the skills lab plays an important role in the learning process of new students who have no contextual cues. As the nursing student progresses through the nursing curriculum to graduation, the role of the skills lab can evolve and change to meet the expectations for learning dictated by the faculty and content objectives. According to Benner, students may progress from novice to the next level of advanced beginner, then to the competent, proficient, and expert levels of nursing ability.

CONDITIONS

The skills laboratory can be used effectively throughout the nursing curriculum. According to Infante (1985), the purpose of a nursing skills laboratory is to offer students the appearance of reality in an artificial environment where the setting is controlled and offers practical application. The students are encouraged to achieve a predefined level of skill competence (Clarke et al., 2002). As skills move from simple, such as bathing, to complex, such as suctioning, the skills lab can be a learning experience that provides for advancing levels of knowledge and abilities.

Faculty involved in undergraduate curricula should identify skills associated with each level of progression to ensure that all necessary content is reflected in the educational goals of the laboratory. In addition, identified skills should be appropriate to the skill level of the student. Typically, nursing education has utilized the skills lab to provide psychomotor skill acquisition at the beginning of the curriculum. However, with technologies used in the lab, such as computer-based interactive case studies and human-patient simulators, new modalities have provided unlimited opportunities for knowledge as well as skill development. Critical thinking scenarios are appropriate and can be facilitated by skills lab experiences.

Learning situations can be enhanced by the contained setting of the skills laboratory. With close supervision and responsive interactions between students and faculty, the students learn in an environment of collaboration and inquiry. Questions about new procedures or concepts can be answered and discussed promptly without the constraints of a fast-paced patient care area. Faculty members act as facilitators and have opportunities to present information regarding advances in evidence-based practice. Students feel confident to try new skills in a low-risk situation without fear of harming patients. Mistakes are excellent sources of learning and do not have to possess penalizing consequences. However, if the skills laboratory is used for mastery performance evaluation of student abilities, the results can be recorded as a component of a course grade or used for remedial identification. Students who have weakness in psychomotor or critical thinking skills can use the environment of the skills laboratory for tutoring assistance from faculty. Through one-on-one interaction, the weak student can practice and receive immediate feedback from a qualified evaluator to gain knowledge and confidence.

TYPES OF LEARNERS

Undergraduate nursing students possess various learning styles. The skills laboratory can provide a rich learning experience for all types of learners. Whether the student learner is self-directed or takes a more dependent approach, the faculty can individualize instruction based on each student's abilities and learning style. (See Chapter 1 for an overview of cognitive styles, learning styles, and learning preferences.) Kolb's theory of experiential learning proposes cycles of learning along a continuum from concrete experience to abstract conceptualization of knowledge (Dobbin, 2001). Nursing students possess a more concrete, active pattern learning style characterized by the need for dynamic involvement when learning new concepts and skills (Schroeder, 2004). According to Dobbin (2001), "learners also can have a preference for reflective observation (watching to learn) or active experimentation (learning by doing)" (p. 5). For example, tactile exploration by touching and manipulating syringes and needles is essential for the concrete learner.

Lecturing has only limited ability to educate in regards to psychomotor skill acquisition. As the student learns new skills in the lab, questions arise and what-ifs are posed to enhance the learning experience. The use of return demonstration strengthens mastery and confidence.

Faculty must ensure that instruction in the skills laboratory is directed to students with a wide range of learning styles. Students may possess any one or combination of the following learning styles: visual (spatial), aural (auditory-musical), verbal (linguistic), physical (kinesthetic), logical (mathematical), social (interpersonal), or solitary (intrapersonal) (Schroeder, 2006). Through the use of simulators, audio-visual software, graphs and diagrams, charts, pictures, demonstrations, practice, discussion, or even music, the skills laboratory can address the needs of all students when acquiring new nursing knowledge. The key to effective teaching in the lab is dependent on the faculty use of a varied and innovative approach to education.

CONDITIONS FOR LEARNING AND RESOURCES

Opportunities for learning skills in the clinical environment continue to dwindle due to fewer clinical placements available in healthcare institutions. With often fierce competition among schools of nursing for optimal student assignments in hospitals and community resources, the skills lab takes on an increased importance for all clinical courses in the curriculum. Skills, which were once discussed and practiced briefly in the lab and then performed on clients, may no longer be practiced in the clinical area due to patient availability and legal ramifications. Practice in the skills lab may be the only opportunity for learning many basic as well as complex skills needed after graduation. Therefore, skills taught in each course must be identified and additional time and supplies allotted for practice in the lab. Skills will not only be taught in isolation with low-fidelity simulators such as static manikins, but can also become a part of scenarios with high-fidelity human patient simulators. These scenarios offer the students opportunities to interact with simulators with specific problems, and the skills learned are carried out as interventions become necessary, rather than in isolation. Thus, scenarios based on learning objectives for each course throughout the curriculum and imbedded with increasingly complex skills become an important avenue for assisting the student in progressing from novice to higher levels of ability. Skills performed within scenarios also allow for the adult learner to apply knowledge and psychomotor ability to immediate learning goals.

Skills labs must take on a new look that parallels the hospital environment as simulators become patients and assist the student in the suspension of disbelief while practicing necessary skills. This environment includes not only sights, but also the sounds that are inherent in a busy clinical area. Labs must include the equipment, technology, and resources that are currently found in the clinical environment. The skills laboratory includes not only typical equipment such as intravenous pumps, but also computers and PDAs with evidence-based resources that will be needed to assist students with problem solving and critical thinking as they work through scenarios. Informatics should be accessible as students must learn to work with databases and documentation software. Labs will need to be designed to provide rooms/bays that are essentially self-contained hospital units for scenarios to be carried out. Although the rooms may be used for a variety of scenarios, different rooms may need to be designed and equipped for areas such as obstetrics, emergency care, acute care, home care, pediatrics, and intensive care units, in addition to ancillary units. As the hospital environment changes and innovations such as telenursing and eICUs become commonplace, skill labs require design elements that provide multiple screen workstations connected to multiple simulators.

USING THE METHOD

Teaching within the new skills lab combines the best of the traditional methods of instructions with the new technological advances. Regardless of the complexity of the skill, acquisition begins with didactic instruction and practice in the lab on low-fidelity manikins. Additionally, students may be provided with kits of equipment and supplies to continue practicing skills at home. These include such things as mock wounds for dressing changes and styrofoam wig heads with tracheotomy tubes for practicing tracheotomy care. As mentioned before, performance of skills at this time is rule governed and inflexible. These skills can then be embedded within a scenario accompanied by the complexity of care based on the course objectives. Three to five students can work through the scenario on a high-fidelity human patient simulator, identifying indicators for various skills, perhaps obtaining orders for the skill, collecting supplies needed, performing the skills, observing the effects, and documenting and reporting the procedure and effects. Although only one student actually performs any one skill, other students actively participate in the skill through discussion and support. The importance of the skill takes on a new meaning as it becomes a part of nursing care for an illness and a patient with specific needs and responses. Communication and professionalism is fostered with other team members, such as healthcare providers, and among other members of the student's peer group. Debriefing following the completion of the scenario should be considered integral to the process. Discussions with the faculty as facilitators can assist the student in applying theory to practice, correcting mistakes, answering questions, identifying learning needs, and making connections to the real world.

The use of appropriate scenarios and all levels of human patient simulators and manikins are invaluable for teaching skills in a safe environment where patient cooperation is not needed, where repetition is essential, and especially where skills could potentially cause harm to the patient. Critical thinking and problem solving, obtaining appropriate supplies, manipulating equipment, looking up resources, performing procedures accurately and safely, and communicating verbally and in writing are all activities that require considerable amounts of time in the novice learner. In the fast-paced clinical environment, time is of the essence, and students are often expected to perform beyond the level of novice learner. Students can move beyond the novice level with the use of credible scenarios and simulated patients in the realistic, transferable environment of the skills lab.

Skill labs may include evaluation of specific skills as a part of outcome measurements at the end of the semester. Students are often evaluated performing a specific skill or skills as the faculty observe and record their performance. Return demonstration to determine mastery of specified skills is an effective method to determine the safety of transition to patient care in the clinical setting. If students demonstrate a poor performance when evaluated, immediate remedial action can be taken to correct deficiencies before exposure to patients. Patient safety must be the overriding consideration when documenting student abilities. For example, if during a lab checkoff, a student draws up 10 cc of a medication instead of the required 3 cc dose, the faculty can reeducate the student immediately, validate that accurate knowledge is mastered, and avert a potential patient injury in subsequent clinical encounters.

Simulated patients also are used in effectively evaluating skills. The required skills are developed in a short scenario. Three to five students care for the patient and perform the skills as the intervention becomes necessary in the scenario. Students should be aware of the criteria and expected behaviors, having practiced all the skills to be evaluated previously. At the beginning of the scenario, students can draw for the skills they are to perform during the scenario. As the scenario progresses, students care for the patient together, except when a specific skill is needed. Peers then become observers as the student who was assigned a skill performs it according to the criteria outlined and is evaluated by the instructor. Peer observers become active learners as they mentally rehearse and evaluate the skills as they are being performed. Once the skill has been completed, the scenario resumes until another skill is needed. The process is repeated throughout the scenario until all students have demonstrated their selected skills. Verbal and/or written feedback can be given to the students individually by the instructor following the scenario. Students may also give their peers feedback about their performance.

Videotaping may be used as an adjunct to learning or evaluation of skills. Students can learn by videotaping and critiquing their own performance or by reviewing the tape and discussing their performance with a faculty member. They can also videotape and submit their tape for evaluation and feedback by a faculty member. However, Miller, Nichols, & Beeken (2000) found that students prefer faculty member presence during skill demonstrations and immediate feedback rather than videotaping and delayed feedback.

POTENTIAL PROBLEMS

A major problem inherent in the development of the modern skills laboratory is the cost to provide the needed technology, supplies, and the physical space to house them. In order for students to practice with the equipment used in the nursing profession, it must be purchased from medical vendors. Supplies are very expensive, especially when they are the most recent equipment used by the clinical agencies. Needles with integral safety devices are often more costly than traditional needle systems. Students must see and practice with the tools that they will use in their clinical experiences, which requires frequent equipment revision in the laboratory. As enrollment in schools of nursing increases due to shortage mandates, the skills lab provides space that is available from early morning to late in the evening for student use.

Skills labs have typically been large rooms with multiple beds and static manikins. Large numbers of students often practice the same skill at the same time. Although this type of space and instruction are a beginning, additional, smaller simulation rooms will be needed for the more costly high-fidelity human patient simulators with all of the equipment, technology, and added supplies needed for implementing simulations. In addition, some labs have a small control room with a one-way mirror attached to each simulation room.

Other problems include lack of faculty willingness to embrace new technology such as high-fidelity simulation, implementing evidence-based case scenarios, and the additional time it takes to have students, three to five at a time, complete the skills within the case scenarios. Learning new simulation teaching strategies and management of the simulators requires additional faculty time and energy. Writing evidence-based scenarios that contain the necessary skills is another time-intensive faculty activity, unless these are purchased.

Skills laboratories are required to follow safety procedures in regard to protection of students from injury or spills. The expense to adhere to federal and local government regulations may prove costly, but are a necessary component of a safe and effective skills lab.

CONCLUSION

The nursing skills laboratory provides an enriched teaching and learning atmosphere that encourages active and involved exploration and mastery of new knowledge and skills to develop competent graduate nurses. Theory is applied to practice and validated in the skills lab through teaching and technology. The faculty member can use unlimited strategies to educate students who have a spectrum of learning needs in order to foster critical thinking. In the protected environment of the skills lab, students learn, make mistakes, question conceptual ideas, practice psychomotor skills, and expand knowledge to a new level of understanding. Students learn by doing through experimentation that would be impossible and dangerous in direct patient care situations. Faculty have direct observation and supervision of all student activities, which is often difficult in a busy clinical agency. Transition to the role of graduate nurse is enhanced by effective and innovative use of the new skills laboratory.

APPLIED EXAMPLES
Comprehensive Nursing Skills Experiences

In a fundamental skills course offered by various disciplines, skills are a primary focus requiring didactic instruction and demonstrations first given in lecture and then reinforced in the skills lab. Skills that are appropriate for beginning nursing students include the complex task of medication administration: obtaining or understanding healthcare provider orders, learning the appropriate dosages and where to research information about the drug, calculating dosages from the correct amount of drug available, safely and competently handling the syringe during drawing up of medication, administration, disposal of the syringe, recognizing appropriate sites for administration (subcutaneous or intramuscular), performing the five rights prior to administration, and recording the medication in the permanent patient record. All these basic skills must be understood and practiced repeatedly by the student. To meet the wide range of learning styles, instruction should include verbal and written material as well as audio-visual demonstrations and one-on-one interactions and demonstrations with the students. Kinesthetic learning is provided by the use of different types of syringes, vials, and pills; and solitary practice is combined with discussion, reflective observation, and active experimentation.

Administering insulin and digoxin can be used as examples for student practice. Sliding scale insulin orders could be written in a mock chart, and students could be given various blood glucose results so that different amounts of insulin would need to be drawn up. In the lab, students practice drawing up insulin, selecting an appropriate site, administering the medication on a manikin, discarding the syringe, and documenting on the mock chart. They should also practice giving oral medications such as digoxin correctly, which would include auscultation of the apical pulse. Not only must they be able to perform the skill of giving the medication correctly, but they would also need to recognize that an apical pulse rate must be taken before administration, under which circumstances the medication should be withheld based on current literature, and when the healthcare provider must be notified for future actions.

Once the skills have been practiced, three or four students are introduced to the high-fidelity simulator. They are presented with the history and physical findings of a patient who is hospitalized with selected clinical problems. A mock chart is available with healthcare provider orders, which include treatment and medication orders. Medications are noted on the medication administration record, including insulin sliding scale, oral medication, and prn medication orders. The students are made aware of the time of day and results of lab studies such as blood glucose readings. Students at this point are assigned selected skills to perform, such as wound dressing change, urinary catheterization, administration of pain medication via the intramuscular route, application of bandages, or performance of a basic head-to-toe assessment. The skills are embedded in the scenario and must be performed according to patient need and healthcare provider orders. The students must prioritize their actions based on the dynamic events unfolding in the patient scenario. This complex situation fosters critical thinking and problem solving to meet patient demands. The faculty member acts as facilitator to encourage competent participation by individual students and provides immediate feedback to correct problems in cognition and performance of skills. As the student progresses in level of learning ability across the curriculum, the faculty member offers less prompting to increase the independence exhibited by the student. By applying adult learning principles, the student is allowed to demonstrate more creativity in a learning environment that supports personal knowledge and meets immediate learning goals.

Evaluation of required skills is an important function of the skills lab. The lab provides unlimited opportunities for faculty to observe and test acquisition of psychomotor skills as well as cognitive processing. For example, the evaluation process in the form of a formalized checkoff can be implemented at the end of a semester to determine mastery of required skills. Before the checkoff is completed, students receive detailed procedural (step-by-step) information or criteria regarding the skills that they must master. By knowing the exact expectation before the evaluation, the anxiety level experienced by the students is decreased, and the faculty member can more easily determine the skill level of an individual student unclouded by psychological barriers. Practice opportunities are provided to reinforce skills the week before checkoff. The lab is arranged to represent the hospital setting with a patient in bed, a medication room, and a supply area. The student receives an assigned skill, reviews the patient's mock chart, assembles the necessary equipment to perform the skill, and prepares the patient for the procedure. The interaction with the manikin should appear as authentic as possible. This situation can be achieved by encouraging the student to communicate with the patient in a normal manner. The faculty member observes the performance of the skill based on the criteria previously provided to the student. A checkoff form is used to document and evaluate the student's actions in relation to the criteria. The faculty member does not interact with or prompt the student in any manner. If the student fails to follow the criteria, points are deducted, affecting the final score. The criteria contains selected critical behaviors that must be accomplished successfully to pass the evaluation. Examples of critical behaviors are contamination of a sterile field or recapping a used needle. If the student fails to acquire sufficient points or neglects to perform critical behaviors, the student fails the check-off and is provided the opportunity for remediation and a repeated attempt. Failure of the course is possible if the student is unable to successfully master the performance of the skill. The skills lab is an excellent venue to assess competency and determine learning needs. By utilizing theory combined with innovative teaching approaches and technological advances in the skills laboratory, faculty members optimize learning opportunities.

REFERENCES

Benner, P. (2001). *From novice to expert: Excellence and power in clinical nursing practice.* Upper Saddle River, NJ: Prentice-Hall Health.

Clarke, D., Davies, J., & McNee, P. (2002). The case for a children's nursing skills laboratory. *Pediatric Nursing, 14*(7), 36–39.

Dobbin, K. R. (2001). Applying learning theories to develop teaching strategies for the critical care nurse: Don't limit yourself to the formal classroom lecture. *Critical Care Nursing Clinics of North America, 13*(1), 1–11.

Duffin, C. (2004). Simulated 'skills labs' to ease pressure on training. *Nursing Standard, 18*(39), 7.

Infante, M. S. (1985). *The clinical laboratory.* New York: John Wiley.

Knowles, M. (1989). *The making of an adult education: An autobiographical journey.* San Francisco: Jossey-Bass.

Miller, H., Nichols, E., & Beeken, J. (2000). Comparing video-taped and faculty-present return demonstrations of clinical skills. *Journal of Nursing Education, 39*, 237–239.

Pravikoff, D. S., Tanner., A. B., & Pierce, S. T. (2005). Readiness for US nurses for evidence-based practice. *American Journal of Nursing, 105*(9), 40–52.

Schroeder, C. C. (2004). *New students—New learning styles.* Retrieved March 19, 2006, from http://www.virtualschool.edu/mon/Academia/KierseyLearningStyles.html

CHAPTER 23

Student Learning in a Faculty–Student Practice Clinic

Jennifer Mackey and Marjorie Nicholas

INTRODUCTION

In the most effective clinical education, students obtain academic knowledge simultaneously with the development of clinical skills. The American Speech-Language-Hearing Association (ASHA) requires that the education of graduate students who are seeking to become speech-language pathologists includes the acquisition of both *knowledge* and *skills* in a variety of content areas (ASHA, 2005). Ensuring that students gain the requisite knowledge base is accomplished primarily via academic coursework. Ensuring that students obtain the necessary clinical skills is often somewhat more challenging.

Like education models in many healthcare professions, most programs in speech-language pathology in the United States utilize a series of clinical externships in which students work in different healthcare settings to acquire the clinical skills they will need to become professional practicing clinicians. Most also have on-site clinics in which students learn the preliminary clinical skills they need before venturing out to their externships. In this chapter, we describe the MGH Institute of Health Professions' faculty–student practice clinic, known as the Speech, Language, and Literacy Clinic. This clinic operates as both an entry-level and an advanced-practice clinic. While the examples we provide will necessarily be related to speech-language pathology, we believe the lessons learned from this clinical educational model are pertinent to a broad range of healthcare professionals.

The model of clinical education we will describe in this chapter is known as the *teacher–practitioner model* (Montgomery, Enzbrenner, & Lerner, 1991; Meyer, McCarthy, Klodd, & Gaseor, 1995; Peach & Meyer, 1996). One of the important features that we will highlight of our implementation of this model is the integration of academic (knowledge-based) with clinical (skills-based) education. We describe both our entry-level and advanced-practice clinics and then discuss the positive outcomes and challenges of using this model.

DEFINITION AND PURPOSE OF THE
TEACHER–PRACTITIONER MODEL

The essential principle of the teacher–practitioner model is that students learn best from individuals who have dual roles as teachers and practicing clinicians. In this model, the supervisor teaches the student in the classroom and also demonstrates clinical interaction with clients in the clinic. In one of the most well-known models of supervision in speech-language pathology (Anderson, 1981; McCrea & Brasseur, 2003), a continuum of skill development is emphasized for both the student and the supervisor. Interaction between the two parties is also a key feature of the continuum model. This interaction and the continuum of skill development are also fundamental features of the teacher–practitioner model. This model is used by many academic institutions and seeks to create a strong linkage between scholarly and professional roles of the supervisor. Students have opportunities to see firsthand how theory relates to their clinical work with individuals with communication disorders. This model is the foundation for our faculty–student practice clinic, which serves two primary purposes: (1) it operates as a site for the education of students, and (2) it provides communication therapy services to the community.

In its main role as a setting focused on student learning, the clinic provides an atmosphere for the integration of academic knowledge and research-based practice in a clinical environment. As a place where supervisors mentor beginning clinicians, an on-site clinic is an ideal environment for linking clinical practice with theory and academic coursework. This setting encourages the development of critical thinking skills as well as the development of students' self-evaluation skills and personal goals for clinical and professional growth. Superficially, it might appear that the best learning atmosphere is a real-world setting, such as a hospital, rehabilitation center, or specialty clinic. While these settings offer diverse, rich, and important experiences, the pressures of productivity, insurance issues, and medically complex patients make these environments exceptionally challenging for beginning clinicians (ASHA, n.d.) Like many healthcare professionals, speech-language pathologists face personnel shortages and increased requirements for documentation. External supervisors, or preceptors, often struggle with the demands of high caseloads and not enough time to teach and support students with limited knowledge and experience. Therefore, these settings are often best suited to advanced students who have already developed a solid basis for the understanding of intervention planning, diagnosis, and professional interaction.

Due to the various financial and time management pressures of off-site healthcare settings, there is a need for clinical training sites dedicated to nurturing beginning students' self-evaluation and communication skills. These settings provide the solid foundation of skills necessary for students as they enter external practicum sites that generally require a more sophisticated and experienced student clinician. Students leave the on-site clinic with a higher degree of self-awareness of personal strengths and areas of weakness. In addition, the development of critical thinking skills gives the student a framework for problem solving and analysis that eases the transition to the new challenges of fast-paced external placements.

A secondary purpose of the faculty–student practice clinic is to provide diagnostic and therapeutic services to community members with communication disorders. Since the faculty–student practice clinic is an integral part of the educational program, the hosting educational institution financially supports the clinic as a place for student learning. Therefore, the clinic is not dependent on outside sources such as state or governmental funding or payments from insurance or private pay individuals. Clients are requested to pay a nominal user fee to support purchase of materials used in the clinic, such as books, diagnostic tests, treatment materials, and software. This fee can be waived or reduced depending on individual circumstances. No client is ever denied services due to the inability to pay this fee. Having a free clinic is possible because of the nature of the integration of academic and clinical resources, including teachers and supervisors. Furthermore, because the clinic is not dependent on outside funding, it is able to provide services to underserved and underprivileged populations.

USE OF THE TEACHER–PRACTITIONER MODEL

The Entry-Level Clinic

The Speech, Language and Literacy clinic was designed as a space for beginning graduate students to work with children and adults with various speech and language disorders, as well as for experienced graduate students to work in a simulated outpatient setting with adults who have acquired language disabilities. The physical layout of the clinic includes six individual treatment rooms and one large group/conference room. Two observation rooms allow parents, caregivers, students, and supervisors to observe treatment rooms through two-way mirrors. All treatment rooms have video cameras that project to a third observation room equipped with television monitors. Supervisors can observe sessions in this room and also have the ability to operate the camera remotely. This gives student clinicians independence in the therapy room while they are carefully observed by a supervisor.

Students are supervised by licensed speech-language pathologists with expertise in their field. These supervisors, often called instructors, mentors, or preceptors, are faculty members in the Communication Sciences and Disorders department. This designation allows the supervisors to voice their ideas and opinions in faculty meetings and to interact regularly with faculty who teach courses. Several of the supervisors also teach academic and clinical courses. This integration of academic and clinical information and experience allows for a unique learning atmosphere for the students, and a rich collegial environment for faculty. This model of blending academic with clinical instruction is the basis of the teacher–practitioner model and allows students to more fully assimilate information from classes into direct therapy with clients.

Students in their first year of the graduate program will have two semesters of clinical experience in the Speech, Language and Literacy Clinic. During one of these semesters, students work with children with spoken language disorders such as toddlers, preschoolers, or early school-age children who demonstrate difficulties in the areas of expressive or receptive language, articulation or phonology, or social communication. These children might also present with a specific diagnosis such as autism, cerebral palsy or Down syndrome, but most often do not have a specific diagnosis. Students also spend one semester with school-age children and adults with reading and writing disorders. Some of these clients may have a diagnosis of dyslexia.

These two semesters of clinical experience occur during the first and second semesters of the students' graduate program. In the first semester (fall), the entire class is divided into two halves and students are assigned randomly to one section: either spoken language or written language. Students move to the alternate section during the second semester (spring) in order to give them experience with another population. Within each section, each student is paired with another student as a dyad partner. Dyad partners share two clients who are each seen twice a week for individual sessions. Each partner is responsible for the creation of weekly lesson plans as well as participating in diagnostic and therapeutic activities. This experience of working with a partner has several benefits and is considered one of the unique qualities of our on-site clinical experience.

Beginning clinical work is often highly stressful for novice clinicians. Some students may have experienced some type of clinical environment during their undergraduate education, but many see the clinical world as foreign and daunting. Pairing students with another beginning graduate student fosters a feeling of companionship and collegiality. Since speech-language pathologists rarely work independently in the healthcare and educational fields, learning how to function as a colleague is a crucial skill. In addition, working in a partnership provides students with direct experiences with more than one client. This diversity of clients leads students to a greater understanding of a variety of disorders and fosters clinical growth in a manner that working independently with only one client would not allow.

In addition to the dyad partnership, students also participate in a weekly case discussion (CD) group. Students are provided written documentation of CD group expectations and responsibilities. These include requirements for case presentation, as well as suggestions for how to lead a successful discussion among peers regarding clinical questions or issues. For example, students are expected to actively participate in group discussions by asking questions, making suggestions, adding information, and using a professional communication style. Each week, students spend 2 hours with a small group of students in a discussion format, facilitated by a clinical supervisor. Therapy sessions are videotaped so that students can then select a video segment to discuss with the group. For example, students might select a clip of a therapy activity that yielded unexpected results, a positive outcome, or perhaps led them toward a question about the client and the therapeutic process. Each student is given time to discuss issues pertaining to his or her client and is also required to participate in discussions regarding other clients. This forum engages each student in a learning process that expands his or her knowledge base beyond a single client. Since multiple clients are represented, students learn about therapy techniques and treatment planning for a variety of disorders. This type of peer group supervision allows students to expand their perspectives to include different viewpoints and to learn from their peers as well as their supervisor (Williams, 1995).

Encouraging active engagement in the learning process as a group facilitates critical thinking and self-evaluation in all members. The goal of supervision should be to assist students in their own development of self-analysis and evaluation as well as problem-solving skills in order for the student to become independent (Anderson, 1988). Active engagement in one's own learning encourages students to maintain an inquisitive nature and nurtures the development of critical thinking (Facione, 2006). These critical thinking concepts and self-evaluation measures are outlined for students in a tool that we developed (see **Table 23-1**) that states the expectations for participation in case discussions, as well as guidelines to help students consider their own development of communication skills and application of theory to practice within the group setting.

This self-evaluation tool uses a directional arrow to illustrate a continuum of development of skills. One would expect a beginning student to be toward the left-hand side of the continuum (or the beginning), with such communication skills as facilitating discussion and using sophisticated vocabulary to discuss a client's strengths and weaknesses. Similarly, one might also expect to see a beginning student at a less developed level in his or her ability to cite resources and theory related to diagnostic and therapeutic application. This continuum allows students to see their own growth as clinicians as a developmental process. Few, if any, students in their first term in graduate school would be at a well developed level for all of these skills.

Table 23-1   Student Self-Assessment Form

Communication Skills	
Skill	**Ranking of performance**
	Well developed
Facilitates discussions (e.g., summarizes information, poses questions, analyzes strengths and weaknesses of session)	———————————————→
Uses professional communication style (e.g., uses appropriate vocabulary, grammar, voice, speech rate, and articulation)	———————————————→
Contributes to group discussion (e.g., asks questions, adds information, makes suggestions, listens actively, uses appropriate code switching)	———————————————→
Comes prepared (e.g., is on time, is organized, has video-tape queued, has handouts prepared)	———————————————→
Application of Theory to Practice	
Skill	**Ranking of performance**
	Well developed
Defines professional terms	———————————————→
Cites theoretical models and research	———————————————→
Analyzes client's response to therapy and evaluation procedures	———————————————→
Explains rationales for therapy plans	———————————————→
Uses data to develop rationales for modifications and extensions of therapy plans	———————————————→

The concept of a continuum gives the students a feeling of acceptance of current skills, with appropriate vision for areas of needed growth. Students are asked to self-evaluate and identify strengths and areas of growth in the beginning of the first term. Students then return to this form to reevaluate their own progress periodically throughout the first and second terms of clinic. Supervisors also look at the student's self-assessment of skills and progress and use this information as a point of discussion during midterm and final evaluations. It is common, for example, for students to either overestimate or underestimate their skill level in a particular area. Discussions between supervisors and students about perceived skills allow for the self-evaluation process to become a part of the supervision process. Supervisors can then guide students in determining appropriate goals and objectives for growth. Students are encouraged to take this self-assessment tool into external practicum experiences and share it with supervisors in these environments in order to continue the learning process with new populations and professional communication situations.

Communication skills are of high importance to anyone practicing in the health professions, yet they do not always come naturally to beginning clinicians. Supervisors seek to encourage students to use both higher level vocabulary and clear definitions when defining diagnostic terms as well as when discussing specific therapeutic strategies and techniques. Within the case discussion group, students have weekly opportunities to orally present information to their peers and supervisor. This develops oral skills of summarization of information, use of clear terminology, and improved professional interaction with colleagues, clients, and caregivers.

Application of theory to practice is not only part of the beginning student's self-assessment process, but a journey for everyone throughout his or her career. Application involves taking information learned from an academic class, a journal article or a professional presentation, and applying it to clinical practice in a meaningful way. This is a skill that all professionals should strive for and is a major component of both the clinical and academic experiences in our program. We believe that the teaching of this skill begins with the individuals who are instructing our students.

Faculty members are often engaged in both the teaching process and the supervision of students in our clinic. Most faculty continue to practice within their field of expertise, which allows individuals to keep in close contact with their populations of interest. Some examples include serving as a consultant in early intervention agencies or schools and working in area hospitals or clinics. This also allows a faculty member to remain clinically active, which, in turn, provides an immediate experience to share with students who are beginning to understand the clinical process. All too often, clinical skills are taught by individuals who have not had an opportunity to practice clinically for many years. The teacher–practitioner model, in contrast, allows students to benefit not only from an instructor's past experience, but also from recent interactions in the clinical field.

Our model encourages faculty to perform in dual roles as clinical supervisors and academic teachers. First of all, new clinical supervisors attend weekly clinical seminars and courses on the theory of speech and language development along with beginning students. This allows new supervisors to understand the perspective and philosophy of the program and to also experience firsthand the coursework required of students. The supervisor can then refer students to readings from class, specifics of class lectures, or comments made by the course professor. Often, the professor of the class will engage the new supervisor in a discussion within the class. Perhaps a particular therapeutic approach is the class topic and the professor might have the supervisor discuss a personal experience or clinical opinion on the use of such an approach. If questions about a particular theory or clinical application arise in a subsequent clinical supervisory session, the professor of the related course can be consulted.

This integration of academic and clinical practice is beneficial to all involved. Students gain a deeper appreciation for course material when it can be applied to clinical experiences. They view the link between information taught in a course and planning for a therapy session as an integration of ideas. Academic information fuels intervention planning and vice versa. Clinical supervisors gain an understanding of the students' academic experience and its relation to current clinical issues. Academic professors find opportunities to link what is taught in the classroom with what happens in the clinical world. This regular interaction among faculty fosters a rich learning environment for students, as well as a rewarding intellectual atmosphere for everyone. The idea that all professionals should continue to explore and grow is an important lesson for students to learn.

The participation of supervisors in academic courses is extended into direct teaching experiences. For example, supervisors might teach a class on a particular topic within a course, or they could teach an entire course in their field of expertise. When clinical faculty teach in academic courses, students benefit from the overt integration of academic information to its practical application to the clinic.

Another way our program uses the teacher–practitioner model is to have primarily academic faculty supervise in the clinic. Professors teaching academic courses also offer professional opinions regarding challenging cases in the clinic. Thus, the program purposely chooses not to draw a clear distinction between faculty who are primarily academic instructors and those who are primarily clinical supervisors.

The Advanced-Practice Clinic

The advanced-practice clinic specializes in providing diagnostic and treatment services to adults with acquired neurogenic speech and language disorders such as aphasia, dysarthria, alexia, agraphia, and other cognitive-linguistic disorders resulting from brain damage. The clinic was started to provide a site for a subset of the second-year graduate students to gain clinical experience working with adults. It is modeled on a typical outpatient rehabilitation clinic that provides speech-language pathology services to stroke patients and other adults with acquired communication disorders. The advanced-practice clinic operates simultaneously with the entry-level clinic, so that both first- and second-year students are seeing clients in the clinic at the same time. Many other speech-pathology graduate programs throughout the country operate on a similar model.

In keeping with the philosophy of the entry-level clinic, clinical supervision is provided in the advanced-practice clinic by faculty members who also teach the acquired communication disorders courses. This allows for a meaningful integration of the academic knowledge students gain in their courses with the mentored clinical experiences they have with actual clients. As we have stated earlier, we believe that this aspect of the clinical education model is perhaps the most important and novel feature of the program.

In addition to providing a clinical practicum experience for a subset of the students, the advanced-practice clinic also allows the students to learn several important realities of the larger healthcare arena. With the high costs of healthcare in the United States and the limited availability of funds to pay for services, many adults with communication disorders no longer qualify for services. The reasons for this are varied, but generally arise from severe limitations in funds for chronic conditions such as aphasia. While a variety of therapies are generally covered by insurance plans in the first few months poststroke or injury, many insurance plans will no longer cover treatments for communication disorders in the chronic phase. As they enter the postacute period, many people with brain injuries from stroke or head trauma are denied further treatment. This is particularly true for individuals with limited means or those without family members to advocate for extended coverage beyond the acute period.

Settings such as the advanced practice clinics in universities and other healthcare education institutions can serve as bridges across this gap in service. Patients can receive the treatments they require and students gain valuable insights into both the nature of chronic impairments and how variably people respond to their chronic conditions.

Individuals in need of services are referred to the advanced-practice clinic, usually by speech-language pathologists at local hospitals and rehabilitation centers. In addition, many clients are self-referred. Like the entry-level clinic, clients are requested to pay the nominal clinic user fee. In the advanced-practice clinic, because the majority of clients are middle-aged or elderly adults who were forced to retire from working because of their strokes or other injuries, most have requested waivers of the fee.

The clinical supervisors in the advanced practice clinic manage all new referrals and discharges of clients. Clients may continue to receive services in the clinic for as long as they are benefiting from the intervention provided. Both impairment-based and life-participation-based treatments are incorporated into the clinical practice model. Impairment-based therapies are those that would be considered standard treatments to improve a specific speech or language deficit that is interfering with communication to some extent. For example, direct treatment targeting impairments in syntax (the rules for combining words in language) would be a type of impairment-based therapy that could be provided. Life-participation-based treatment approaches are attempts to take a step further to address the effects the communication impairment has on an individual's quality of life.

In their academic coursework covering acquired adult language disorders, students learn about the life participation approach to aphasia, or LPAA (Chapey et al., 2001). A group of practitioners adhering to the LPAA has published a set of core values that stress that services should be provided to people with aphasia as long as they are needed, that the explicit goal of intervention should be the enhancement of life participation, and that both personal and environmental factors should be the targets of intervention. Similarly, the National Aphasia Association has recently published its "Aphasia Bill of Rights," which stresses similar values (National Aphasia Association, n.d.). Students learn about this approach and other recent advances in their academic coursework, but experiencing them firsthand in the advanced-practice clinic makes them come alive for the students.

Students have experiences providing both impairment-based therapies in individual treatment sessions and focusing on life participation enhancements with each client. For example, there is a bagel shop adjacent to the clinic where many clients meet to have lunch prior to the weekly aphasia support group meeting. Within the model of the LPAA, an appropriate intervention target would be to work with the staff at the bagel shop to educate them about aphasia and to teach them strategies to maximize communication interactions with people who may have communication impairments. Another target might be to work with the bagel shop to encourage them to have aphasia-friendly menus and signs that had pictures in addition to words. These actions would result in an improved quality of life for our clients, even though the clients themselves did not receive the interventions directly.

Each semester, in addition to developing and carrying out individualized treatment plans, the students are also required to assist with the aphasia support group and help plan group outings into the community. These outings have included events such as lunch at a nearby restaurant, seeing an Imax movie at the local science museum, and attending a major league baseball game. Making the arrangements for these events has forced the students to think about how their clients must cope with physical, cognitive, and language disabilities in everyday life situations. As a result of their participation in these events, every student in the advanced-practice clinic has commented on how inspired they have been by these experiences.

Students may also gain research experience in either the entry-level or advanced-practice clinic. They have an option to complete a master's thesis during their 2-year program, and many have completed projects either fully or partially within the on-site clinic. Individual case studies, small-group assessment studies, and short-term treatment studies are possible types of projects that can be conducted within the clinic. In planning and conducting their research, students become familiar with the process necessary to complete a research project, from the initial step of getting approval from an institutional review board (IRB) to the final stages of data analysis and interpretation. While students are not required to do their research projects in the clinic, the availability of subjects of all ages with a variety of communication disorders on-site makes the process easier to accomplish for many students.

Students who elect not to do a master's thesis have been able to gain research experience by participating in various faculty members' projects. For example, one of the clinical supervisors had an ongoing project investigating the efficacy of an alternative communication treatment software program. Students assisted in the project by delivering the treatments according to the research protocol and conducting the periodic assessment sessions.

Having the advanced-practice clinic on-site at the institute operating year-round also provides opportunities for first-year students to observe second-year students, as well as opportunities for students from other programs (e.g., nursing, physical therapy) to watch sessions. In addition, students are assigned projects in their academic coursework that require them to observe a treatment session and carefully document what they observed and to determine what they think the treatment goals were in that session. Individual clients with aphasia and other neurogenic communication disorders have also been invited to be guest speakers in the class on aphasia. While students have many opportunities to watch videotaped examples of people with aphasia, they find that live interactions with people are even more valuable.

Finally, the mix of clients in our waiting areas, who are attending either the entry-level or the advanced-practice clinic, has resulted in some interesting learning experiences pertaining to living with disabilities among our students, faculty, clients, and their families. For example, we observed children attending the clinic reading books with an adult with aphasia in the waiting room. Young children have direct observation of individuals with disabilities and adult clients have opportunities to interact with young people in a social communication situation that might not otherwise be available to them. Similarly, students, faculty, and staff members benefit from the environment. For example, students in the entry-level clinic have the opportunity to interact with adults who have aphasia in the social environment of the waiting room before they have the course on aphasia. This gives the students initial exposure to a population that they will learn about later in their education.

TYPES OF LEARNERS

A faculty–student practice clinic can support a wide range of student learning styles and needs, including students who have little experience with clinical application as well as those who are moving toward independence. Using the teacher–practitioner model, supervisors can often be matched to students with specific needs. For example, an instructor who is an expert writer might supervise a student who needs assistance with the development of clinical writing skills. This model also facilitates the learning styles of students who lack confidence, as well as those who may be considered overconfident.

It is common for students facing their first clinical encounter to feel unprepared, anxious, and frightened. Although many of these students find they are able to move beyond this fear and quickly become acclimated to the clinical environment, some students continue to lack confidence in their clinical and interpersonal skills. The teacher–practitioner model allows the instructor to approach this type of student in a positive, supportive manner. Supervisors might spend time in the therapy room with the student clinician in order to model techniques and strategies before moving outside of the room to observe via camera. Students are encouraged to use self-evaluation and peer discussion as a means of improving self-confidence and awareness of areas of strength.

Likewise, students who have exaggerated perceptions of their knowledge and clinical skills (Dowling, 2001; Brasseur, McCrea, & Mendel, 2005) can also be supported in a faculty–student practice clinic. It is for these students that the development of self-evaluation skills is most critical prior to sending a student into an external placement. Analysis of a videotape postsession can be useful in order for the student to have a more objective view of what occurred in the session. For example, a supervisor might assist a student in analyzing a video clip of a session where a client's desired behavioral objective was not met. The supervisor can then help the student identify clinical and personal skills that need to be further developed.

CONCLUSION

Many positive outcomes have emerged as a result of this clinical training model. First, the teacher–practitioner model has allowed our students to be highly prepared when entering external practicum experiences. In fact, many external supervisors report that students are good critical thinkers and adopt professional roles easily. As a result, our students receive multiple job offers upon graduation and have become highly successful professionals in the field. The emphasis on self-assessment throughout the program allows students to become lifelong learners who see their professional growth as a continuum of development. Many alumni currently volunteer to precept our students in their clinical settings and several former students have returned to our program to teach courses and supervise students in our on-site clinic.

The on-site clinic is a student learning environment that enhances the integration of academic and clinical experiences and provides a rich atmosphere for the sharing of knowledge and expertise among faculty and students. The use of peers as dyads during the students' first year fosters personal growth in a collegial, supportive environment. Students learn to work as team members and to interact with a variety of clients as they learn to apply academic knowledge to clinical practice.

Some challenges of this model are common to many clinical education settings. These include logistical matters such as coordinating academic and clinical schedules with students, faculty, and clients, space management, parking, and maintenance of clinical materials. Another challenge is ensuring the right mix of clients each semester for our student clinicians. Clients with complex communication disorders who require expert therapeutic intervention may not be appropriate for a clinic geared towards the education of beginning clinicians. Similarly, clients with mild disorders are often challenging for novice clinicians because mild disorders are sometimes difficult to perceive. Therefore, finding clients who will benefit from working with graduate students is an important consideration when planning a faculty–student practice clinic.

It is crucial that faculty have time built into their schedules to meet and discuss student issues, academic planning, and coordination of course topics with clinical needs. For example, conducting a class about how to use diagnostic materials is especially helpful if this class comes before a student needs to test a client in the clinic. This is one example of how the teacher–practitioner model can function at its highest level.

This model in a faculty–student practice clinic allows for the integration of academic knowledge with the application of clinical skills. The on-site practice clinic is focused on the needs of student learners as they develop self-evaluation, critical thinking, and professional communication skills. Students benefit by having many immediate opportunities to apply their newly acquired knowledge to clinical situations with a variety of clients. Faculty members benefit from opportunities to engage in scholarly activities and from continued involvement in clinical practice. The use of the teacher–practitioner model in a faculty–student practice clinic results in an optimal environment for student learning as well as patient care.

REFERENCES

American Speech-Language-Hearing Association. (n.d.). *Responding to the changing needs of speech-language pathology and audiology students in the 21st century.* Retrieved January 20, 2006, from the American Speech-Language-Hearing Association web site, http://www.asha.org/about/credentialing/changing.htm

American Speech-Language-Hearing Association. (2005). *Standards and implementation procedures for the certificate of clinical competence.* Retrieved January 20, 2006, from the American Speech-Language-Hearing Association Web site, http://www.asha.org/about/membership-certification/handbooks/slp/slp_standards.htm

Anderson, J. (1981). Training of supervisors in speech-language pathology and audiology. *ASHA, 23,* 77–82.

Anderson, J. L. (1988). *The supervisory process in speech-language pathology and audiology.* Boston: College-Hill Press.

Brasseur, J., McCrea, E., & Mendel, L. L. (2005). Remediating poorly performing students in clinical programs. *Perspectives on Issues in Higher Education, 9*(2), 20–26.

Chapey, R., Duchan, J. F., Elman, R. J., Garcia, L. J., Kagan, A., Lyon, J. G., & Simmons-Mackie, N. (2001). Life participation approach to aphasia: A statement of values for the future. In R. Chapey (Ed.), *Language intervention strategies in aphasia and related neurogenic communication disorders.* Philadelphia: Lippincott Williams & Wilkins.

Dowling, S. (2001). *Supervision: Strategies for successful outcomes and productivity.* Boston: Allyn & Bacon.

Facione, P. A. (2006). *Critical thinking: What it is and why it counts.* California Academic Press, Insight Assessment. Retrieved July 8, 2006, from http://www.insightassessment.com/pdf_files/what&why2006.pdf

McCrea, E. S., & Brasseur, J. A. (2003). *The supervisory process in speech-language pathology and audiology.* Boston: Allyn & Bacon.

Meyer, D. H., McCarthy, P. A., Klodd, D. A., & Gaseor, C. L. (1995). The teacher–practitioner model at Rush-Presbyterian–St. Luke's Medical Center. *American Journal of Audiology, 4,* 32–35.

Montgomery, L., Enzbrenner, L., & Lerner, W. (1991). The practitioner–teacher model revisited. *Journal of Health Administration Education, 9,* 9–24.

National Aphasia Association (NAA) Aphasia Bill of Rights. (n.d.). Retrieved January 20, 2006, from http://www.aphasia.org/aphasianews111105.php

Peach, R. K., & Meyer, D. H. (1996, April). The teacher–practitioner model at Rush University. *Administration and Supervision Newsletter*, 9–13.

Williams, A. L. (1995). Modified teaching clinic: Peer group supervision in clinical training and professional development. *American Journal of Speech-Language Pathology, 4,* 29–38.

CHAPTER 24

The Preceptored Clinical Experience

Brian M. French and Miriam Greenspan

The preceptored clinical experience provides an opportunity for students, new graduate clinicians, experienced clinicians new to a work setting or practice area, or others to work with an experienced staff member in order to begin socialization and role transition, as well as gain exposure to the healthcare arena. This experiential teaching and learning methodology provides clear benefits to the learner, preceptor, school, and healthcare setting.

DEFINITION AND PURPOSES

In 15th century England, the word *preceptor* was first used to identify a tutor or instructor. The term first appeared in the nursing literature in the mid-1970s (Peirce, 1991). The more recent use of the term *preceptorship* denotes an experience lasting a designated period of time, during which an experienced clinician or preceptor enters into a one-on-one relationship with a novice clinician learner (the student, preceptee, or orientee) to assist the novice in the transition from learner to practitioner (Baggot, Hensinger, Parry, Valdes, & Zaim, 2005; Benner, Tanner, & Chesla, 1996; Marcum & West, 2004; O'Malley, Cunliffe, Hunter, & Breeze, 2000). The preceptorship is a process during which the preceptor, through role modeling, information sharing, coaching, and direction, teaches the preceptee the art of professional practice. The precepted clinical experience is a planned and organized instructional program with specific objectives and goals. It can be useful in supporting the learning process of students at all levels during a clinical, management, education, or research practicum. Other uses include orienting new graduate clinicians or experienced clinicians transferring between clinical areas. Visitors to the clinical area, such as clinicians from another country seeking exposure to the American healthcare system and roles, can also benefit from being precepted.

Student-precepted experiences typically take place within a capstone clinical course during the later part of the curriculum. Such a course might be designed to promote synthesis of theoretical knowledge, allow for more in-depth study of a specific patient population, and apply evidenced-based research to the clinical practice area. In addition, preceptors can assist students to demonstrate leadership and collaborative skills and provide experiences to enhance understanding of organizational behavior as well as ethical, legal, economic, and political issues.

Preceptorship is often used as a way of facilitating the role transition of novice clinicians. Preceptorship can also be used as a methodology for orienting experienced clinicians who are new to a particular patient population or institutional setting. This offers the clinician learner the opportunity to apply previously acquired knowledge in an experiential manner while safely accumulating new knowledge and experiences for future reference (Benner et al., 1996). During the preceptorship, a partnership is formed between the preceptor and the preceptee, in which both contribute to the outcome (Godinez, Schweiger, Gruver, & Ryan, 1999; O'Malley et al., 2000). The partnership becomes an ongoing mutual exchange between the preceptor and the learner, in a mutually trusting, supportive environment. The preceptor offers information, direction, and feedback, and the preceptee offers insight about personal goals, learning needs, and learning styles. During the preceptorship, both the student and the graduate clinician learn the rules, language, and behaviors of the work environment (Godinez et al., 1999; Horsburgh, 1989; O'Malley et al., 2000; Tradewell, 1996).

The preceptored experience differs from spend-the-day shadowing experiences or informal pairing relationships that are typically geared toward providing a broad exposure to the healthcare environment or to promote individual career awareness or understanding of the clinician role. It also differs from the mentor-mentee experience, which is generally a more long-term relationship designed to promote career growth and development and may be mutually supportive and collaborative in nature (Alspach, 2000).

The preceptorship is the opportune time for the novice to be socialized into the new work setting. In the case of students, it may be the first exposure to the roles, responsibilities, and accountabilities of the clinician role. For the graduate clinician, the preceptorship serves as a period of transition from the role of student to that of professional. The experienced clinician moving into a new work setting also requires assistance with socialization, and must adjust previous experiences to fit into the current work setting with new rules, new languages, and new patient populations.

THEORETICAL FOUNDATIONS

Socialization has been defined as the passing of a role from one person to the next, the process by which a person acquires and internalizes new knowledge and skills (Horsburgh, 1989; Santucci, 2004; Tradewell, 1996). Socialization enables the transition from previous roles to new roles, and from familiar to unfamiliar work environments. Tradewell also states that socialization occurs through observing the preceptor role model behaviors and language as well as by exposure to incumbent staff as they reflect on their practice through stories of their own work experiences. Santucci states that the socialization period involves the learning of work systems, staff roles, and employer expectations for students and new employees alike. The preceptor informs, guides, and supports the clinician in navigating the social mores of the workplace and applying knowledge gained from past clinical and classroom experiences to the technological and physiological aspects of patient care in the new setting.

During this period, preceptees may experience a loss of self-confidence in their abilities to perform skills and think critically. For experienced clinicians entering a new practice arena, the loss of their self-confidence is particularly difficult. In their previous work settings, they have been capable, experienced practitioners, relying on past experiences and intuition to function effectively. They were comfortable in their practice and felt knowledgeable about the expectations of the work environment, resources, and sources of support. In the new work environment, their self-image has changed as they find themselves unsure of how to behave or practice and lacking in knowledge regarding resources and support systems. This unfamiliarity engenders a self-image or vision that is difficult to accept, even if the period is transient.

During the transition, the preceptee begins to leave behind previously learned beliefs and behaviors and integrates new standards and expectations into her practice. Kramer (1974) described this difficult process as reality shock, a period in which the learner begins to recognize differences and inconsistencies in the new environment, in comparison to the old environment. Students transitioning to the professional role are exposed to the realities and contradictions of the real world, as compared to the known and ordered world of academia. The preceptee may question the value of what was learned, as well as the ethics of what is observed in the workplace. Finding a balance and learning to mesh the academic and work environments in a way that is acceptable for the learner may be difficult and emotionally stressful as familiar support and social systems are left behind. The work of learning, performing in a new role, balancing new and old roles, and making meaning of new work is an exhausting process that requires high-energy consumption by the learner and significant support from the preceptor.

Communication and feedback are the backbone of the preceptor-preceptee relationship. Open, honest, compassionate, and timely feedback is valued by the preceptee. Such communication requires mutual trust and respect. While it takes time to develop this trust, the reality of the preceptorship experience is that it is of the moment, existing only within a limited time frame. It is critical that an initial meeting between the learner and preceptor include a discussion of their past experiences, expectations and goals for the relationship, and personal work, learning, teaching, and communication styles. This conversation sets the stage for a successful, sharing relationship.

The preceptor is called upon to be teacher, counselor, and clinician, to guide the preceptee through this complex transition (O'Malley et al., 2000). A safe, supportive, and informative environment is vital during this period (Goh & Watt, 2003). While the key relationships are between preceptor and preceptee, supportive faculty and unit staff is critical. Faculty, managers, and clinical specialists must meet with preceptors to describe the course or orientation program objectives and enlist the assistance of other staff as necessary to assist in designing the preceptorship. In this way, there is an investment in and support for the program from the beginning. Consideration should be given to the kind of support that will be given to the preceptors throughout the experience. Support can be in the form of public acknowledgement of their work, scheduled meetings with the preceptor to ascertain whether assistance is needed, or with the preceptor and preceptee to discuss progress, support for the types of assignments the preceptor selects, and possible schedule adjustments for the preceptor to enhance the learning experience.

TYPES OF LEARNERS

Whether the individual involved in the precepted experience is a student, new graduate, experienced clinician, or a temporary visitor, all are adult learners who actively participate on some level in the identification of their individual learning needs and designing or choosing learning experiences intended to meet those needs. The precepted experience takes place in a complex and dynamic clinical environment with the preceptor facilitating the learning. The experience is enhanced by learners who exhibit well-developed adult learning characteristics. This includes an independent self-concept, willingness to freely share life experiences with others, active engagement in the process in order to meet learning goals, an openness to learning opportunities regardless of when they occur in the experience, and a problem-centered approach to learning.

CONDITIONS FOR LEARNING

The two most commonly named goals for the preceptored learning experience reported in the literature include the facilitation of socialization into the work setting and role transition from student to graduate clinician, or from newly hired orientee to staff member (Gaberson & Oermann, 1999; Guhde, 2005; Smith & Chalker, 2005). Gaberson and Oermann also reported benefits for students in terms of the ability to integrate classroom theoretical knowledge with actual clinical practice within a healthcare organization. In addition, the preceptor has the ability to provide individualized attention and guidance to the learner and improve the learner's clinical competence and confidence. The schools also benefit from preceptored experiences as students have less dependence on faculty, because preceptors serve in the educator role. In this way, a faculty member can more effectively manage a group of students through collaborative relationships with preceptors.

From the organizational perspective, student-preceptored clinical rotations may assist in meeting mission statement goals, such as a commitment to educating future clinicians. In addition, preceptorships may facilitate recruitment of employees as the learner has a relationship within the organization and is exposed to the workplace and staff. The supportive relationship between an orientee and preceptor may also impact new employee recruitment, job satisfaction, and retention rates (Casey, Fink, Krugman, & Propst, 2004; Gaberson & Oermann, 1999).

RESOURCES

Although the preceptored experience may take place in any organization that delivers health care, it is important to ensure that the clinical environment matches the goals of the experience from either the course and student or program and orientee perspective. The length of the experience is dependent on the goals to be achieved. In short, the experience can be of any length but must be long enough to provide the varied clinical exposure and experiences to ensure achievement of course or orientation objectives.

Whether it is a student or orientee experience, the preceptor and learner will benefit from contact and guidance from a faculty member or organization-based educator, clinical specialist, or manager. Preceptors should have access to a student's goals and objectives or an orientee's competency checklist in order to facilitate planning, tracking of achievements, and evaluation of performance.

Organizations that provide clinical placements to student clinicians require qualified staff to precept. In addition, they require qualified staff to precept new or transferring employees. Depending upon the staff mix in a given clinical area, there may not be an adequate supply of interested, committed, and educationally prepared staff to serve in the preceptor role, and this could be a rate-limiting factor for the numbers of students or new hires a unit or department is able to absorb. This is particularly true if the unit or department also welcomes groups of students with clinical instructors at the same time, thus creating competition for patient assignments. Staff may view the role of preceptor and the teaching and evaluation responsibilities as added work, and this may also limit the number of students or orientees for a given clinical area. All of these scenarios require commitment on the part of the unit or department manager, clinical specialists, educators, and faculty to creating a learning environment that supports staff throughout the process so that they are prepared to serve and feel valued in their roles as preceptors.

Recognition for clinicians who are preceptors can take many forms. Schools may appoint preceptors to adjunct faculty status, provide access to continuing education programs, provide certificates of appreciation or recognition receptions, and in some cases, provide vouchers for free or reduced tuition for selected courses. Although these recognition and reward efforts may have a budgetary impact on the academic institution, benefits may also be realized through recruitment of preceptors to enroll in academic programs. Healthcare organizations may or may not provide similar incentives for staff who are preceptors, including certificates of appreciation, preceptor awards, luncheons, less off-shift or weekend scheduling, lighter than usual patient assignments, or pay differentials. Again, these methods of recognizing staff for their roles as preceptors may have a budget impact but may also encourage staff to participate in this key role and contribute to job satisfaction and retention through recognition of their hard work. Speers, Strzyzewski, and Ziolkowski (2004) report that nonmaterial benefits had greater relative importance for staff in their decision to serve in the preceptor role.

USING THE METHOD

Under the guidance of an experienced clinician preceptor, the student or novice clinician begins to apply the knowledge and theory learned in the classroom to the reality of patient care and begins to transition from learner to professional. It is equally important that the environment is one in which the novice feels safe enough to ask questions and take risks. Having clear expectations for the precepting experience for both the preceptor and the novice further contributes to a successful experience. Faculty should review the goals prior to the experience if the novice is a student. If the novice is a new graduate clinician or an experienced clinician new to a particular work setting, he/she should come with expectations for the precepting experience and be prepared to discuss them with the preceptor. The preceptor, working with unit-based leadership, should also develop a set of goals and expectations for the precepting experience. During the initial meeting between the preceptor and the preceptee, goals and expectations for the experience should be shared and reworked into a mutually agreed-upon plan with time frames for achievement.

The preceptor is the key to the success of this experience. When designing the precepting experience, time and attention should be paid to the selection, preparation, and ongoing support of the preceptor. Attention should also be given to the roles and responsibilities of the learner, the clinical faculty, and the unit leadership in this learning experience.

The Preceptor

Precepting requires an individual who is committed to nurturing and teaching the next generation of professionals, someone who is both caring and clinically competent. On occasion, preceptors are selected based on their availability, convenience, and clinical abilities, but an outstanding clinician does not always translate into a skillful preceptor. There are four criteria for selecting a qualified preceptor. The first criterion in selecting a preceptor should be the clinician's interest in and willingness to assume the role in addition to his or her patient care responsibilities.

The second criterion is ensuring a positive relationship between the preceptor and the preceptee. The relationship must include trust and understanding if learning is to take place. Factors that can facilitate this trusting relationship include ensuring that the preceptor reviews written goals and objectives for the experience to facilitate up-front planning; reviewing preceptor and preceptee expectations for communication, behavior, and timelines for goal achievement; and providing time for meetings for discussion, reflection, and feedback throughout the experience. Other factors that may influence the relationship include involving the potential preceptor in the interview process for a new staff member and having a manager or clinical specialist choose a preceptor who matches her perceptions of the preceptee based on her knowledge of both individuals, including such factors as communication and learning and teaching styles.

Clinical knowledge, skill, and ability are the components of the third criterion for choosing an ideal preceptor. A practitioner with a depth of understanding of the patient population and a high level of technical skill is necessary when selecting a preceptor. Benner et al. (1996) state that the competent practitioner often provides the best guidance for the new clinician. The competent practitioner is adept at assessing and diagnosing patient needs in a step-by-step fashion. This attention to detail and use of a logical and orderly process is useful when teaching the student or novice practitioner. Proficient, expert clinicians have a breadth of knowledge and intuition not possessed by the competent practitioner but their skill often proves to be too abstract for the novice and therefore may not be the best choice to serve as a preceptor. As a task-focused learner, the novice is more comfortable with the more concrete precepts of the competent practitioner.

The ability to listen and communicate with respect describes the fourth criterion for the preceptor. During the transition from student or orientee to practitioner, the amount of new information, new experiences, and new responsibilities may be overwhelming. Students and orientees may experience a range of emotions from excitement and eagerness to anger and frustration during the transition period. The preceptor will need to be attuned to these reactions and adapt the learning experience accordingly. In order to manage this, the preceptor will need to be able to listen closely and assess the needs of the preceptee, much as they assess the needs of the patient.

The preceptor's role will be multifaceted. As teacher and guide, the preceptor will be introducing the novice to clinical practice (Godinez et al., 1999). In the first meeting between the preceptor and preceptee, the preceptor will discuss the goals for the precepting experience. The preceptor will also determine the preceptee's learning needs and learning style. This can be done by simply asking how the preceptee learns best (e.g., visual, auditory, audiovisual, verbal, or kinesthetic) or through a more formal assessment process using any of a number of standardized tools such as Kolb's learning style inventory (Kolb, 2005; Kolb & Kolb, 2005).

Role modeling patient care skills from interpersonal interactions to assessment and diagnosis and finally to intervention and evaluation will be the initial primary method of teaching. Ongoing explanations for each action will inform the learner of the reasons for the choices the preceptor makes. In addition to modeling practice at the bedside, the preceptor will model skills in communication with the interdisciplinary team involved in patient care, as well as with the patient and family.

In the early phase of the precepted experience, the novice will observe and listen to the preceptor role model. As the experience progresses, the role of the preceptor will move to teacher, as the preceptor instructs the learner in providing direct patient care, using technology, interacting with the multidisciplinary team, and accessing the resources available within the work environment.

The preceptor will spend time coaching the preceptee by role-playing interactions before they occur. For instance, the preceptor may have the preceptee practice reviewing the plan for participating in patient care rounds before they occur or giving a clinician-to-clinician report before the shift ends. The skill of the preceptor will be called into action, knowing when to hover close by the preceptee as he or she provides direct care, and knowing when to allow the learner to practice more independently. As the patient dynamic changes, so will the choices the preceptor makes relative to the autonomy of the novice. When the patient's condition is acute or changes unexpectedly, the preceptor will work closely with the learner as he or she provides care, makes assessments, and plans with other members of the healthcare team. When the patient is well known to the preceptor and learner, with a stable or improved condition, the preceptor may choose to review the care plan with the learner and then observe and evaluate the learner's ability to implement the plan.

Along with the responsibility for teaching at the bedside, the preceptor must introduce and socialize the preceptee to the work environment in order to assist in the transition from student or orientee to professional clinician. It is incumbent upon the preceptor to introduce the preceptee to the culture of the unit, the values of the staff, the formal and informal roles occupied by members of the staff, and the formal and informal rules by which the unit functions. Preceptors will need to explain basics such as how the schedule works and how to manage the hospital's communication system, as well as how to cope with the realities of the healthcare environment. The preceptor becomes a guide to the learner who has left behind familiar environments and support systems and must form a new and stable base on which to grow as a clinician.

When working with new clinicians, the preceptor, with support from unit leadership, should attempt to carve out some time for reflection. While this is challenging in today's fast-paced clinical environment, it does serve several important purposes. Time away from the clamor of the unit allows the preceptor and learner to review the patient experience and to discuss in greater depth how and why specific patient care decisions were made. Perhaps most importantly, this time provides a safe space for the learner to reflect on his or her own thoughts and feelings about what has occurred with the patient and how he or she has performed. Through these discussions, the relationship between the preceptor and preceptee is built, trust is developed, and communication is enhanced. This is vital for later discussions as they evaluate the success of the practicum or process of orientation and each person's behavior in the process. Most likely, students will be familiar with this time for reflection as this is common practice in an instructor-led clinical practicum.

The Preceptee

The preceptee is an active participant in the precepting experience and must assume a leadership role in ensuring the success of the experience. In addition to the initial sharing of goals for the experience, the learner is responsible for informing the preceptor when the goals are not being met, when new lessons are not clear, or when he or she is uncomfortable performing a new skill. Feedback from the learner helps the preceptor adapt and adjust the experience in a meaningful way that leads to a successful outcome. Without feedback, the preceptor will only be making assumptions, which may not always be correct. The learner is also accountable for following through on the suggestions and recommendations made by the preceptor. This may include practicing a skill, researching an unfamiliar aspect of clinical care, or reading a suggested article or chapter about a particular patient condition.

The Faculty and Unit Leadership

The role played by faculty and unit leadership will vary depending on the level of experience of both the preceptor and preceptee. If the preceptor is new to the role, then the faculty or unit leadership will play a mentoring role in the process and may need to provide more guidance to ensure success. As the preceptor gains experience in the role, faculty and unit leadership may only need to meet with the preceptor and preceptee occasionally to monitor the process or consult on more complex issues that the preceptor is unable to solve independently. Regardless of the experience level of the preceptor, faculty or unit leadership must maintain open communication and monitor the experience on some level to ensure objectives are met and intervene if there are issues that arise in the preceptor-preceptee relationship. Such support can be offered in direct discussions that occur periodically throughout the preceptorship or by phone or e-mail when specific questions or concerns arise.

Evaluating the Preceptored Clinical Experience

Ideally, evaluation should be a formative and ongoing process, part of the daily communication between preceptor and preceptee. Discussion and feedback about skill performance, assessment and diagnosis, and bedside interactions should be part of the regular communication of each day. By incorporating this process into the routine of the day, it becomes a respectful, helpful activity, and one that moves the precepting experience continuously forward. Competency-based tools, timelines, or lists of objectives can serve as valuable guidelines for such discussions. If goals have been set at the beginning of the precepting experience, discussion can be based on how closely the experience has come to meeting those goals. Asking simple questions such as "How do you think you performed today? Is there anything you would do differently? And how close are we to reaching each goal?" provide a basis for self-reflection and allow the preceptor to evaluate the learner's understanding of his or her performance. The preceptor can then compare his assessment of the preceptee's performance with the learner's self-assessment and provide constructive feedback to support or improve the preceptee's performance. If only summative evaluation is used to evaluate the precepting experience, the learner will not benefit from the preceptor's suggestions and recommendations since it has not been provided in a time-sensitive or event-sensitive manner. Many schools and clinical units have created evaluation tools that consider the preceptor's actions, the preceptee's actions, or both. For the new clinician, such tools most often follow a competency-based format that covers the various aspects of caring for a particular patient population, including skill acquisition, problem solving, and decision making. For the student, tools generally focus on goal attainment and the overall clinical experience, including the effectiveness of the preceptor. Preceptors may use a self-evaluation model focusing on the various aspects of the preceptor role, or they may receive feedback from the preceptee, faculty, or unit leadership using a more inclusive method. Faculty or unit leadership should participate in the evaluation process periodically during the precepting experience. They can offer objective insight into the progress being made and make recommendations gleaned from their expertise in patient care and teaching. They can also serve as a role model and support the preceptor in handling more complex feedback issues that might occur during the precepting experience. Preceptors take their roles very seriously and may feel they are solely responsible for the outcome of the experience. Active and timely faculty or unit leadership involvement will help the preceptor manage some of the perceived burden of that responsibility.

POTENTIAL PROBLEMS

In order for a successful partnership to develop, consistent, interested, capable preceptors are necessary (Boychuck, 2001; Boyle, Popkess-Vawter, & Taunton, 1996; Casey et al., 2004; Oermann & Moffitt-Wolfe, 1997). On the other side of the equation, there must be an engaged, participative preceptee (O'Malley et al., 2000).

The challenges described by students and new graduates during this transition include being able to set priorities and organize patient care needs, acquiring time management skills, a fear of communicating with physicians, a lack of confidence in their performance, and struggles with dependence and independence in the preceptor-preceptee relationship (Casey et al., 2004, Oermann & Moffitt-Wolfe, 1997). The issue of independent practice is a dilemma for preceptors as well as preceptees. Knowing when to allow the preceptee to practice more independently or when to step in and actively guide and participate in the patient care is subjective and varies from moment to moment. An event that can be handled by a preceptee in one instance may require the direct involvement of the preceptor in another case because of the impact of individual patient characteristics. This seeming inconsistency in preceptor behavior may contribute to the preceptee's issues of self-confidence and highlights the need for open, honest communication between preceptor and preceptee.

Potential problems can arise in the preceptorial experience due to factors related to the preceptor, the learner, or the process. The importance of formal training in preparing a staff member to function effectively as a preceptor is well documented in the literature (Alspach, 2000; Neumann et al., 2004; Speers et al., 2004). Although clinicians chosen to be preceptors are typically well prepared to care for their patients, in order to be effective as staff preceptors, they must also be knowledgeable regarding the principles of adult education and adult learning, learning styles, planning and implementing learning experiences, reality shock, and the principles of evaluation and providing constructive feedback. Faculty, managers, clinical specialists, and staff educators must provide opportunities for advanced education in these areas in order to adequately prepare clinicians to serve in their assigned role and to maximize the potential success of the preceptor-preceptee relationship and achieve a positive outcome. In addition, staff preceptors should have periodic contact with faculty and their managers, clinical specialists, and educators throughout the preceptorship in order to enhance communication, problem solve, and continue their development as preceptors through evaluative feedback of their performance. For preceptors, the sense of responsibility they feel for the experience extends beyond the clinical teaching that occurs. They often feel responsible for diagnosing and resolving all problems that occur, even those that are beyond their scope to manage. Frequent involvement of faculty or unit leadership helps to establish a relationship in which the preceptor feels comfortable sharing concerns and seeking an expert's advice.

The learner must receive clear, up-front communication regarding his or her responsibility for the learning process, achievement of outcomes, preceptor expectations and what he or she can expect of the preceptor, as well as practical issues such as adhering to assigned schedules and completion of assignments. This helps avoid misunderstandings about his or her role as learner and the goals of the experience. It also removes the primary responsibility for the success of the experience from the preceptor and ensures that the preceptee is aware of his or her accountability for successful outcomes.

Beyond preparation of both preceptor and learner, other issues internal to the individual must also be considered as affecting the relationship. There are many potential causes for perceived or real personality conflicts between a preceptor and preceptee, but many arise when there is a clash of values and beliefs that can occur between different age groups. The need to manage generational issues in the workplace is well documented in the literature (Gerke, 2001; Weston, 2001). Differing worldviews, personal motivating factors, preferred work environments, perceptions of work-life balance, and individual strengths and differences can create conflicts between a preceptor of one generation and a preceptee of another. Awareness and understanding of these different generational values, behaviors, and expectations is the first step in working towards a successful preceptor-preceptee relationship. Integration of this information into preceptor preparation programs is key to assisting with the teaching and learning challenges created by a multigenerational workforce.

Preparation of preceptors and preceptees requires a structure to support expected outcomes. Educational preparation of preceptors to serve in that role, orientation of learners as to what to expect in the clinical setting, written course or orientation program objectives, competency or skill checklists, articulated time frames for outcome achievement, appropriate matching of preceptor and learner, appropriate scheduling, and identification of resources to assist in the process are all aspects of a well- planned and organized preceptorship. Effective planning and creation of tools to support the process allow the preceptor and learner to focus on the learning process within the context of the busy clinical environment.

The acuity and pace of the current clinical environment provides unique challenges for the preceptor and student or orientee. The preceptor is no longer serving in one role, that of caregiver and coordinator of care, but also as a teacher of caregiving and care coordination (Alspach, 2000). The challenge of teaching while providing high quality care requires the preceptor to balance these roles. Most often, the student or new orientee has less clinical knowledge and skill than the more experienced preceptor. The preceptor must consider the rights of the patients and adhere to the ethical standard of beneficence, the duty to help, to produce beneficial outcomes, or at least to do no harm within the context of the teaching and learning process (Gaberson & Oermann, 1999). Patients must be aware that a learner is involved in their care as part of informed consent and preceptors should ensure that the learner has demonstrated the knowledge and skill to provide care safely prior to doing so independently. The challenge for the preceptor is to achieve not only the desired patient clinical outcomes but also the desired educational outcomes for the student or orientee. The preceptor's judgment must be used exquisitely to determine when a learner can provide care safely and learn safely to achieve both goals.

CONCLUSION

The preceptored clinical experience is a valuable teaching and learning methodology with clear benefits for academic institutions and healthcare organizations alike. Students and orientees who are in the preceptee role benefit from the real world experience of seasoned clinical staff preceptors. Preceptors benefit by adding this credential to their experience and learn new and valuable teaching, communication, and evaluation skills. Planning and communication are the keys to ensuring a successful period of socialization and role transition for the preceptee.

EXAMPLE
New Graduate Critical Care Program

The New Graduate Critical Care Program (Mylott & Ciesielski, 2003; Mylott & Greenspan, 2005) is a 6-month orientation and continuing education program designed to develop and support baccalaureate-prepared, new graduate registered nurses in the acquisition of experiential nursing knowledge and the application of theory and research in the care of critically ill patients. Using concepts developed by Benner (1984) and Benner et al. (1996) that explicate the development of novice nursing practice, the program combines participative and reflective didactic sessions with a preceptored clinical practicum in the intensive care unit of hire. Preceptor development is facilitated through group workshops and individual consultation. Seven intensive care units participate in the program, including medical, surgical/trauma, cardiac surgery, neurological, pediatric, burn, and coronary care. A team of central and unit-based critical care nurse managers, clinical nurse specialists, educators, and human resources staff meet regularly to provide program oversight and development.

The program is 6 months in length and the majority of participants complete it within the allotted time. Formal didactic instruction is completed within 5 months and the last month is class-free to allow for immersion in practice. This approach serves as a transition period to full professional responsibility. This time frame is consistent with the literature on similar programs, and the nursing leadership believes that a 6-month orientation is needed for the new graduate to acquire the experiential knowledge and clinical skills to practice safely and independently. Preceptors and leadership believe that much of the variation in readiness to practice occurs in the last 2 months, when the work is largely about becoming an independent clinician.

PARTICIPANT CHARACTERISTICS

Through experience, the leadership group has identified several attributes that are associated with success. These attributes include experience working as a nursing assistant in critical care; passing the NCLEX registered nurse licensing exam on the first attempt; and a committed desire to practice in critical care.

The average age of the program's new graduate nurse participants is 24 years as compared with an average age of over 46.8 years for the general nursing population in the United States (HRSA, 2004). Implications for a growing proportion of younger nurses in the practice environment are described within the literature (Nursing Executive Center, 2002). In response, the program planners have implemented a workshop on generational differences as an intervention to facilitate communication and the development of positive relationships between preceptors and new graduates (Tyrrell, 2005). Program evaluations are positive to date.

To evaluate the professional development of the new graduate participants, e-mail surveys with questions targeted towards their achievements were sent to participants in the first four classes (n=24) who are currently employed at the institution. An 88% response rate (n=21) was achieved, and collated responses indicate that respondents have accomplished much professionally and are highly involved in professional development activities. In addition to the items cited in **Table 24-1**, five respondents have served as preceptors to subsequent new graduate program participants.

CURRICULUM

The curriculum addresses the learning needs of both the new graduate preceptees and the experienced nurse preceptors. A variety of learning options and supports are offered throughout the 6-month experience. For the preceptees, a variety of learning options and supports are offered throughout the 6-month experience. The style of teaching is case

Table 24-1   Professional Development Survey Responses

Professional development indicators	% Affirmative response	N
Enrolled in graduate school	37	8
CVVH competent	94	20
Serves as unit resource nurse	59	12
Have passed CCRN exam or completed review course with intent to take exam	37	8
Clinical advancement program participation	10	2
Project Hope humanitarian effort participation	6	1

based, including simulation, narrative, and discussion sessions. Topic areas cover pathophysiology encountered in critically ill children and adults and interventions for each illness discussed. Content focuses on managing the patient requiring mechanical ventilation as well as patients requiring close cardiac monitoring, invasive hemodynamic monitoring, and neurological monitoring. Simulation sessions include respiratory distress and failure, shock, and cardiopulmonary arrests. These sessions require participants to work as a team to assess the patient, identify actual and potential problems, communicate and collaborate with various members of the health care team to identify and initiate interventions, and evaluate outcomes.

The preceptors are offered a workshop prior to participating in the program. The content includes new graduate behavior as described by Benner et al. (1996), teaching strategies, learning styles, communication and feedback skills, and interventions for precepting challenges. Techniques include case-based discussions, reflection, and role modeling. There is a panel discussion with experienced preceptors. Throughout the course of the 6-month program, preceptors are offered the opportunity to meet and discuss challenges with their peers.

The program's effectiveness is evaluated using a variety of measures. A focus group of preceptors and orientees is held in the fifth month to review the effectiveness from the participant's perspective. An evaluation tool is given to both preceptors and orientees to determine program effectiveness and areas in need of change. The tool's elements require both preceptors and orientees to evaluate the orientees' readiness to practice independently. In addition, both preceptors and orientees complete self-evaluations of how they fulfilled their program roles, as well as evaluations of their partner's effectiveness in fulfilling program roles. Finally, a postprogram review of each orientee's capabilities is done using standards agreed to by the intensive care unit leadership. The standards include participants' ability to:

- manage patients requiring invasive, closely monitored treatments such as continuous venous-to-venous hemodialysis;
- serve as a resource nurse responsible for managing the flow of patients and staff during a work shift;
- function as a program preceptor within 2 years of program completion.

NEW GRADUATE IN CRITICAL CARE PRECEPTOR NARRATIVE

The following is an adaptation of a narrative written by an experienced staff nurse preceptor (Albert, 2004). It describes the events of a typical day spent orienting a new graduate nurse participating in the hospital's new graduate critical care program. The narrative was submitted as part of a portfolio in support of the preceptor's nomination as the first Norman Knight Preceptor of Distinction Award. Nominees are asked to submit a narrative that illustrates their abilities as a preceptor. The author of the narrative, Jennifer Albert, RN, BSN, a staff nurse in the surgical/trauma intensive care unit, received the award. Awardees receive funds to attend a graduate course of their choice or protected paid time to complete a course of study with a clinical nurse specialist in their area of interest. An annual ceremony is held to announce the award and is followed by a reception for the hospital community and invited guests. A plaque that describes the award's purpose and lists the names of awardees is prominently displayed on the first floor of the hospital. The names of the patient and preceptee used in the narrative have been changed to ensure anonymity.

I am a staff nurse in the Surgical Intensive Care Unit where I have practiced for the past seven years. My nursing career began in 1989, six months before graduating from nursing school. As part of my senior practicum, I spent twenty hours per week working one-on-one with an experienced nurse on the surgical/trauma floor. I was blessed with a preceptor who was warm and welcoming, patient and professional, and who, above all, had the desire to share her knowledge and expertise with me, the neophyte nurse. I credit this positive experience with my willingness to take the challenge of reciprocating two years later when I was approached about precepting a student nurse from my alma mater. I was a bit apprehensive, as I had no previous teaching experience. What I did have however, was the desire to share my newly acquired knowledge and to make this a fulfilling experience for this student, just as had been done for me two years previously.

Since my first experience in 1991, I have had the opportunity and privilege to serve as a preceptor for over a dozen nurses, all with varied levels of experience. My intent here is not to sound boastful, but rather, grateful. For, it is I who has truly been enriched both professionally and personally by each of these individuals whom I've had the opportunity to precept over the years.

Presently, I am nearing the halfway mark in a six-month orientation process with my preceptee, Sue, a new graduate nurse enrolled in the critical care program. The narrative that follows is a glimpse into one of our days together.

Andy is a thirty-nine-year-old with a history of psoriases who had presented to an outside hospital with diffuse erythema extending from his thigh to his ankle, fever, and worsening renal failure and mental status, despite having received a dose of IV antibiotics in this hospital the previous night. His symptoms were most likely the result of either renal failure or profound sepsis. He was transferred to our hospital for further evaluation and his admitting diagnosis was necrotizing fasciitis. Andy would most likely be the most challenging and complex patient Sue had cared for thus far. Yet, as a preceptor, I knew the circumstances couldn't be more ideal because Sue had already had some exposure to this patient, as she had had the opportunity to observe his surgery, as well as participate in admitting him to our unit.

We assemble outside of Andy's room at 7:00 am with the flow sheet to get report from the night nurse. I make the calculated, but hopefully inconspicuous decision to move my seat, so that I am sitting next to Sue so that she is sandwiched between the night nurse and me. A few years ago, it never would have occurred to me that where I sat during report had any relevance. Yet, one of my former orientees commented to me one day, "Have you ever noticed that during report they (the nurses giving report) tend to always address you?" Frankly, I had never made this observation, but as I watched over the next few months, it became apparent that this was indeed true. My colleagues had the tendency to talk directly to me, almost turning their backs toward my orientee at times. To prevent this, I began to position myself directly next to my orientee, so that there was no confusion and we were both being addressed during report.

We were told that Andy was started on Xigris. Other critical pieces of data we receive during report are that his platelet level has fallen to 40,000, his hematocrit is trending down, and his leg dressing, which had not been bloody during the night was now saturated with blood, only one hour after the surgeons had changed it.

We enter the room together and Sue begins the morning routine of zeroing and leveling transducers, setting alarms, checking drug doses, and infusion rates. I note, but choose not to yet verbalize my own observation—that there is heparin in all of the transducer bags. I quietly wonder if Sue has made the same observation, and if she has, will she make the connection that even this small amount of heparin could be contributing to Andy's thrombocytopenia and therefore needs to be removed from the transducers. Sue begins a thorough physical assessment. Andy's neurological status is difficult to assess since he is heavily sedated. Recalling that with previous patients we had shut off the propofol drip in order to get a more thorough exam, Sue questions whether we should do this with Andy. Sue's ability to incorporate previous experiences is becoming evident and I support her plan, but cautiously remind her about what had been relayed to us in report—that Andy becomes dysynchronous with the ventilator and tends to drop his oxygen saturation when awake or under-sedated. My role as preceptor is to help Sue anticipate this potential instability and I do so by questioning her about how she plans to react and what interventions she plans to employ should Andy become unstable. With an action plan in place, Sue moves ahead.

Having completed her physical exam, Sue discusses her findings and observations. She is particularly concerned and focused on the continued bleeding from Andy's leg. His dressing is now saturated with blood. At this point in her orientation, Sue has no previous experience to draw on that would allow her to differentiate normal from excessive bleeding. I attempt to coax from her what she might expect to see in a patient who had lost significant blood volume by asking "How might the patient's hemodynamic profile change?" "What lab values would be of particular concern?" and "What medications might be contributing to this ongoing bleeding?" Together we explore the answers, examining the most recent vital signs, interpreting the reading from the Swan Ganz catheter, and discussing the signs of hypovolemia. Lastly I prompt Sue about the medication that may be contributing to the patient's condition. She reviews Andy's medication list, but is unable to identify the two drugs that I find concerning. I suggested that she take a close look at the transducer bags. I immediately see the smile go across her face as she identifies her earlier oversight, even before actually looking at the bags. Sue removes the heparin from the transducers and I recommend that she take a ten minute break to read about Xigris, knowing that once she does, she will be able to identify my second concern—that this medication increases the risk of bleeding and is contraindicated with acute bleeding.

Sue is far enough along in her orientation that she has begun to take a more active and participatory role in rounds. Today I will take a back-seat role and allow her the primary role of interacting with the physicians during rounds. In preparation for this, I assist her in generating a list of questions in regards to the bleeding that she might want to have answered or addressed. Rounds begin and I step back into the patient's room, far enough away so that I can hear the discussion, yet not directly involved in it. This will allow Sue the opportunity to independently interact with the physicians, while providing her with the security of knowing I am close by should she need my assistance. Following rounds, I have Sue reiterate the plan for the day, which she may think is redundant, but I need to know she has extrapolated the correct information from rounds and that she is clear on how we are to proceed (Albert, 2004).

UNBUNDLING THE NARRATIVE

Ms. Albert's narrative provides an insightful view into the thinking and practice of an expert preceptor. She chose to become a preceptor based on her own positive experience working with a caring and skilled preceptor, her wish to continue that experience for others, and finally her realization of the rewards of precepting through her own personal and professional sense of enrichment. Ms. Albert's passion for the role comes through clearly in the course of the narrative.

The expertise of precepting is apparent from the way Ms. Albert introduces the patient she selected for the shift. She was thoughtful and goal directed in the choice of patient assignment and gave specific reasons for her selection. She also displayed her awareness of the level of acuity this patient presented and the challenge this would be for Sue, her preceptee. Ms. Albert's clinical expertise is woven throughout the narrative, as she is able to guide her preceptee while anticipating potential patient problems and possible interventions.

Ms. Albert describes the importance of having a sharing, respectful relationship with a preceptee. When a preceptee she had worked with previously presented her with a critical observation regarding staff behavior toward preceptees during report, Ms. Albert felt compelled to follow up to confirm. This resulted in a decisive change in her personal placement during report, underscoring her openness as a preceptor. She mirrors this behavior later in the narrative when she describes her placement in the background during rounds with the physician staff. Ms. Albert never leaves Sue completely alone, but choreographs her presence such that it won't prevent other healthcare team members from treating the preceptee as the patient's nurse.

Ms. Albert's awareness of the new graduate's need for routine is clear as she describes the daily regimen Sue must follow when starting the shift. She is constantly aware of the patient and his needs and is thinking many steps ahead of the preceptee, but allows the preceptee time to think through and problem solve for herself. Rather than specifically telling Sue directly what to look for, she coaches, provides clues, and asks thoughtful questions to guide her. In so doing, Ms. Albert teaches and informs the preceptee while preparing her to begin her own critical thinking process. Ms. Albert uses this process several times during the shift to help Sue identify actual and potential clinical issues and also to help her devise a plan for intervention. The tactic is also utilized to prepare Sue to participate in rounds with the healthcare team. Prepping the preceptee is another example of how an expert preceptor teaches and helps build the new graduate's self-confidence and self-esteem.

Finally, Ms. Albert is tuned into her preceptee's own needs. When she provides time for Sue to review Xigris, she is aware of her preceptee's informational needs, but also her need to step back and consider all that had occurred to that point in the day. The same holds true when Ms. Albert reviews the discussion from rounds, which creates an opportunity for Sue to not only review the care plan, but also to ask questions or clarify the points discussed. Finally, Ms. Albert is aware of how Sue may feel about this process and is prepared to explain her reasons for engaging in such a manner.

Ms. Albert's narrative exemplifies the characteristics of an expert preceptor, starting with her commitment to precepting, extending through her own clinical expertise, and concluding with her ability to teach, coach, and guide her preceptee in a compassionate, respectful, yet structured manner.

REFERENCES

Albert, J. (2004, March 4). Preceptor narrative. In S. Sabia (Ed.), First annual Norman Knight preceptor of distinction award. *Caring Headlines*, *1*, 4–5.

Alspach, J. G. (2000). *From staff nurse to preceptor: A preceptor development program, instructor's manual* (2nd ed., p. 11–13). Aliso Viejo, CA: AACN.

Baggot, D., Hensinger, B., Parry, J., Valdes, M. S., & Zaim, S. (2005). The new hire/preceptor experience: Cost-benefit analysis of one retention strategy. *Journal of Nursing Administration*, *35*(3), 138–145.

Benner, P. (1984). *From novice to expert: Excellence and power in clinical nursing practice*. Upper Saddle River, NJ: Prentice Hall.

Benner, P., Tanner, C., & Chesla, C. (1996). Entering the field: Advanced beginner practice. In P. Benner, C. Tanner, & C. Chesla (Eds.), *Expertise in nursing practice: Caring, clinical judgment, and ethics* (pp. 48–77). New York: Springer Publishing Company.

Boychuck, J. (2001). Out in the real world: Newly graduated nurses in acute-care speak out. *Journal of Nursing Administration*, *31*(9), 426–439.

Boyle, D. K., Popkess-Vawter, S., & Taunton, R. L. (1996). Socialization of new graduate nurses in critical care. *Heart and Lung*, *25*(2), 141–154.

Casey, K., Fink, R., Krugman, M., & Propst, J. (2004). The graduate nurse experience. *Journal of Nursing Administration*, *34*(6), 303–311.

Gaberson, K., & Oermann, M. H. (1999). *Clinical teaching strategies in nursing*. New York: Springer.

Gerke, M. L. (2001). Understanding and leading the quad matrix: Four generations in the workplace: The traditional generation, boomers, gen x, nexters. *Seminars for Nurse Managers*, *9*(3), 173–181.

Godinez, G., Schweiger, J., Gruver, J., & Ryan, P. (1999). Role transition from graduate to staff nurse: A qualitative analysis. *Journal for Nurses in Staff Development*, *15*(3), 97–110.

Goh, K., & Watt, E. (2003). From 'dependent on' to 'depended on': The experience of transition from student to registered nurse in a private hospital graduate program. *Australian Journal of Advanced Nursing*, *21*(1), 14–20.

Guhde, J. (2005). When orientation ends . . . Supporting the new nurse who is struggling to succeed. *Journal for Nurses in Staff Development*, *21*(4), 145–149.

Health Resource, and Services Administration. (2004). Preliminary findings: 2004 national sample survey of registered nurses. Retrieved July 19, 2006, from http://bhpr.HRSA.gov/healthworkforce/reports/rnpopulation/preliminaryfindings.htm

Horsburgh, M. (1989). Graduate nurses' adjustment to initial employment: Natural field work. *Journal of Advanced Nursing*, *14*(8), 610–617.

Kolb, A. Y., & Kolb, D. A. (2005). *The Kolb learning style inventory—version 3.1: 2005 technical specifications*. Boston: Hay Resources Direct.

Kolb, D. A. (2005). *The Kolb learning style inventory—version 3.1: Self scoring and interpretation booklet*. Boston: Hay Resources Direct.

Kramer, M. (1974). *Reality shock: Why nurses leave nursing*. St. Louis, MO: C V Mosby.

Marcum, E. H., & West, R. D. (2004). Structured orientation for new graduates: A retention strategy. *Journal for Nurses in Staff Development*, *20*(3), 118–124.

Mylott, L., & Ciesielski, S. (2003, May 12). It takes a village: New graduate nurses enter critical care at Massachusetts General Hospital. *Advance for Nurses*, *32*, 29–30.

Mylott, L., & Greenspan, M. (2005, May). *MGH-IHP New Graduate in Critical Care Program Annual Report.* Executive summary presented to the Vice President for Patient Care and Chief Nurse, Massachusetts General Hospital and the Director, Graduate Program in Nursing, MGH Institute for Health Professions, Boston, MA.

Neumann, J. A., Brady-Schluttner, K. A., McKay, A. K., Roslien, J. J., Twedell, D. M., & James, K. M. G. (2004). Centralizing a registered nurse preceptor program at the institutional level. *Journal for Nurses in Staff Development, 20*(1), 17–24.

Nursing Executive Center. (2002). *Nursing's next generation: Best practices for attracting, training, and retraining new graduates.* Washington, DC: The Advisory Board Company.

Oermann, M. H., & Moffitt-Wolfe, A. (1997). New graduates' perceptions of clinical practice. *The Journal of Continuing Education in Nursing, 28*(1), 20–25.

O'Malley, C., Cunliffe, E., Hunter, S., & Breeze, J. (2000). Preceptorship in practice. *Nursing Standard, 14*(28), 45–49.

Peirce, A. G. (1991). Preceptorial students' view of their clinical experience. *Journal of Nursing Education, 30*(6), 244–249.

Santucci, J. (2004). Facilitating the transition into nursing practice: Concepts and strategies for mentoring new graduates. *Journal for Nurses in Staff Development, 20*(6), 274–284.

Smith, A., & Chalker, N. (2005). Preceptor continuity in a nurse internship program: The nurse intern's perception. *Journal for Nurses in Staff Development, 21*(2), 47–52.

Speers, A. T., Strzyzewski, N., & Ziolkowski, L. D. (2004). Preceptor preparation: An investment in the future. *Journal for Nurses in Staff Development, 20*(3), 127–133.

Tradewell, G. (1996). Rites of passage: Adaptation of nursing graduates to a hospital setting. *Journal of Nursing Staff Development, 12*(4), 183–189.

Tyrrell, R. (2005). *Understanding and leading a multigenerational workforce.* Boston, MA: Massachusetts General Hospital.

Weston, M. (2001). Coaching generations in the workplace. *Nursing Administration Quarterly, 25*(2), 11–21.

RECOMMENDED READING

Baltimore, J. (2004). The hospital clinical preceptor: Essential preparation for success. *Journal of Continuing Education in Nursing, 35*(3), 133–140.

Flynn, J. P., & Stack, M. C. (Eds.). (2006). *The role of the preceptor: A guide for nurse educators, clinicians, and managers* (2nd ed.). New York: Springer Publishing Company.

Johnson, S. A., & Romanello, M. L. (2005). Generational diversity: Teaching and learning approaches. *Nurse Educator, 30*(5), 212–216.

Yonge, O., & Myrick, F. (2004). Preceptorship and the preparatory process for undergraduate nursing students and their preceptors. *Journal for Nurses in Staff Development, 20*(6), 294–297.

CHAPTER 25

Service-Learning

Hendrika Maltby

INTRODUCTION

Students in clinical placements are expected to acquire skills, problem solve, and prepare for future employment in professional fields. Many courses also require students to reflect on their practice—what went well, what did not, and how practice could be improved for the future. Experiential learning and reflection are two of the components of service-learning. The involvement of the agency as a true partner in the meeting of agency needs and student learning adds the third component. The focus needs to be on both the students and the recipients of care in partnership (Bailey, Carpenter, & Harrington, 2002). That is, meeting community needs, students' learning objectives, and formal reflection of the experience are the components of service-learning. This chapter describes the use of service-learning in the health professions.

DEFINITION AND PURPOSE

The Community-Campus Partnerships for Health (CCPH) organization has defined service-learning as:

> A structured learning experience that combines community service with preparation and reflection. Students engaged in service-learning provide community service in response to community-identified concerns and learn about the context in which service is provided, the connection between their service and their academic coursework, and their roles as citizens (Seifer, 1998, p. 273).

Using this definition, healthcare professions have discovered that there are many opportunities to work with communities in enhancing health, as well as working with each other. "Service-learning not only connects theory with application and practice but also creates an environment where both the provider of service and the recipient learn from each other" (Norbeck, Connolly, and Koerner, 1998, p. 2). This ties in with the philosophy of a liberal education, common in North American universities:

> [Liberal education] has always been concerned with cultivating intellectual and ethical judgment, helping students comprehend and negotiate their relationships with the larger world, and preparing them for lives of civic responsibility and leadership. It helps students, both in their general-education courses and in their major fields of study, analyze important contemporary issues like the social, cultural, and ethical dimensions of the AIDS crisis or meeting the needs of an aging population. (Schneider & Humphreys, 2005, p. B20)

Service-learning operationalizes liberal education. Its purpose is to involve students in the community to provide a service that is determined by the community and connected to learning objectives in a course. Students begin to "understand that the people of a community are the true experts in knowledge of their community, because both the problems and the assets belong to them" (Mayne & Glascoff, 2002, p. 194).

THEORETICAL FOUNDATIONS

Service as a concept in the community has been implemented since ancient times, when people provided support and care to families (Cohen, Johnson, Nelson, & Peterson, 1998). John Dewey was one of the first champions of service-learning in the early 1900s, when service and educational goals were connected (Bailey et al., 2002). Over the years, various American presidents have established a variety of organizations that provided service to communities, such as the Peace Corps, VISTA volunteers, the Foster Grandparents program, and the Office of National Service.

Increasingly, community partnerships and interdisciplinary education are coming to the forefront of health professional education. In the Pew Health Commission's 1998 final report, a number of recommendations were made and a set of 21 competencies for the 21st century for health professionals that transcend disciplinary differences was outlined (Bellack & O'Neil, 2000). A main recommendation of this report was the requirement that all health professionals have interdisciplinary competence. This incorporates the competencies of partnering with communities to make healthcare decisions and working in interdisciplinary teams. More recently, the Institute of Medicine (IOM) has made recommendations for education of public health professionals for the 21st century, citing that "effective interventions to improve the health of communities will increasingly require community understanding, involvement, and collaboration" (IOM, 2003, p. 15). Service-learning is part of this education.

Community-Campus Partnerships for Health (CCPH) is a nonprofit organization founded in 1996 that assists in fostering health-promoting partnerships between communities and health professional schools (CCPH, 2006a; Seifer & Vaughn, 2002). It is a "network of over 1000 communities and campuses throughout the United States and increasingly the world that are collaborating to promote health through service-learning . . . partnerships . . . for improving health professional education, civic engagement and the overall health of communities" (CCPH, 2006a). Seifer (1998) also clarifies the differences between service-learning, traditional clinical education, and volunteerism. In service-learning, there is a balance between service and learning objectives, and an emphasis on reciprocal learning, developing citizenship skills, and achieving social change, reflective practice, addressing community-identified needs, and the integral involvement of community partners. Seifer emphasizes that service-learning is not required volunteerism, which lacks reciprocity and reflection and may not be connected to course objectives.

Using service-learning in nursing and other health professions enables the development of perceptions and insight as described in cognitive learning theories in the opening chapter (Bradshaw, 2007). Developing a variety of teaching strategies to complement student learning styles is necessary to enhance this development. Students in health professions are usually practice oriented and want to do something that relates to the adult learning principles of Knowles (1975) of recognizing the meaning or usefulness of the information learned. Service-learning allows the student to implement classroom learning objectives while providing a wanted service to a community.

TYPES OF LEARNERS

Service-learning is suitable for any level of student in any program. Diversity and cultural understanding can be key elements. The Corporation for National and Community Service (2006) released a strategic plan for 2006–2010 with four focus areas. Focus three describes the elements for engaging students in their communities with the following goals: "engage 5 million college students in service, up from 3.27 million in 2005; and ensure at least 50 percent of America's K–12 schools incorporate service-learning into their curricula" (p. 21). Chapdelaine, Ruiz, Warchal, and Wells (2005) found that approximately 500 college and university presidents have signed the Declaration on the Civic Responsibility of

Higher Education, which challenges higher education to become engaged with the community so that the knowledge gained by the students can benefit society. Service-learning has been added to courses and programs outside of health care, such as geography, political science, education, and mathematics (C. Williams, personal communication, University of Vermont, Community University Partnership and Service-Learning office, January 14, 2006).

Examples in health care include a variety of professions in multiple settings. Cashman, Hale, Candib, Nimiroski, and Brookings (2004) had medical and nurse practitioner students provide depression screening at a community clinic through the application of service-learning, providing a mutually beneficial opportunity. Chabot and Holben (2003) integrated service-learning into dietetics and nutrition education. Graduate rehabilitation students worked with inner-city seniors to provide primary prevention through service-learning and also learned about interdisciplinary roles and advocacy for those in need (Hamel, 2001). Occupational and physical therapy students provided service at a child care facility (Hoppes, Bender, & DeGrace, 2005). The nursing profession uses service-learning in partnership with many community agencies, including a sheriff's department (Fuller, Alexander, & Hardeman, 2006), a tuberculosis screening clinic (Schoener & Hopkins, 2004), a women's health center (Callister & Hobbins-Garbett, 2000; Mayne & Glascoff, 2002), a community health improvement center (Carter & Dunn, 2002), and a variety of community health agencies (Mallette, Loury, Engelke, & Andrews, 2005; Redman, 2002; Simoni & McKinney, 1998). Service-learning has also been used as a tool for developing cultural awareness with prenursing students in a first-year experience course (Worrell-Carlisle, 2005).

All of the examples cited previously use service-learning; students provided a necessary service that was tied into the coursework they were undertaking. Reflection on the service and the process was a key element. Students were able to examine issues such as homelessness in the elderly (Hamel, 2001), disabled children (Hoppes et al., 2005), social justice (Redman & Clark, 2002), underserved rural populations (Simoni & McKinney, 1998), financially disadvantaged people (Scott, Harrison, Baker, & Wills, 2005), and culture (Worrell-Carlisle, 2005). Additionally, students had their worldviews challenged and often changed them in the process.

CONDITIONS FOR LEARNING

Service-learning courses can be placed anywhere in the curriculum, and students can be partnered in groups or as individuals working with homeless people, those with diabetes, in residential living centers, health departments—in fact, almost anyone and anywhere. The learning environment becomes very broad and not bound by classroom walls. The first step is to build partnerships with community agencies that match course goals and objectives.

Prerequisites include teaching students what service-learning is and the difference from volunteerism. Outlining reflection requirements and how to incorporate this component is essential as reflection helps students to connect the service to course objectives and to understand why service is important. Reflection can be done in a variety of ways, such as in-class writing assignments, final papers, or journals.

RESOURCES

Resources can be as much or as little as needed, depending on partnerships. Many placements will be able to provide necessary supplies for projects while others may rely on students providing the materials they need. For example, the agency may be able to fund clinics (screening for tuberculosis, cholesterol, etc.); other funding may be found through other sources such as area health education centers (AHECs) or the university. AHECs were begun by the American government in the late 1970s "to address health staffing distribution and the quality of primary care through community-based initiatives . . . designed to encourage universities and educators to look beyond institutions to partnerships that promote solutions which meet community health needs" (University of Vermont, College of Medicine, 2006). Research grants can also be applied to incorporate service-learning into the curriculum and to evaluate partnerships.

One of the major requirements is time, particularly when developing partnerships. Partners can be found anywhere. This may be through a partnership-type office at the educational institution that keeps a list of partners and their needs, for example, a town planning office might be looking for geography students. The faculty member may have contacts via other courses, clinical experiences, service, or research in which the faculty member is involved.

Students also need time to provide the service. For example, a three-credit-hour course takes about nine hours of preparation time for students outside of class; therefore the service can be a part of the nine hours. Time can range from 10–15 hours over a semester to a concentrated 90–135 hours. The revision of assignments for the course can also incorporate the service-learning projects. Suggested web sites that may serve as a resource for faculty are discussed at the end of this chapter.

USING THE METHOD

Health seldom takes place in a vacuum. It requires the efforts of the individual, family, group, university, and community working in partnership. Service-learning works to address the needs identified by a partner. Therefore, one of the first essential steps is to identify a partner. This can be done over a summer, the semester prior to the service-learning, or at the beginning of the course. Maurana, Beck, and Newton (1998) have outlined some principles of good partnerships, including common goals, mutual trust and respect, building on strengths, clear communication, and continuous feedback. They list three key themes in building successful partnerships: "1. Always remember that community members are experts in their community, 2. Promise less and deliver more, and 3. Be committed for the long haul" (p. 51). Once the partner has been identified, the contract can be as informal as a verbal agreement: 'students will help . . .,' or it can be a formal written agreement outlining the roles and responsibilities of faculty, students, and partners. Web sites provided at the end of the chapter provide examples of different types of contracts. Partnerships can become one of the strengths of the course and can be utilized each time the course is offered.

The course syllabus needs to incorporate service as part of the course and not as a "mere sidebar" (Heffernan, 2001, p. 1). Heffernan describe six models of service-learning (**Table 25-1**). The model of service-learning chosen for the course will depend on the goals and objectives that students need to meet.

Decisions on the partners and model of service-learning lead to the other required components that should be included in the syllabus. How are the stu-

---

Table 25-1   Models of Service Learning

1. Pure service-learning where the service is the course content.
2. Discipline-based service-learning which make the link between content and experience explicit.
3. Problem-based service-learning in which students may act as 'consultants'.
4. Capstone courses usually offered to students in their final year.
5. Service internships, intense experiences with regular and ongoing reflection.
6. Community-based action research (or community-based participatory research) using research to act as an advocate for the community.

Source: Heffernan, K. (2001). *Fundamentals of service-learning course construction.* Providence, RI: Campus Contact.

dents going to engage with the partner? Will students work individually or in groups? Will the partner be a guest speaker in the class? Will students meet partners on their own or will the faculty arrange formal meetings? Will projects be outlined in the syllabus or will the partner and student(s) decide on this together? Will the projects be presented?

The reflection on service in conjunction with course objectives needs to be clear. How are these reflections going to be done (in-class writing assignments which are announced or unannounced, final paper, etc.)? How will they be graded? Are there specific criteria to be used? Will students have a grading rubric? Ash and Clayton (2004) provide an articulated learning structure for reflection through four questions: What did I learn? How did I learn it? Why does this learning matter? In what ways will I use this learning? Similarly, Kuiper (2005) suggests prompts for reflection such as: The problems I encountered . . . , I think I solved them by . . . , When I had difficulty I . . . . Using prompts guides students to critically reflect on the experience and how it affects both the partners and themselves. **Table 25-2** is an example of a grading rubric.

Finally, how will reciprocity be accomplished? Usually evaluations by and of all partners (the community, the students, the faculty) are necessary. These can be formal or informal. Shinnamon, Gelmon, and Holland (1999) have developed evaluation of service-learning tools for students, faculty, and community partners

---

Table 25-2 Grading Rubric

Health Promotion Across the Lifespan: In-Class Reflections:
There will be *FOUR* in-class writing assignments based on the readings and your work to date. A question will be posed during the class. You will need to tie in your reading and other work in the response. These will be assessed by how well you link the readings to your work and your thoughts about the two. They will be short and unannounced ahead of time (five marks each).

Community/Public Health Nursing

Journal
Students will complete a journal entry every two weeks (for a total of six) throughout the semester. The journal will be submitted electronically to the clinical faculty with whom you are working.

You will need to address the following items:
1. Summary and reflection of practice: This is a general overview of activities over the previous two weeks including your thoughts, feelings, judgments, and

Table 25-2   Grading Rubric (*continued*)

an evaluation of your experience to this point. It should consist of no more than one to two pages (typed).

2. Describe how you used previous knowledge and experience during the previous two weeks. Link experiences to specific course objectives. For example, if you are teaching children about asthma, you would incorporate child development, teaching and learning strategies, coping skills, respiratory diseases, chronic illness, environmental issues, etc. By the end of the semester, you need to have addressed all course objectives. Be sure to include the ethical standards.

3. What research and/or practice questions can you generate based on your previous two weeks' experience? What additional knowledge do you require for your practice in the next two weeks? How will answering these questions improve your practice?

4. Discuss one research-, practice-, or theory-based article that relates to each question in No. 3 and reflects evidence-based practice. How does what you learned from the article relate to your practice?

5. Describe the value of activities to your individual learning and meeting personal objectives.

6. Discuss the impact on your personal beliefs about nursing, health care, the nurse in community and public health, and community partnerships.

Topic (possible marks)	Your mark
Summary (5):	
Previous knowledge/course objectives (5):	
Question/additional knowledge improvement for practice (10):	
Article and relation to practice (10):	
Value of activities (5)	
Impact on personal beliefs (5)	
Total (40)	

and ask questions about attitude, experiences, and influence on future work using a Likert scale. Evaluations help to create better relationships and a stronger experience. Showcasing service-learning projects during class presentations or a campuswide poster presentation contributes to reciprocity by recognizing the work of the students and the partners.

POTENTIAL PROBLEMS

Teaching in and the facilitation of a service-learning course takes time, so a major potential problem is lack of time. Time is required to form partnerships, prepare students, and involve partners in the design and implementation of the course. Another potential problem is the lack of preparation of the students (partnerships, reflection). The information needs to be in the course syllabus and class time needs to be devoted to describing service-learning, explaining reflection, and the process of partnership. It is recommended that faculty teach only one service-learning course at a time.

Lack of involvement of community partners in the design and implementation of the service-learning projects can be a potential problem. Because one of the components of service-learning is reciprocity, involvement of community partners is mandatory. This can be remedied by clear and open communication. Regular contact with faculty is necessary so that issues can be dealt with early.

Another potential issue that has arisen is presenting service-learning work for promotion and tenure. CCPH (2005) has developed a scholarship toolkit to provide health professional faculty with a set of tools to carefully plan and document their community-engaged scholarship and produce strong portfolios for promotion and tenure.

CONCLUSION

Service-learning provides students the opportunity to develop transferable skills such as "the ability to synthesize information, creative problem solving, constructive teamwork, effective communication, well-reasoned decision making, and negotiation and compromise . . . and an increased sense of social responsibility" (Jacoby, 1996, p. 21). Service-learning fits well with health professional education. Students need to get out of the classroom and become more involved in the community and with each other in order to make knowledge come alive and to experience the context of that knowledge. This strategy can provide students with insight into community conditions; community collaboration is lived, not just talked about in class.

APPLIED EXAMPLES

Health Promotion Across the Lifespan

The Health Promotion class is a junior nursing class and is now service-learning (SL) based. The semester-long SL project produces 30-second public service announcements (PSAs) to meet the course objectives of family education strategies, to learn to give concise messages, and to realize that health education could be more than handing out pamphlets. Our community partner is the regional educational television network (RETN), the local producer and provider of media for learning, as well as a public service organization. The production coordinator came to the class to teach the basics of developing and producing the PSAs. Groups of four to six students (78 students altogether, in 14 groups) chose a health promotion issue for a particular age group and drafted a script and storyboard. This was approved by faculty and RETN. Although this sounded simple, it actually took more time than we anticipated. Having both faculty and RETN approve the scripts enabled students to incorporate their advice without stifling creativity. For example, one group that developed its PSA on toddler poisoning had the child carry the mock poison bottle rather than be seen drinking from the bottle. Once the scripts were approved, groups videotaped their PSAs with equipment borrowed from the university. It took about an hour of videotape to edit down to a 30-second message. Editing was done by RETN. The outcome was 14 health messages that were shown throughout the state over several months. Reflection on the process was done through in-class writing assignments (unannounced); and outcomes indicated that the students learned about communication, the value (and difficulty!) of providing short messages, and found this a very enjoyable experience in which to learn about health education.

Community/Public Health Nursing

Vermont has been pioneering a community partnership model since 1992, with a statewide system of 12 regional partnerships to improve health indicators, social well-being, and quality of life at the community level (Vermont Agency for Human Services [VAHS], 1999). These collaborative groups make decisions for the development and implementation of local strategies to achieve well-being outcomes developed in coordination with the state team for children, families, and individuals (VAHS, 1999; 2001). The People in Partnership (PIP) group in Lamoille Valley (Lamoille County and Southwest Orleans County) includes community members and a variety of agencies and organizations including the health department, home health department, parent-child center, women's shelter, the hospital, school districts, social services, substance abuse prevention council, and higher education partners. These partners meet every 2 weeks to share information and to coordinate and improve supports, services, and resources to reflect the needs of their community. VAHS publishes annual community profiles that outline over 60 health indicators across 10 outcomes of well-being for a wide range of populations at the community level. PIP's diverse membership uses the profiles to monitor community conditions, formulate strategies to improve troublesome indicators, and evaluate changes, which gives them a good grasp of the community health issues. The nursing students in the

Lamoille Valley are involved in projects that are developed by the partnership group. For example, a group of students developed a short course on nutrition, exercise, and stress reduction to teach fourth-grade students about being fit and healthy, as well as to prepare them for standardized testing. The nursing students developed a manual with all of the teaching plans and resources so that other teachers can now use the information. Another group is working with the drug and alcohol program to organize a community forum on underage drinking. Reflection through journals helps to put this experience into context. Students discovered that public health is more complex than originally thought, and partnering within the community provided insights that they had overlooked.

REFERENCES

Ash, S. L., & Clayton, P. H. (2004). The articulated learning: An approach to guided reflection and assessment. *Innovative Higher Education, 29*(2), 137–154.

Bailey, P. A., Carpenter, D. R., & Harrington, P. (2002). Theoretical foundations of service-learning in nursing education. *Journal of Nursing Education, 41*(10), 433–452.

Bellack, J. P., & O'Neil, E. H. (2000). Recreating nursing practice for a new century: Recommendations of the Pew Health Professions Commission's final report. *Nursing and Health Care Perspectives, 21*(1), 14–21.

Bradshaw, M. J. (2007). Effective learning: What teachers need to know. In M. Bradshaw & A. Lowenstein (Eds.), *Innovative teaching strategies in nursing and related health professions* (4th ed., pp. 3–18). Sudbury, MA: Jones and Bartlett Publishers.

Callister, L. C., & Hobbins-Garbett, D. (2000). Enter to learn, go forth to serve: Service learning in nursing education. *Journal of Professional Nursing, 16*(3), 177–183.

Carter, J., & Dunn, B. (2002). A service-learning partnership for enhanced diabetes management. *Journal of Nursing Education, 41*(10), 450–452.

Cashman, S. B., Hale, J. F., Candib, L. M., Nimiroski, T. A., & Brookings, D. R. (2004). Applying service-learning through a community-academic partnership: Depression screening at a federally funded community health center. *Education for Health, 17*(3), 313–322.

Chabot, J. M., & Holben, D. H. (2003). Integrating service-learning into dietetics and nutrition education. *Topics in Clinical Nutrition, 18*(3), 177–184.

Chapdelaine, A., Ruiz, A., Warchal, J., & Wells, C. (2005). *Service-learning code of ethics*. Bolton, MA: Anker.

Cohen, E., Johnson, S., Nelson, L., & Peterson, C. (1998). Service-learning as a pedagogy in nursing. In J. S. Norbeck, C. Connolly, & J. Koerner (Eds.). *Caring and community: Concepts and models for service-learning in nursing* (pp. 53–63). San Francisco: American Association for Higher Education.

Community-Campus Partnerships for Health. (2005). Community-campus partnerships for health. Retrieved October 15, 2005, from http://depts.washington.edu/ccph/index.html

Corporation for National and Community Service. (2006). Strategic plan 2006–2010. http://www.nationalservice.gov/pdf/strategic_plan_web.pdf

Fuller, S. G., Alexander, J. W., & Hardeman, S. M. (2006). Sheriff's deputies and nursing students: Service-learning partnership. *Nurse Educator, 31*(1), 31–35.

Hamel, P. C. (2001). Interdisciplinary perspectives, service learning, and advocacy: A nontraditional approach to geriatric rehabilitation. *Topics in Geriatric Rehabilitation, 17*(1), 53–70.

Heffernan, K. (2001). *Fundamentals of service-learning course construction.* Providence, RI: Campus Compact.

Hoppes, S., Bender, D., & DeGrace, B. W. (2005). Service learning is a perfect fit for occupational and physical therapy education. *Journal of Allied Health, 34,* 47–50.

Institute of Medicine. (2003). *Who will keep the public healthy? Educating public health professionals for the 21st century.* Washington, DC: Author.

International Service Learning. (2006). *Who we are.* Retrieved January 6, 2006, from http://www.islonline.org

International Partnership for Service Learning and Leadership. (2006). *Uniting study abroad and volunteer service.* Retrieved December 28, 2005, from http://www.ipsl.org

Jacoby, B. (1996). *Service-learning in higher education: Concepts and practices.* San Francisco: Jossey-Bass.

Knowles, M. (1975). *Self-directed learning: A guide for learners and teachers.* New York: Cambridge.

Kuiper, R. A. (2005). Self-regulated learning during a clinical preceptorship. *Nursing Education Perspectives, 26*(6), 351–356.

Maurana, C. A., Beck, B., & Newton, G. L. (1998). How principles of partnership are applied to the development of a community-campus partnership. *Partnership Perspectives, 1*(1), 47–53.

Mallette, S., Loury, S., Engelke, M. K., & Andrews, A. (2005). The integrative preceptor model: A new method for teaching undergraduate community health nursing. *Nurse Educator, 30*(1), 21–26.

Mayne, L., & Glascoff, M. (2002). Service learning: Preparing a healthcare workforce for the next century. *Nurse Educator, 27*(4), 191–194.

National Service-Learning Clearinghouse. (2006). *The national site for service-learning information.* http://temp.servicelearning.org/hehome/index.php

Norbeck, J. S., Connolly, C., & Koerner, J. (1998). *Caring and community: Concepts and models for service-learning in nursing.* San Francisco: American Association for Higher Education.

Redman, R. W., & Clark, L. (2002). Service-learning as a model for integrating social justice in the nursing curriculum. *Journal of Nursing Education, 41*(10), 446–449.

Schneider, C. G., & Humphreys, D. (2005). Putting liberal education on the radar screen. *The Chronicle of Higher Education.* Retrieved December 28, 2005, from http://chronicle.com/weekly/v52/i05/05b02001.htm

Schoener, L., & Hopkins, M. L. (2004). Service learning: A tuberculosis screening clinic in an adult residential care facility. *Nurse Educator, 29*(6), 242–245.

Scott, S. B., Harrison, A. D., Baker, T., & Wills, J. D. (2005). Interdisciplinary community partnership for health professional students: A service-learning approach. *Journal of Allied Health, 34*(1), 31–35.

Seifer, S. D. (1998). Service-learning: Community-campus partnerships for health professions education. *Academic Medicine, 73*(3), 273–277.

Seifer, S. D., & Vaughn, R. L. (2002). Partners in caring and community: Service-learning in nursing education. *Journal of Nursing Education, 41*(10), 437–439.

Shinnamon, A., Gelmon, S. B., & Holland, B. A. (1999). *Methods and strategies for assessing service-learning in the health professions.* San Francisco, CA: CCPH.

Simoni, R. S., & McKinney, J. A. (1998). Evaluation of service learning in a school of nursing: Primary care in a community setting. *Journal of Nursing Education, 37*(3), 122–128.

University of Vermont, College of Medicine. (2006). *What is an AHEC?* Retrieved January 6, 2006, from http://www.med.uvm.edu/ahec/TB8+BL+I.asp?SiteAreaID=91

Vermont Agency for Human Services. (1999). *A guide to state, regional, and community partnerships with Vermont's children, families, and individuals.* Montpelier, VT: Author.

Vermont Agency for Human Services. (2001). *Serving Vermonters in the new millennium.* Montpelier, VT: Author.

Worrell-Carlisle, P. (2005). Service-learning: A tool for developing cultural awareness. *Nurse Educator, 30*(5), 197–202.

RESOURCES

One major resource is the Community-Campus Partnerships for Health web site (http://depts.washington.edu/ccph/index.html). It contains a plethora of information, including sample syllabi that include service-learning to provide assistance to faculty who want to use this methodology.

There is also a National Service-Learning Clearinghouse (NSLC) web site (http://temp.service learning.org/hehome/index.php). This has a range of information for elementary, high school, and tertiary education settings. It includes information on national and international conferences and an invitation to join an electronic mailing list forum for "discussion on such issues as, curriculum requests, class assignments and the institutionalization of service-learning as they pertain to the Higher Education service-learning community" (NSLC, 2006). This site has a link to the Corporation for National and Community Service (http://www.nationalservice.gov), which lists opportunities in a variety of organizations. Access for the strategic plan is also through this web site; it provides further information on service-learning from kindergarten to graduate school.

Service-learning is being used for international projects, such as faculty-led study-abroad courses. "International Service Learning (ISL) is incorporated as a non-profit organization in Costa Rica and operates under Good Samaritan Missions, a 501c3 non-profit organization, in the United States. As an international educational agency, ISL provides medical and educational teams of volunteers to provide services for the underserved populations of Central and South America, Mexico, and Africa" (ISL, 2006). The International Partnership for Service Learning and Leadership (IPSL) is another organization that links academic programs and volunteer service, giving students a fully integrated study abroad experience. "The service enlivens the formal learning, and the learning informs the service. Both students and the host communities benefit from the substantial service each student gives. By studying at a local university and serving 15–20 hours per week in a school, orphanage, health clinic or other agency addressing human needs, students find their knowledge of the host culture—and of themselves—take on greater depth and meaning" (IPSL, 2006). Faculty who want to incorporate service-learning into study-abroad options will need to consult with their own institution's international offices.

CHAPTER 26

Nursing Process Mapping Replaces Nursing Care Plans

Charlotte James Koehler and Kristina Gilden Bowen

INTRODUCTION

Concept mapping, also known as *mind mapping*, is a means by which students can better understand key relationships within a complex system such as the human body or a healthcare organization. Concept mapping has found a useful place in nursing education as an alternative strategy to the linear, rote organization of information through the nursing process. To better help educators understand the use of this strategy, the phrase *nursing process mapping* is used in this chapter.

DEFINITION AND PURPOSES

The *nursing process mapping* format is a tool to assist nursing students to organize their thoughts and actions and to communicate these ideas to their clinical instructor. It can be used in conjunction with an in-depth assessment database and is used instead of a traditional nursing care plan. Schuster (2002) and Baugh & Mellott (1998) are among several authors who recognize the use of mapping as an effective method of planning nursing care. Kinchin and Hay (2005) found that concept mapping can be used as a tool to promote meaningful learning. They also found that concept maps could form the rationale for encouraging students to work in groups to maximize learning.

Mapping is defined as a graphic pictorial tool to arrange key concepts. As used in nursing education, the key concepts are nursing diagnoses and related assessment data that students collect through their clinical experience. The map develops as students diagram schematically the relationships among various clinical data. This process assists the student to visualize complex relationships and to apply theory to the clinical area. In some areas of nursing care, for example, labor and delivery, posting assignments for students ahead of time is illogical due to the time frame of patient stay. *Nursing process mapping* can be used as a tool to prepare the student to care for the typical laboring patient.

Traditional nursing care plans have been with us for a long time and have served a much-needed purpose. However, with the growth of nursing knowledge and the continuous reassessment of the role of the nurse comes evaluation of tools and ways of accomplishing tasks. In evaluating the traditional nursing care plan, as used by students, several problems come to mind. To begin with, it is rarely used as a plan, but it is frequently used in retrospect and developed almost completely after the care has taken place. To call it a care plan is a misnomer. Format rather than substance is often emphasized. For example, clinical instructors spend many hours ensuring that the student knows what column the information goes in and how to phrase the information correctly, rather than focusing on the thought processes the student uses in developing the "plan."

Another problem with the traditional nursing care plan is the use of documenting rationale that often becomes an all-consuming task. In the early stages of nursing care plans this was important. The profession was building a scientific base, and nursing textbooks provided very little nursing care documentation. Today information on nursing care is in all nursing textbooks, is accessible through Internet resources, and is covered thoroughly in nursing education programs. Students know to use ice to reduce swelling of an incision—it is common knowledge—but they spend time finding the correct page and line to reference this information when this time could be spent thinking about what is happening with the patient, selecting important information, and relating the material. Another situation that often occurs with students is the ready access of care plans from texts, hospital computers, and the Internet. It is not unusual for the student to select a few appropriate diagnoses and then incorporate them into their care plan with very little thought.

The purpose of mapping nursing practice in nursing education is to have the student develop critical thinking skills. The process allows the student to assess the patient, gather information from the literature, select relevant points, relate all of this information to the care of the patient, and illustrate the information graphically.

Castellino (2002) found that when compared to traditional nursing care plans, mapping decreased tedious paperwork and represented a more holistic view of the patient. Traditional nursing care plans are formatted using a linear approach to organize the assessed data and selected diagnosis. Mapping uses a nonlinear approach to this process, so students are better able to integrate and understand relationships between patient problems. Both faculty and students found mapping to aid in the development of critical thinking.

THEORETICAL RATIONALE

Constructionist theory (Hughes & Hay, 2001) states that the main role of teachers is to encourage active learning and construct knowledge based on previous experiences. They stated that concept mapping was built on the learner's perception and would increase learning and understanding. Concept mapping has been well documented for many years in education literature, especially in the fields of math and science. It has been used in a variety of settings and with students who have different educational and experiential backgrounds.

Several authors have discussed using concept mapping as a tool to link nursing theory and clinical practice. Kathol, Geiger, and Hartig (1998) state that using mapping provides students with an ability to visualize components of the nursing assessment and to help them visualize the interrelatedness of the multiple aspects of patient care. In this study, the maps were used for clinical preparation, and students developed a map from a case study as part of the final exam.

In another study (Baugh & Mellott, 1998), concept mapping was used with case studies in small groups during an advanced medical-surgical course. These maps were updated as students continued to increase their theoretical knowledge and clinical experience. Beitz (1998) discussed concept mapping in relationship to classroom nursing education and as preparation for examinations. Maps can show content inadequacies as well as illogical associations presented. They can also help decipher what concepts are most important.

Hsu and Hsieh (2005) concluded that using case studies in classroom environments and then having students develop a concept map assists the student to incorporate new nursing concepts and provides an arena in which to assess student misconceptions. They also discuss how students learn to define problems, connect theory with case studies, and develop appropriate interventions.

CONDITIONS

Mapping is a versatile technique that can be used in a variety of situations. The process requires instructor flexibility and students whose anxiety level is low enough to be introduced to something new and different. Since mapping is a process, it can be used in a variety of ways and can be very simplistic or developed to a very complex format. Because this process is so adaptable, it can be used with a learner of almost any age and in a variety of situations. The application is limited only by the imagination of the user.

Planning and Modifying

Teachers who are new to this technique can become more familiar and comfortable with it by using it in a structured classroom setting. Mapping can be used in lecture to represent a concept or idea (Wager, 1994), such as the relationships among information, psychomotor skills, cognitive skills, and attitude as they relate to competence in giving nursing care. It is used more informally to organize thoughts for a classroom presentation. Devising interesting but familiar ideas for students to map as a classroom activity is one strategy for introducing the mapping process.

Mapping can be a successful tool in leading and guiding discussions during postconferences. This is especially appropriate with a complex patient with whom many students have been involved. The greater the number of students who can participate in the mapping process, the more meaningful the discussion will be. Students can assist each other to draw relationships among large amounts of data and to eliminate data that is irrelevant.

The mapping of clinical concepts also assists the beginning nursing student to prioritize assessment data and develop meaningful and relevant nursing diagnoses. Ling and Suh-Ing (2005) found students needed time to develop their mapping skills, but once the skills were mastered, the students were able to interpret problems systematically, identify priority problems, and find proper interventions.

TYPES OF LEARNERS

Mapping is appropriate for undergraduate and graduate students. It is adaptable to independent learning, small group work, and very large classroom situations. Critical thinking, which is required for this process, helps students assimilate the interrelatedness of new information. Simple or complex, mapping varies widely to suit many learning situations. It is important to introduce this process in a way that students with a variety of experiences and knowledge relate to and in a way that allows them to see its usefulness.

Many theorists have described various learning styles and learning preferences that would fit well with the use of concept mapping. Gardner and Hatch's (1990) discussion of visual/spatial form of intelligence emphasizes the ability to visualize and create mental images. Students who have strengths in this form of intelligence find mapping to be an easy and fulfilling method of relating their understanding of clinical situations. The ability to spatially describe the clinical situation helps them to better comprehend all aspects of patient care. Kelly and

Young (1996) noted that a connection between experiences brings about meaningful learning. Only simplistic connectedness exists in nursing care plans, whereas the premise of mapping is to show the relationship of each domain of the patient and to unify it into a whole. This allows maximal student learning.

Nursing faculty need to enable the students to become more aware of their own personal learning styles and to offer varied experiences to facilitate different learning styles. Concept mapping is one avenue to learning that will assist with different types of learners as well as allow faculty and students to become more creative in teaching and learning.

RESOURCES

Mapping can be used in almost any setting and requires few resources. A paper and pencil are the only necessary supplies. Wycoff (1991) states that color activates the brain and helps us think better; adding colored pens and colored paper could help the student be more creative and enjoy the exercise. Wycoff also states that music increases right brain activity and helps turn on our thinking process, which assists the development of mapping. Using one or both of these strategies would be helpful if it is appropriate to the setting.

In *Concept Mapping: A Critical-Thinking Approach to Care Planning* (Schuster, 2002), there are many examples and guidelines to assist in the use of mapping in the classroom and clinical areas.

USING THE METHOD

Becoming familiar with the process and planning how to use mapping in individual situations is most important to overall effectiveness. Using mapping as visual aids in class and in handouts is an effective way to introduce the concept. This is done without labeling it or calling attention to the method, but just as a way of graphically representing information that one wants the student to comprehend. Open discussion framed around a structured way of thinking, such as the nursing process, in combination with student creativity, helps the students understand how information, skills, and attitudes learned from life, prerequisite courses, and clinically based courses are all necessary and important in reaching the aspiration of competence in practice.

A way of further involving the students is to have them use the technique personally and in a nonthreatening way. Wycoff (1991) suggests that the students be provided selected background music, colored pens, and paper and then asked to write a specific word or draw a representation of the word on the center of the paper. Starting with something as concrete as "desk" or "chair" and moving to something more related to nursing, such as "injection" or "bed bath," can be easy for students to relate. The students are to spend no more than 5 minutes on any one map. They are instructed to write down all thoughts and words that come to mind and to write as fast as they can. These ideas should flow from the central word or picture with ideas that generally relate to each other on branches. Remind the students that this is a process and that whatever they put on their map is okay. There are no right or wrong answers.

Once students become familiar with the concept of mapping, they can be directed to specific uses for communicating nursing assessment, care, and evaluation. This is a creative process, and giving the students a great deal of direction stifles this creativity; the process once again will become focused on form rather than substance. Giving this type of guidance without structure allows the student to think critically about the patient, focus on important assessment information, choose appropriate nursing interventions, and visualize the interrelatedness of the process that is nursing care.

A more guided approach to use concept mapping is to provide the students with a more concrete guideline. The clinical reasoning web in **Figure 26-1** is an example of this. It incorporates the nursing process as it challenges students to think critically about how each nursing diagnosis and interventions relate to each other to create a picture of the patient's care. The student begins by collecting data about the client's medical diagnosis and placing the information in the center of the clinical reasoning web. Next, priority nursing diagnoses are selected to address these medical diagnoses. Cues that would provide evidence that this nursing diagnosis is present are recorded on the web. Then the student assesses for the presence or absence of the cues to confirm that the nursing diagnosis is valid. Once the nursing web is complete, the student looks for relationships among the nursing diagnoses. This enables the student to identify the keystone issue, the nursing diagnosis that seems most influential in supporting the other diagnoses. Interventions aimed at the keystone issue will also address and help resolve other problems. This increases the efficiency of nursing care.

The second part of the clinical reasoning web consists of the evaluation. Students record their expected outcome for caring for this client, the measurable criteria, and the test used to determine if the expected outcomes are met. The measurable outcome criteria are the positive form of the negative cues that led to the diagnosis, something the student should expect the client to work toward for improvement. Once the outcome is specified, nursing interventions are selected to achieve the outcome. The test is simply a statement of how the criteria will be measured.

Figure 26-1   Clinical reasoning web.

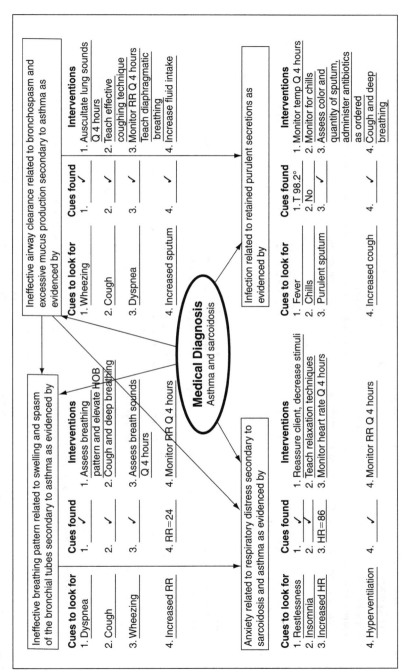

Source: Adapted with permission from Wager, W. (1994, August). *Teaching/Learning Process.* Paper presented at Teaching Skills for Health Professions Educators, St. Simons Island, GA.

continues

Figure 26-1   Clinical reasoning web. (*continued*)

Priority diagnosis _____   **or keystone issue** Respiratory status

Outcome (with measurable criteria)	**Test(s)**	**Evaluation/testing** of patient response to interventions and progress toward outcome

By the end of the clinical day, the client will have increased airway clearance as evidenced by _____

	Test(s)	Evaluation/testing
1. No wheezing	Monitor	Wheezing heard upon auscultation.
2. Effective and productive cough	Observe	Effective and productive cough and deep breathing observed.
3. Absence of dyspnea	Monitor	Client complained of shortness of breath. O_2 sat 97%, RR 25.
4. Increased sputum expectoration	Assess	Increased expectoration of brownish sputum.

Was outcome met? _partially_

Outcome (with measurable criteria)	**Test(s)**	**Evaluation/testing** of patient response to interventions and progress toward outcome

By the end of the clinical day, the client will maintain an optimal breathing pattern as evidenced by _____

	Test(s)	Evaluation/testing
1. Absence of dyspnea	Monitor	Client complained of shortness of breath. O_2 sat 97%, RR 25.
2. Effective, productive cough	Observe	Effective and productive cough and deep breathing observed.
3. Absence of cyanosis	Monitor	Skin and mucous membranes were pink.
4. RR of 12 to 20 bpm	Assess	RR 25.

Was outcome met? _partially_

Judgment: ____ Continue care plan _✓___   Modify ____   Discontinue ____

Why? (rationale, explain your judgment)
The client has shown some improvement with this plan of care and the plan should be continued to continue improvement.

Key lab tests:	**Results**	**Nursing indications**
1. $PaCO_2$	29.7	Have client breathe into paper bag to slow respirations.
2. WBC	6.8 (Normal)	If abnormal, administer antibiotics as ordered.
3. pH	7.46	Have client breathe into paper bag to slow respirations.

Figure 26-1 Clinical reasoning web. (*continued*)

Priority diagnosis		or keystone issue ___Respiratory status___
Outcome (with measurable criteria)	**Test(s)**	**Evaluation/testing** of patient response to interventions and progress toward outcome

By the end of the clinical day, the client will have a calm appearance and verbalize reduced anxiety as evidenced by _____

1. Decreased restlessness	Monitor	Client appears calm and quiet, did not report anxiety.
2. Uninterrupted sleep	Observe	Client reported insomnia last night.
3. HR between 60 and 100 bpm	Monitor	Heart rate is 86 bpm.
4. RR between 12 and 20 bpm	Assess	RR 25.

Was outcome met? __partially__

Outcome (with measurable criteria)	**Test(s)**	**Evaluation/testing** of patient response to interventions and progress toward outcome

By the end of the clinical day, the client will have no signs of infection as evidenced by _____

1. Absence of fever	Monitor	Temperature 98.2°, client remained afebrile during the clinical day.
2. Absence of chills	Observe	No chills observed.
3. Decreased purulent sputum	Assess	Increased expectoration of brownish sputum.
4. Effective, productive cough	Observe	Effective and productive cough and deep breathing observed.

Was outcome met? __partially__

Judgment: Continue care plan ✓   Modify _____   Discontinue _____

Why? (rationale, explain your judgment)

The client has shown some improvement with this plan of care and the plan should be continued to continue improvement.

Key lab tests:	**Results**	**Nursing indications**
1. PaCO$_2$	29.7	Have client breathe into paper bag to slow respirations.
2. WBC	6.8 (Normal)	If abnormal, administer antibiotics as ordered.
3. pH	7.46	Have client breathe into paper bag to slow respirations.

Evaluation of the nursing interventions is a two-step process. First the student must use the test to determine if the outcome was achieved. The student compares the client's current state to the outcome criteria and determines if the outcome was fully met, partially met, or not met. Second, the student must make a clinical judgment, based on the test results, of what to do next. Some possible judgments might be to continue the interventions another day, change the interventions, discontinue care, continue care but at a lower level of intensity or discontinue care but establish an "at risk for" diagnosis because vigilance is still necessary (Herman, Zager, & Manning, in press).

Student examples of mapping (see **Figures 26-2** through **Figure 26-5**) show how maps vary tremendously in format and terminology, but the thought and insight needed to care for patients is evident much more so than in traditional nursing care plans. These maps used a comprehensive database. On the reverse side the students included a brief (two or three sentences) evaluation of the care that they gave during the clinical setting, a brief evaluation of how they are meeting course objectives, and a general reference statement (i.e., author or lecturer). They were also required to attach a copy of a nursing journal article. They were encouraged to use a nursing research article, but a clinical article was accepted. They underlined portions of their article that helped them to better care for their patient.

CONCLUSION

When asked a few simple questions about this process, students were overwhelmingly positive. They stated that the process of using concept mapping made them think through patient problems on their own, personalize the process of caring for the patient, and not just copy a care plan out of the book. Students also commented that when using this method, they were better able to see the interrelatedness of the entire nursing process. It was also easier to use concept mapping and less time consuming than traditional nursing care plans.

Faculty using the form assessed that it communicated more succinctly what care was given and what thought process was used by the student. It was easier to read and evaluate, as well as being interesting.

Anytime something new is used, there is a potential for problems. Questions to ask those involved are will all students be able to use and feel comfortable with a nonguided format? and will faculty feel comfortable with the evaluation? The most important question to ask about mapping is will mapping facilitate the learning process? These questions will be answered as the mapping process is used. Perhaps the most important question of all is does our current method facilitate learning?

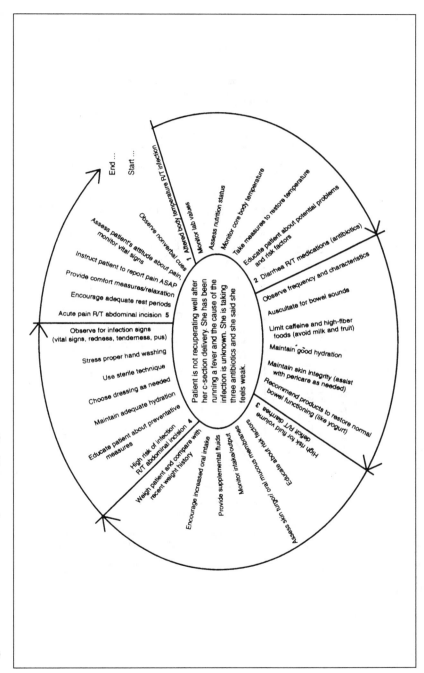

Figure 26-2 Student example of mapping.

Figure 26-3   Student example of mapping.

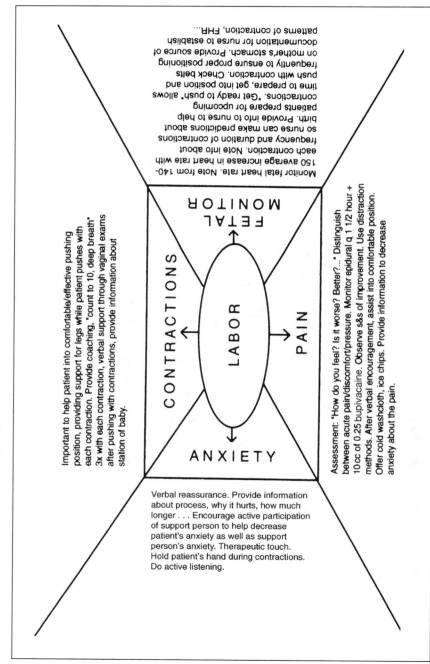

Important to help patient into comfortable/effective pushing position, providing support for legs while patient pushes with each contraction. Provide coaching, "count to 10, deep breath" 3x with each contraction, verbal support through vaginal exams after pushing with contractions, provide information about station of baby.

Monitor fetal heart rate. Note from 140-150 average increase in heart rate with each contraction. Note info about frequency and duration of contractions so nurse can make predictions about birth. Provide info to nurse to help patient prepare for upcoming contractions. "Get ready to push" allows time to prepare, get into position and push with contraction. Check belts frequently to ensure proper positioning on mother's stomach. Provide source of documentation for nurse to establish patterns of contraction, FHR...

FETAL MONITOR

CONTRACTIONS

LABOR

PAIN

ANXIETY

Verbal reassurance. Provide information about process, why it hurts, how much longer . . . Encourage active participation of support person to help decrease patient's anxiety as well as support person's anxiety. Therapeutic touch. Hold patient's hand during contractions. Do active listening.

Assessment: "How do you feel? Is it worse? Better?..." Distinguish between acute pain/discomfort/pressure. Monitor epidural q 1 1/2 hour + 10cc of 0.25 bupivacaine. Observe s&s of improvement. Use distraction methods. After verbal encouragement, assist into comfortable position. Offer cold washcloth, ice chips. Provide information to decrease anxiety about the pain.

Figure 26-4   Student example of mapping.

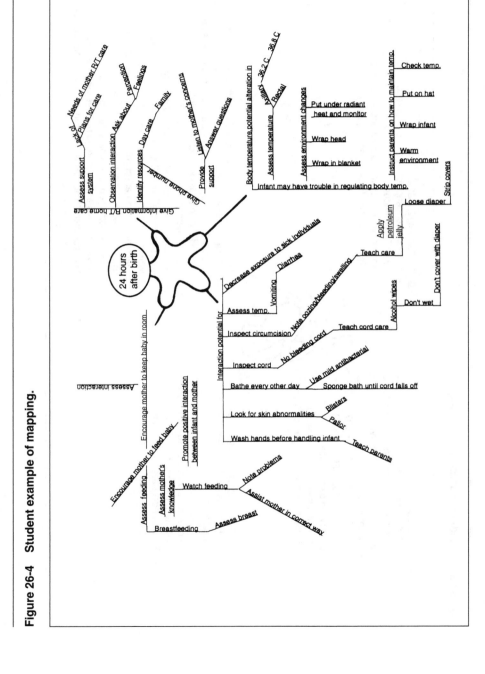

Figure 26-5   Student example of mapping.

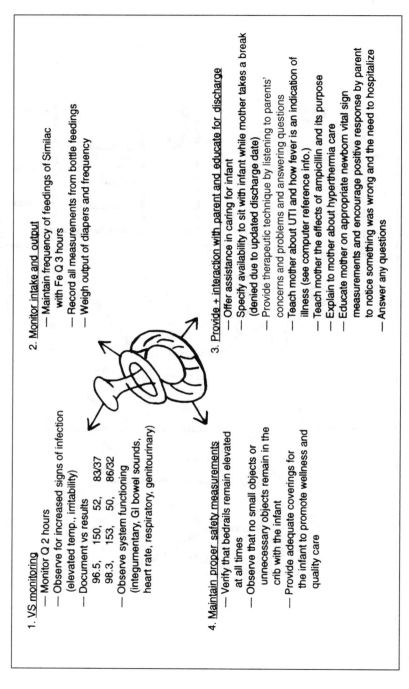

1. VS monitoring
   — Monitor Q 2 hours
   — Observe for increased signs of infection
     (elevated temp., irritability)
   — Document vs results
     96.5,   150,   52,   83/37
     98.3,   153,   50,   86/32
   — Observe system functioning
     (integumentary, GI bowel sounds,
     heart rate, respiratory, genitourinary)

2. Monitor intake and output
   — Maintain frequency of feedings of Similac
     with Fe Q 3 hours
   — Record all measurements from bottle feedings
   — Weigh output of diapers and frequency

3. Provide + interaction with parent and educate for discharge
   — Offer assistance in caring for infant
   — Specify availability to sit with infant while mother takes a break
     (denied due to updated discharge date)
   — Provide therapeutic technique by listening to parents'
     concerns and problems and answering questions
   — Teach mother about UTI and how fever is an indication of
     illness (see computer reference info.)
   — Teach mother the effects of ampicillin and its purpose
   — Explain to mother about hyperthermia care
   — Educate mother on appropriate newborn vital sign
     measurements and encourage positive response by parent
     to notice something was wrong and the need to hospitalize
   — Answer any questions

4. Maintain proper safety measurements
   — Verify that bedrails remain elevated
     at all times
   — Observe that no small objects or
     unnecessary objects remain in the
     crib with the infant
   — Provide adequate coverings for
     the infant to promote wellness and
     quality care

REFERENCES

Baugh, N., & Mellott, K. (1998). Clinical concept mapping as preparation for student nurses' clinical experiences. *Journal of Nursing Education, 37,* 253–256.

Beitz, J. (1998). Concept mapping: Navigating the learning process. *Nurse Educator, 23,* 35–41.

Castellino, A. R. (2002). Outcomes management: Evaluation of outcomes in nursing students using clinical concept map care plans. *Nurse Educator, 27,* 149–150.

Gardner, H., & Hatch, T. (1990). *Multiple intelligences go to school: Educational implications of the theory of multiple intelligences* (Technical Report No. 4). New York: Center for Technology in Education.

Herman, J., Zager, L., & Manning, L. (in press). *The eight step approach to leading learning.* Bossier City, LA: ICAN Publishing Inc.

Hsu, L., & Hsieh, S. (2005). Concept maps as an assessment tool in a nursing course. *Journal of Professional Nursing, 21,* 141–149.

Hughes, G., & Hay, D. (2001). Use of concept mapping to integrate the different perspectives of designers and other stakeholders in the development of e-learning materials. *British Journal of Educational Technology, 32,* 557–559.

Kathol, D., Geiger, M., & Hartig, J. (1998). Clinical correlation map: A tool for linking theory and practice. *Nurse Educator, 23,* 31–34.

Kelly, E., & Young, A. (1996). Models of nursing education for the 21st century. *Review of Nursing Research in Nursing Education, vii,* 1–39.

Kinchin, I., & Hay, D. (2005). Using concept maps to optimize the composition and collaborative student groups. *Journal of Advanced Nursing, 51,* 182–187.

Ling, H., & Suh-Ing. (2005). Concept maps as an assessment tool in a nursing course. *Journal of Professional Nursing, 3,* 141–149.

Schuster, P. M. (2002). *Concept mapping: A critical thinking approach to care planning.* Philadelphia: F. A. Davis.

Wager, W. (1994). *Teaching/Learning Process.* Paper presented at the Teaching Skills for Health Professions Educators conference, St. Simons Island, GA.

Wycoff, J. (1991). *Mindmapping: Your personal guide to exploring creativity and problem solving.* New York: Berkeley Books.

CHAPTER 27

Issues in Clinical Teaching: Cautionary Tales for Nursing Faculty

Patricia Christensen

INTRODUCTION

"My patient doesn't have an apical pulse!" declared the sophomore nursing student to her instructor.

"Really?" the wary instructor asked as she and the student headed toward the patient's room.

Once at the bedside of a smiling, very alert elderly woman, the student indicated to her clinical professor the spot where she was attempting to auscultate the heartbeat at approximately the level of the small intestine. "You said we should listen one inch below the nipple line," she said, as she indicated the area of the sagging breasts.

This situation is just one of the hilarious anecdotes reported by a nursing faculty member in the *Journal of Nursing Jocularity*. "I could write a book" can be heard around the tables in the faculty lounge at most nursing schools. Nursing students are nowhere a greater challenge than when they attempt to demonstrate their newfound knowledge in the clinical area on real, live patients. Thankfully, most of the students' mistakes do not have dire consequences, but the supervision of students raises issues that are of concern. Long gone are the days when a doctor told a patient—and the patient bought the story—that her shaved head was "part of her treatment," this after a horrified student nurse discovered that she had prepped the wrong patient for a craniotomy! This true story illustrates how far accountability for mistakes has evolved. Patients today would not accept that story—nor should they.

In the dynamic environment of clinical teaching, issues and events occur unexpectedly. Although one cannot accurately know all eventualities, it is wise for nursing faculty members to be aware of and plan for student clinical errors and

393

problems. Presented here are vignettes of clinical situations—all true—that may be useful to faculty members to explore as they venture forth with neophyte nurses-to-be.

CASE HISTORY 1: PROTECTION OF
PATIENT AND STUDENT SAFETY

Approximately 3 hours into a busy clinical day on an obstetrics unit, Rhonda, a junior nursing student, approached her clinical instructor. "I don't feel so good," Rhonda said. "I have this fever and my neck is all swollen."

"What?" her instructor exclaimed. "What are you doing here with a fever?"

"I didn't want to miss a clinical day. You said we should make sure to meet all our clinical objectives," the student responded.

The student was immediately sent home and the patient was reassigned to a staff nurse. The clinical instructor reported the incident to the nurse manager and finished the clinical day. The faculty member had practically forgotten the incident when, 2 days later, the student called and reported, "Guess what? I have the German measles." The faculty member thought back on the patient this student had cared for on that day. With a sickening feeling, she remembered that the student had cared for the only antepartal patient on the unit—a patient in early pregnancy with hyperemesis gravidarum. What if the student had infected the pregnant woman? Immediately, the faculty member called the patient's doctor and reported the ghastly coincidence. After a quick check of the patient's file, it was established that the patient had already been immunized for rubella, so there was no further cause for concern.

Today, with students required to show proof of immunizations, this particular case probably would not occur. Students can still report to the clinical area with a wide array of possible infectious processes, however. For example, a common cold sore can infect a newborn with the herpes virus, which can prove deadly to the baby; or a student infected with flu or cold germs could pass that infection to clients and staff members alike. With clinical time at a premium in most facilities, the students are frequently warned not to be absent for clinical days. Clinical absences can mean the loss of valuable experiences and faculty scrambling to make up labs at semester's end. Although no faculty member would suggest that a student come to clinical practice sick, faculty members can send a message that clinical days are so valuable that students had better not miss them. Students, often conscientious and not wanting to miss valuable clinical time, may underreport or minimize an illness.

Conversely, it is important to note that patients can infect students and faculty members. One scenario that was communicated to this author from a clinical specialist illustrates this point. Frequently, hospitalized patients with a communicable disease (HIV, AIDS, hepatitis, and meningococcal meningitis, for example) are not immediately diagnosed nor are the diseases suspected; thus the patients are not automatically isolated. Consequently, once the diagnosis is confirmed, care givers may have to be identified, and follow-up blood work and medication needs to be initiated in the event of exposure. If the patient was cared for by a student for a 4–8 hour time span before the diagnosis is made, this may or may not be identified when the manager reviews work schedules of possible infected individuals. For this reason, instructors need to be on guard for suspect diagnoses and follow up to assure the student is part of that investigational process. If faculty members spent time in the room with the student and client, they may also be affected (B. McCracken, personal communication, June 16, 2005).

CASE HISTORY 2: THE STUDENT NURSE UNCOVERS A SCANDAL

Helen, a senior nursing student in her last semester before graduation, was attempting to complete the assignments for the nursing management practice. As part of her requirements, she had to assess an organizational unit independently, including leadership style, structure, strengths and weaknesses of the unit, and so forth. She had been assigned to a community long-term care facility, where she also worked as a patient care technician. The student was having difficulty completing the assessment because she had become aware of some very disturbing incidents that were occurring at the nursing home, and she was unclear how to handle them. Serious suspected problems such as patient abuse, employees reporting to work inebriated, and inadequate supervision of unlicensed personnel were among the student's concerns. In her clinical conference, the instructor cautioned the student to report only her observations and not to draw conclusions, but nevertheless, the instructor was concerned. When the student submitted her final report on the facility, the instructor was aghast to read what the student had reported. Although the student had, in some instances, reported naive conclusions, the student had also undoubtedly made some astute observations of real problems—suspicious bruises on elderly patients' arms, the smell of alcohol on an employee's breath, and the absence of licensed personnel at certain times.

Armed with this information, the faculty member requested a conference with the dean of the nursing school to discuss the legal and ethical responsibilities of the student, the instructor, and the school in this case. Likewise, the dean was alarmed and deemed it imperative to include the university's attorney in the conference. After careful consideration, the attorney determined that most of the damning information in this case had been obtained while the student was an employee of the institution, not as a student. Therefore, the school's responsibility lay in urging the student employee to report her suspicions to her supervisor. The student did this with very unsatisfactory results—denial by the supervisor of any trouble and an accusation that the student was mistaken. The student subsequently resigned from that nursing home; no further attention was given to her suspicions. The nagging doubts remained, however, in the minds of the student, the instructor, and the dean—were patients in that facility at risk, and what should have been done?

This case illustrates the real dilemma faced by nursing faculty members when students observe reportable conditions—things such as child abuse and neglect—but that the nursing instructor does not witness. Do the faculty member and the school of nursing have a responsibility to report these cases? All states have laws that govern reportable incidents by health professionals, and it is incumbent upon faculty members to explore these issues. Consultation with the state board of nursing, the state department of social services, and the university attorney may be indicated in these cases.

CASE HISTORY 3: SAFEGUARDING OF NURSING STUDENTS

In the community health course, junior nursing students were assigned to various agencies within the health department and assigned as well to visit homes of families in the community. Many of the homes were in poor, neglected, crime-ridden areas. (All students had been cautioned about safety concerns while in dangerous neighborhoods and were encouraged to go in pairs on their home visits.) The instructor took turns going with each student, but for most of the semester, the students had to make their home visits without the instructor.

Nursing student Rebecca was assigned to Ms. Wilson, a new, single mother, and her infant in a government housing project. On the scheduled home visit day, Rebecca was unable to arrange to visit with another student and so proceeded to the client's home alone. While walking toward the new mother's apartment, the student's progress was impeded by a group of five young men who were loitering around the project. As Rebecca attempted to make her way down the walkway, the young men made lewd and suggestive remarks to her. Eventually, the men surrounded the student but did not touch her. The remarks included, "Hi, baby, whatchoo doin' here?" "Can we help you?" and "Man, you are some chick." The student attempted to retain her composure, but she later stated that she was very afraid. With as much confidence as she could muster, she told the group that she was a nurse and she came to take care of Ms. Wilson's baby. As she spoke, she continued to walk toward her client's home. She was able to reach the client's apartment and complete her assessment of the newborn, but she dreaded returning to her car. She wanted to call her instructor, but the young mother did not have a phone. Rebecca waited in the apartment until the young men moved on and then made a quick walk to her car and sped away. She was unhurt, but the episode was very unsettling for her, and later for her instructor, whom she told about the incident at the clinical conference.

This encounter was reported to the program director and the dean, and a committee was formed to study the issue of student safety in the community health course and to formulate policies and procedures to deal with these potential problems. Among the recommendations were that students were never to make home visits alone. At least one other student, public health nurse, or the instructor must accompany each student. Additionally, students and faculty members were issued beepers so that their whereabouts could always be determined.

Student safety is a major issue on college campuses today. Families have the right to expect that their sons or daughters will be safe while at that school. Nursing students, especially in community health courses, are often exposed to environments such as the one described previously. The schools of nursing must take extra precautions while students are out on clinical experiences. Not only are students sent to unsafe neighborhoods, but they are also often en route in other students' vehicles. Insurance coverage must be adequate to cover all eventualities. A system must be put in place to ensure that students and the school are adequately served in the area of student safety.

CASE HISTORIES 4 AND 5: STUDENTS AS POLICE

Nursing professionals, including students, are often confronted with situations where liability for reporting to authorities is unclear. For example, where is the line between child abuse and discipline as understood by parents and nurses? Is a smack on a child's face by a parent, in the presence of a nurse, child abuse or the parent's usual mode of discipline? Situations like this can and do arise in the course of clinical experiences. The following two vignettes illustrate some examples.

Case History 4

Betty, a senior nursing student, was assigned to a welfare mother and her two children for home visits as part of the requirements for the child health course. She was supposed to make a series of visits to assess the children's growth and development, their immunization status, and other aspects of primary care.

In the state where Betty practiced, it was unlawful for women to receive welfare benefits if they were living with, or being supported by, a man in the house. Welfare fraud had become a major issue in the state, and all abuse of the system was to be reported. On several of her visits, Betty observed a young man, who the mother stated was the father of her children, playing with and caring for the children. Betty also observed that the father kept his clothes and personal effects in the trailer he shared with the young family. The dilemma that confronted Betty was, should she report this case? Betty consulted with her clinical instructor and together they attempted to analyze as many aspects of this case as possible, with the overriding question being, what was best for these children?

On the numerous occasions that Betty had been at the home, she had observed the father interacting lovingly with his children and providing much-needed help with their care. Betty did not ask directly, nor was it ever mentioned by the parents, the exact circumstances of the man living with the family. The two small children appeared to be benefiting from the relationship, and it appeared that the family badly needed the consistent financial support of welfare.

A central question appeared to be, should nurses be part of law enforcement? Was this a case of fraud or a matter of client confidentiality? After careful consideration, Betty and her instructor decided to just leave well enough alone and not report that the children's father probably lived in the home. This was a case where the nurse did not feel it to be her responsibility to report a suspected violation of policy or law. Would the situation have been different if the children were not being cared for as well? Another case of a student nurse in a difficult clinical situation shows a different perspective.

Case History 5

Philip, a senior nursing student, was assigned to a single-parent family in his community health course. In the home lived a 22-year-old mother, a 3-year-old girl, and an infant boy 6 months of age. Also, it appeared that different men lived with the mother occasionally. Philip found the public housing apartment to be extremely dirty and untidy on all occasions when he made home visits. The children were often hungry and poorly dressed, but no one had observed the mother or the various men abusing the children, nor were they left alone. Frequently, however, no one would answer the door when the student knocked. One Sunday morning, the clinical instructor read in the paper that the woman who was Philip's client had been arrested for prostitution and was suspected in the death of a man who had come to the apartment for sex. After verifying that, indeed, the woman reported in the paper was the children's mother, the question arose, was there an obligation to report possible child neglect? After careful consideration, the student and the clinical instructor decided that, in this case, it would be prudent to report to the social services authorities that the children needed further evaluation of the home to be safe from abuse and neglect.

Both of these cases illustrate the need for careful analysis of cases on an individual basis. Most families, especially poor ones, have very complex relationships that can either hinder or enhance the well-being of children. If nurses are seen as agents of law enforcement, then they may lose the confidence and rapport that has been fostered over many years of public health tradition. More important, if nurses are not trusted, poor, vulnerable families may lose the care that they so desperately need.

CASE HISTORY 6: THE INCOMPETENT STUDENT

Eleanor, a second-semester junior student, was the daughter of a trustee of the university where she attended nursing school. She appeared to be an average student in her class work, but her clinical skills were incompletely assessed. In her first 2 years of clinical courses, her final evaluations reflected that she had met the objectives, but lacked confidence and was reluctant to ask for assistance. Eleanor was very open about being the daughter of a trustee and made numerous remarks about her influential father and their discussions of her nursing school experiences.

One clinical day in her parent–child course, Eleanor was assigned to a young woman in labor. All students had been assigned readings and audiovisual aids to see before they attempted patient care in the hospital. The objectives for that clinical laboratory were to provide comfort measures, to assess the progress of labor, to provide psychological support, and to observe and report any possible signs of complications. Although a staff nurse was also assigned to the patient, that staff nurse was very busy that day and did not stay in the room with the patient at all times.

About 4 hours into labor, the fetal monitoring strip of the unborn baby began to show decelerations (slowing heart rate), and on several occasions the mother stated that she felt "faint and dizzy." Eleanor, who was in the room alone with the patient for approximately 20 minutes, did not assess the fetal monitoring strip, take the vital signs of the mother, or report to the nurse or her instructor what the patient stated. On entering the labor room, the instructor immediately observed the slow fetal heart rate and promptly turned the mother on her side and took her blood pressure. Within a few minutes, the fetal heart rate was within normal limits and the mother was comfortable. Her blood pressure, which had been 90/48 when the instructor entered the room, rose to her baseline reading of 128/78.

On interviewing the student about the situation, it became clear to the instructor that Eleanor lacked even basic judgment and knowledge about the relationship among vital signs, patient well-being, and indicated nursing actions. Somehow, through copying other students' and published care plans and being quiet and unobtrusive, Eleanor had progressed through 2 years of clinical courses with minimal clinical skills. The question lingered in the instructor's mind: had other clinical faculty been intimidated—perhaps unconsciously—by the student's father's influence in the university? On careful evaluation, the instructor determined that Eleanor would receive a failing grade for the clinical course.

When the student was informed of her grade, she stated that she thought it was unfair and said, "I'll tell my father." After several conferences with the program director and the dean, it was determined that because the student had passed other clinical courses and was allowed to progress in the program, she was entitled to extra tutoring and could not be failed at that time. Vast amounts of faculty time were spent in extra tutoring for Eleanor. After she graduated with her class, Eleanor took the NCLEX exam on two occasions and failed both times.

In subsequent faculty discussions, there was always the issue lurking: how had this student been allowed to progress and graduate? In an effort to ensure that a similar situation did not occur, stricter and more objective clinical evaluation methods were instituted. These methods included objective clinical exams, as well as tests of performance. In addition, a policy was adopted that did not permit progress in the program after a clinical failure. Also, a warning system of identifying and reporting students at risk for failure was instituted.

CASE HISTORY 7: THE PEANUT BUTTER SCARE

As part of a family nursing course, students were enthusiastically planning for a teaching program on healthy snacks for a group of elementary school students. The nursing students worked diligently on a poster and handouts for the young children. They planned for an enthusiastic and interactive teaching project, which would involve the children. Among the planned activities was the serving of healthy snacks. There were many suggestions, such as "ants on a log" (peanut butter in celery ribs with raisins as the "ants"), cheese and crackers, carrots, apples, and other fruits and vegetables. The students made arrangements to buy the food and prepare the snacks.

The day of the teaching project, the students met at the school and assembled the snacks. The teaching project went well, with a lot of interaction occurring between the nursing students and the children. The children enthusiastically identified the cutout pictures of healthy snacks on the colorful poster. They outlined the coloring sheets with bright crayons. As the snacks of fruit, "ants on a log," and milk were put out, the children clamored for their healthy snacks. Each of the children came forward and eagerly accepted the paper plates with the equal portions of fruit, celery sticks with peanut butter, and a small cup of milk. One child, a small 8-year-old girl, tugged on a student nurse's shirt and shyly asked if there were any other snacks she could have.

The student said, "No, these are all we have. Don't you like fruit and peanut butter?" The little girl turned away with her plate and sat at her desk.

While the other children ate their food, this young girl just looked at her plate. Another one of the nursing students noticed this behavior and approached the child. "What's the matter? Aren't you hungry?"

"My mommy won't let me eat peanut butter. It makes me sick," the little girl responded.

Just then, the girl's teacher came to the class. "Oh, no!" she exclaimed. "Judy can't eat peanut butter. She is very allergic. She can go into shock."

The nursing student realized with a sudden rush of anxiety that a major disaster was narrowly averted. She immediately took the plate away and apologized to the girl. As a substitute, she gave the child an extra helping of apple and orange slices on a clean plate.

During postconference with her instructor and the other students, the student relayed the scary experience. The nursing faculty member realized at once that somehow, in the planning and implementation of the learning experience, the risk of food allergy had not been adequately addressed.

Increasingly, there are reports of severe allergic reactions among all segments of the population, including children. Many of the culprits are well-loved and frequently consumed foods such as peanut butter. Other sensitivities that are of concern include latex products, including examining gloves, foods with dyes or other additives, and common household products. The list of possible antigens is long and diverse. What implications does this reality have for nursing education? Most nurses are mindful of allergies among hospitalized patients because these conditions are assessed and noted prominently on the patients' charts, but what about community clients? How can these risks be minimized in that population? The answer lies in two major strategies—assessment and informed consent.

As a result of the peanut butter episode, the faculty members formulated and implemented a policy that all community clients must be assessed for allergies and sign an informed consent form. In the case of children, permission forms are to be distributed to parents and returned to the school or other setting. The forms not only ask for allergies but also grant permission for the child to participate in a health project. Although it may be difficult to implement, only those children whose parents have given permission will be allowed to participate in clinical experiences with nursing students. Unfortunately, the risks to children and the financial liability of the school must limit the participation of children who do not obtain permissions in advance from parents and guardians.

CASE HISTORY 8: SUBSTANCE ABUSE OF THE STUDENT NURSE

Nancy, a student nurse, had come under the scrutiny of faculty members because she was suspected of being anorexic. She appeared to have lost a great deal of weight over four semesters. At the beginning of Nancy's final semester, her faculty advisor asked her directly if she was eating properly. Nancy vehemently denied that she was anorexic or having any problems at all. The faculty advisor made a referral to the university counseling department and gave all the pertinent information to Nancy with the advice that she seek assessment and guidance. Nancy did not follow up on this advice and continued her studies.

Nancy was within 2 weeks of graduation when she came to her clinical area, the emergency department of a large, urban hospital, after drinking the night before. Since she was anorexic and didn't metabolize well, the alcohol was still present in her system. When she went to her leadership practicum that morning (which she could have rescheduled with her preceptor), she smelled of alcohol. She was working in the clinical area with an unconscious patient. The staff members thought initially that the patient was the source of the smell of alcohol. However, one of the nurses realized it was the student who smelled like alcohol. The nurses called the instructor, who called the department chair of the school of nursing. The instructor went to the clinical site immediately. The administrators of the clinical site asked the student to consent to a blood alcohol test. Following the test, it was determined that the student was positive. The nursing instructor called the student's family to come and drive the student home. Subsequently, the student was expelled from the nursing program. It was the recommendation of the board of nursing based on the principle that the student had jeopardized patient safety (C. Dyches, personal communication, June 20, 2005).

CASE HISTORY 9: THE DISHONEST STUDENT

Cynthia, a senior student, had to fulfill 120 hours of clinical experience with a preceptor to complete the requirements of her final nursing course. The course faculty members conducted phone conferences and mail communications with the preceptors to monitor student progress. Cynthia avoided the phone conference between the student, preceptor, and instructor throughout the semester.

Eventually, the instructor had a conversation with the student, and supposedly the preceptor. The instructor later noticed that the signature on the evaluation form did not match the signature on the original contract. This raised her suspicions that there was something improper in this student's clinical documentation. The instructor identified the preceptor through her license and contacted her at home. The preceptor related that she had worked at the location, but had since resigned. She stated, further, that she had never agreed to serve as the preceptor. The preceptor's information was correct such as educational degrees, settings, and so forth.

Evidently, the student had gained access to personnel files from someone else. The student was confronted by the instructor and eventually confessed that she had not completed the clinical hours with that preceptor. The faculty and dean of the school of nursing contacted the board of nursing for advice. The issues centered on both the dishonesty of the student's clinical performance and the breach of personnel records at the site. The board of nursing recommended that the student be expelled. An RN who had participated in the student's fraud had her license suspended. In addition, the board of nursing reviewed the site and contacted the necessary authorities. Furthermore, it was found that the "preceptor" was within her rights to bring charges against the student for identity theft (C. Dyches, personal communication, June 20, 2005).

GUIDELINES FOR FACULTY

Although problems such as the ones reported here are unpredictable, clinical nursing faculty members would be wise to consider some contingency plans for the unexpected. One of the most important considerations in protecting the student, the patient, and the school is open communication. An ongoing and supportive relationship between the school of nursing and the respective state board of nursing is essential. Additionally, an open communication line with the university attorney (or an attorney consultant) can provide essential legal guidance. Paramount in these relationships is the need for immediacy in replies. Often, situations that demand a quick answer occur. Relationships must be forged on a trusting basis that allows for on-the-spot consulting.

Another dimension of open communication centers on informing students of their rights and responsibilities while attending the school of nursing. A student handbook is often an avenue for distributing such information. A written account, such as a handbook, can serve as a contract for students. A student handbook should be specific enough to be useful, but not so specific as to limit the school in a changing environment. For example, it is not possible—or desirable—to attempt to list every eventuality that may occur. Pertinent information can be catalogued under headings such as "Uniform Policy," "Student Illness in the Clinical Area," and "Student Safety in the Clinical Area." Likewise, consequences of "Unsafe Behavior" can be addressed in a way that does not limit the school policy.

Another avenue of student information can be a complete and mandatory student orientation. There is often a need to convey information to students that is more fluid and changing than can be covered in a handbook—for example, the location of an agency, parking, contact persons in the clinical area, and so forth. In many cases, having students sign for written information can form a "contract of understanding." Under no circumstances can school officials assume that students have essential information upon entry into the program or course. A certain amount of redundancy in student expectations for each course is to be expected.

The relationships among the schools of nursing and the clinical agencies need to be initiated, fostered, and evaluated on a regular basis. The mutuality of these relationships cannot be overstated. The process of supporting these relationships includes:

1. All agencies need current copies of all class and clinical syllabi distributed to all units where students practice.
2. Orientation of faculty and clinical practitioners must be conducted in collaborative sessions. Thus, the professionals in the clinical agencies have a clear picture of the student objectives and their role in supporting those objectives. Conversely, faculty need thorough orientation to the clinical agencies' policies, procedures, chain of command, risk management, and so forth.
3. Contact people for each agency and each faculty member should be distributed to all affected parties with a chain of command and agency and faculty office phone numbers. In addition, students need contact lists of faculty and clinical agencies.
4. The process of mutual evaluation of the school of nursing and the clinical agency needs to be in place and used each term. Also, contingency plans for bad weather and emergencies should be thoroughly explained. Copies of this document need to be distributed to all faculty members and appropriate agency personnel.

The National League for Nursing Accreditation Commission, Inc. (NLNAC), the American Association of Colleges of Nursing (AACN), and program nurse consultants at all state boards of nursing can provide guidance to schools on the formation of student policies and handbooks. It is advisable to have policies and handbooks pilot-tested and read by students, faculty, and parent groups for clarity and meaning before officially disseminating them to students and faculty. This author also advises a legal opinion on policies.

In the dynamic environment of clinical teaching, events that are unpredictable and troublesome occur. Although no one can accurately know all eventualities, nursing faculty members should be aware of, and plan for, student clinical errors and problems. The careful and judicious formulation of student policies and handbooks and open and ongoing communication with students, faculty, state officials, and legal consultants will diminish the chances of dire consequences arising from student mishaps.

RECOMMENDED READING

Carroll, M., Morin, E., Hayes, R., & Carter, S. (1999). Assessing students' perceived threats to safety in the community. *Nurse Educator, 24*, 31–35.

Edmond, C. (2001). A new paradigm for practice education. *Nurse Education Today, 4*, 251.

Ellerton, M. (2003). Preceptorship: The changing face of clinical teaching. *Nurse Educator, 5*, 200–201.

Erickson-Owens, D. (2001). Fostering evidence-based care in clinical teaching. *Journal of Midwifery & Women's Health, 46*, 137–145, 121–125.

Johnson, C. (1999). Evaluating preceptorship experiences in a distance nursing program. *Journal of National Black Nurses' Association, 2*, 65–78.

Kotch, J. (1997). *Maternal and child health, programs, problems, and policy in public health.* Gaithersburg, MD: Aspen Publishers.

Mellon, S., & Nelson, P. (1998). Leadership experiences in the community for nursing students: Redesigning education for the 21st century. *Nursing and Health Care Perspectives, 19*, 120–123.

Melrose, S. (2004). What works? A personal account of clinical teaching strategies in nursing. *Education for Health, 2*, 236–239.

Morin, K. (2002). Selected factors associated with students' perceptions of threat in the community. *Public Health Nursing, 19*, 451–459.

Sawin, K. (2001). Teaching strategies used by experienced preceptors. *Issues in Interdisciplinary Care, 3*, 197–206.

Shoultz, J., & Amundson, M. (1998). Nurse educators' knowledge of primary health care: Implications for community-based education, practice, and research. *Nursing and Health Care Perspectives, 19*, 115–119.

Tang, F. (2005). Students' perceptions of effective and ineffective clinical instructors. *Journal of Nursing Education, 44*, 187–192.

SECTION VI

EVALUATION

The final section of this text presents a brief glimpse at a key aspect of any educational program: evaluation. Whereas the importance of evaluation is often overlooked, it is an essential part of the teaching-learning process. Educators predominately think of evaluation either in the form of testing and grading or in clinical evaluation. Two chapters in this section describe innovative strategies by which the faculty can conduct student evaluation.

The final chapter is a fitting conclusion to this book. Evaluation of education in the health professions starts at the lower levels of evaluation of learning to indicate how well students are meeting outcomes of the course and the program. Instructors customarily use data such as results on exams and clinical performance. Feedback from students, as consumers, provides useful, practical information. This information then feeds into the total program evaluation and provides data on the curriculum, teaching effectiveness, and the use of learning activities. A thorough evaluation provides information for the future.

CHAPTER 28

Evaluation of Programmatic Learning Outcomes

Jill M. Hayes

INTRODUCTION

The role of faculty in a collegiate setting involves a complex set of expectations that vary depending on the institutional mission and the type of program. Regardless of the institutional mission, all educational institutions have a focus on teaching and student outcomes.

The teaching role of the faculty includes all aspects of facilitating student learning, including evaluation of learning. However, evaluation of learning is only one component of evaluation associated with the faculty role. Faculty members are also involved in evaluation of teaching, evaluation of their peers, and evaluation of the program. Therefore, an understanding of evaluation as it relates to programmatic evaluation is important.

So what makes the evaluation component of education so important? There is a growing demand from consumers and stakeholders of education that colleges and universities be more accountable for the product they are graduating. Mandates from accrediting associations and education commissions state that effectiveness of educational programs be addressed, placing an emphasis on measuring student learning and documenting student learning outcomes. Historically, quality of educational programs has been measured in terms of resources, program offerings, faculty qualifications, and student services. However, these definitions of quality are being challenged, and educators are being charged with the task of documenting program effectiveness in terms of learning. Program evaluation is defined as assessment of all components from planning to implementation of the educational experiences for the purpose of measuring program effectiveness (Chen, 1990). The evaluation plan serves as a blueprint for the evaluation of a specific program.

FOUNDATIONAL CONCEPTS

Before addressing specific aspects of evaluation, a brief introduction to some basic concepts of evaluation is included. These concepts are universal in nature and are applicable to any type of evaluation.

Definition

Evaluation is traditionally defined as "a means of appraising data or placing a value on data collected" (Bourke & Ihrke, 2005, p. 443). It involves collecting data to determine if what is observed is different than what was expected. Therefore, evaluation is conducted for the purpose of making decisions. Evaluation, as it is related to the teaching-learning environment, is defined as the process used in determining the effectiveness of teaching and/or the value of a learning opportunity in assisting students to achieve the goals of education. The inherent purpose of educational evaluation is to provide valid data on which to make educational decisions related to the program of study. Therefore, evaluation and teaching become a synergistic process in which each influences the other.

It is important to distinguish between the roles of evaluation and the goals of evaluation. The goal of evaluation is synonymous with the definition of evaluation: to determine the worth of something through the collection of data. A common mistake in evaluation is not clearly identifying or articulating the purpose of the evaluation. Defining the goal involves specifying what is to be accomplished, what decisions need to be made, and who are the intended audience or stakeholders. For example, the goal of evaluation in a school of nursing or any professional discipline is to determine the effectiveness of the program.

The roles of evaluation depend on what that something is that is being evaluated and on whose standards of value the results will be analyzed. Therefore, the role of evaluation is situational and specific. Because of this, one must be clear in the role of evaluation and the expected outcomes of conducting the evaluation. For example, one role of evaluation would be to inform students of their progress in mastering the content included in a specific course. Another role of evaluation would be to provide faculty members with feedback concerning the effectiveness of their teaching. Both roles provide data associated with the overall goal of measuring program effectiveness.

Clarification of Terms

The terms *assessment of learning* and *measurement of learning* are sometimes used mistakenly instead of *evaluation*. Assessment of learning is defined as an appraisal of changes in learner knowledge, skills, attitudes, and ways of thinking (Bourke & Ihrke, 2005) and is the first step of the evaluation process in learning. Evaluation is the compilation of information from various sources and is ongoing. These data are interpreted to determine the extent to which identified actions were successful. Assessment is different from evaluation in that evaluation is the process of making value judgments based on available information and conclusions for the purpose of improvement or revision.

Similarly, measurement differs from evaluation in that no value judgments are made. Measurement is the process of assigning a quantitative or qualitative description to what is being evaluated. It helps with the value judgment by answering the question of how much? The purpose of measurement is to provide a reference point on which to make value judgments on collected data. The concept of measurement in learning is extremely critical because faculty do not have a meter (machine) that attaches to the learner to demonstrate the level of learning that is occurring. Therefore, because this process is not observable, educators must design a situation in which the desired behavior may be observed or assessed. This situation is termed *measurement*. It is a designed situation, thus the designer (evaluator) is making some assumptions. In the best constructed situation, because of the assumptions that precede the development of that situation, the measurement is only a method of estimating what the learner has learned and unfortunately is often imprecise (Van Hoozer, Ostmoe, Weinholtz, Craft, Gjerde, & Albanese, 1987). Therefore, more than one type of measurement must be used when conducting evaluation.

There are two major ways of interpreting test scores and other types of measurement used in evaluation: norm-referenced and criterion-referenced interpretation. A norm-referenced interpretation focuses on how learners' results compare with those of their peers. Norm-referenced data are reported in terms of percentiles, using relative standards, and they allow comparisons using group or national norms. Therefore, when using norm-referenced measurement, the characteristics of the comparison group need to be clearly defined.

Criterion-referenced measurement involves interpretation based on present criteria, not in relation to another group. The focus is on the performance level of the learners and describes how well the student performs in relation to the set criteria. Criterion-referenced assessment must be based on a preestablished performance level.

Systematic Evaluation

Programmatic evaluation is intrinsic to programs of nursing education and the entire academic arena (Gard, Flannigan, & Cluskey, 2004). To be effective, the evaluation should be based on established standards, which for nursing are most often set by external accrediting agencies. Inherent in the evaluative process is decision making relative to program outcomes, based on the evaluative findings. Reliability and validity of the findings are strengthened through the application of a systematic approach to the evaluation, guided by established guidelines, and implemented by a formalized group of faculty and/or administrators, with expertise in the process of evaluation.

Because the process of decision making is inherent in evaluation, valid and reliable data must be collected. Validity and reliability can be obtained only through a systematic approach to evaluation. A systematic approach can be ensured when an evaluation design is used to guide the process. An evaluation design is defined as a plan that identifies what decisions will be made, when and from whom data will be gathered, as well as what instruments will be used to obtain the data. General considerations include what evaluation model will be used, what type of data needs to be collected, how the data will be analyzed and by whom, and how the evaluation results will be disseminated. Deliberate decisions about the evaluation design ensure that the evaluation plan is valid, reliable, timely, pervasive, and credible.

EVALUATION MODEL

Different models of evaluation exist. However, most models are based on a decision-facilitating model that evolved from the prototype context, input, process, and product (CIPP) model by Daniel Stufflebeam (1980). This evaluation model is a comprehensive model based on the assumption that evaluation is a continuing process. The CIPP model consists of four types of evaluation that facilitate four types of decisions. The first type of evaluation is *context evaluation*. Context evaluation involves studying the environment associated with the program, such as what clinical experiences exist to enhance the educational process in nursing education. It compares the actual conditions with the desired ones. Context evaluation has been described as a situation analysis or the diagnostic stage of evaluation. During this stage of evaluation, planning decisions are made. Data collected during this type of evaluation include that which answers the following questions: What is the purpose of this service? What is to be achieved? Is there a need for this service? The key concept associated with context evaluation is that it is a continuous process providing information throughout the evaluation design and not a one-time activity.

The second stage of the model, *input evaluation*, is designed to provide information for determining how to utilize the resources to meet the program outcomes. Input evaluation is necessary in making structural decisions in which one determines the actual and potential resources, facilities, and strategies available to the system. Structuring decisions to determine the required sources of support are made during this stage of evaluation. Data collected during this evaluation phase help to determine what resources are available. For example, the number of faculty available and/or the number of faculty positions that are filled. In addition, this evaluative step should explore the credentials and/or the experience level of available faculty. How will the planned change affect the ongoing components and processes in the current structure? Input evaluation can be relatively simple or extremely complex depending on the magnitude of the program.

Process evaluation is the third stage of the CIPP model. This stage of evaluation addresses the implementation of the program and identifies the congruency between the planned and actual situation. Examples include the overall curricular design, sequencing of courses within the curriculum, and the established timeline for students to complete the stated learning outcomes. Therefore, implementing decisions is associated with this stage of evaluation. Data that describe the actual functioning of the system as well as identify areas of weakness are collected. Data are collected on the following questions: is the program being implemented as it was planned? and have problems developed that were not anticipated in the original plan? Process evaluation has been described as a piloting project to identify the glitches in the program so that changes can be made before the final outcome.

Product evaluation, more currently called outcome evaluation, provides data for recycling decisions. This evaluation determines if the outcomes produced have met the objectives of the program. Evaluation data helps determine whether the program benefited those intended, and whether the program has attained its goals. Within the context of this evaluative process, the competencies of graduates would be compared to the needs of the healthcare industry and the success of graduates on required certification examinations would be examined. In addition, questions would explore whether the outcome of the program was worth the investment. A systematic evaluation design includes these four components of evaluation, each occurring at different times.

An additional evaluative model that may also be characterized as decision facilitating, and that is useful in the measurement of program effectiveness, is the discrepancy evaluation model (Herbener & Watson, 1992). This model examines intended or actual program outcomes and focuses on one or more of the following potential discrepancies in program structure: between program design and actual program operations, including planned curriculum content compared with actual content presented. A second area of discrepancy to be explored would be between predicted program outcomes relative to the students' success on end-of-program standardized examinations and actual student success/pass rate. Third, a program might examine discrepancies between student achievement in key program outcomes such as critical thinking and desired standards or benchmarks of competency. Additional program evaluation examines discrepancies between the value judgments of groups regarding the purpose and effectiveness of the educational program, such as between the service sector and the academic environment (referred to in the CIPP model as context); multiple offerings of the same course, by different faculty, with differing emphases placed on content; and program objectives, instructional strategies, and measurements of students' progress. This model points to a need for the evaluation plan to be standardized with realistic achievable benchmarks and the need to be consistently applied.

TYPES OF EVALUATION

In addition to the evaluation terminology mentioned previously, two other terms are used to describe the types of evaluation: *formative* and *summative*. Formative evaluation is the gathering of data to make decisions during the planning, development, and implementation of the program. Formative evaluation is frequent and periodic and provides feedback while the program is being implemented. The purpose of formative evaluation is to assist in making changes to achieve the goals of the program or to refine or improve the outcome. Therefore, formative evaluation is considered diagnostic in nature.

Summative evaluation is utilized to determine the effectiveness of a program after the program has been implemented. Summative evaluation measures final outcomes or results and occurs at the end of the evaluation design. Conclusions are made and information is gathered for future decisions.

Historically, early evaluation methods focused on the articulation of learning objectives, the development of measurement tools, and the measurement of student learning to determine if objectives were met—a summative evaluative process. In the 1960s, formative evaluative processes came into popularity, as the public sector began to require more accountability of education programs receiving federal funding. Outcome evaluation became the focus of programmatic evaluation in the later part of the 20th century and was advanced when the National League for Nursing adopted this form of evaluation into their accrediting process and a majority of educational programs adopted this format. This trend continues today, and most programs of postsecondary education, including nursing education, design their evaluation plans to incorporate both formative and summative evaluation in an attempt to determine the measure of students' success in meeting stated program outcomes.

FACULTY RESPONSIBILITY IN EVALUATION

The faculty member has responsibilities in the following types of evaluation: program evaluation, teacher evaluation inclusive of both self and peer, and evaluation of student learning, each of which will be discussed briefly.

Program Evaluation

A systematic evaluation design in education usually is referred to as program evaluation. Bevil (1991) defines program evaluation as the systematic and continuous process of gathering and analyzing data about all dimensions of the program and then using this information for decision making about program quality and effectiveness. The key concepts in this definition are continuous process and decision making. Program evaluation is a decision-support activity that extends beyond data collection, measurement, and dissemination of the evaluation results. It is a circular process that involves people who will assess and deliberate the findings to make program decisions, implement these decisions, and reevaluate the results (Oermann & Gaberson, 1998).

As mentioned previously, because of the circular nature of program evaluation, it should be an integral part of any educational institution. The purposes of evaluation are to diagnose problems, assess strengths and weaknesses, and test new approaches for accomplishing and advancing the school's philosophy and outcomes. It should be practical, yielding information that is reliable and useful to the decision makers and to the stakeholders. More specifically, program evaluation helps faculty and administrators account for scarce fiscal resources, make administrative and curricular decisions, appraise faculty and staff development needs, examine both intended and actual effects of the program within the community, and provide a mechanism to ensure fulfillment of accreditation requirements.

Program evaluation includes all of the internal and external forces and constraints that impinge upon a nursing education program. It involves both a review of past practices and a prediction of future practice. It looks at the environment, needs, resources, and deficiencies of the institution. An educational program evaluation collects data about the organization and administration, faculty, students, curriculum, and resources. Some examples of data include:

- assessment of the curriculum
- functions of the organization
- faculty roles within the program
- faculty qualifications
- assessment of faculty teaching, scholarship/service
- assessment of the behavioral outcomes of graduates
- comparison of graduates with past graduates and with graduates of other comparable programs
- library resources and technology
- classroom, laboratory, and clinical practice resources

Although faculty involvement in the evaluation process is an important variable in program evaluation, the designation of a formalized group/committee structure to consistently guide and direct the systematic plan of evaluation is essential. This committee or designated group must be well versed in the evaluation plan and guide the processes of data collection, analysis, interpretation, and storage, as well as the reporting of the findings to appropriate individuals, including faculty. The first and most obvious role of the evaluation committee is in providing appropriate data as specified by the evaluation plan. The validity of the evaluation findings depends on the validity and reliability of the data collected. Other faculty responsibilities include participating in determining the type of evaluation, suggesting appropriate tools of measurement, and revising the evaluation design as the organization changes.

An important faculty role in program evaluation is participating in the analysis of data and making appropriate recommendations. It is important to objectively analyze evaluation data to prevent the formation of false assumptions. Thus, it may be necessary in the analysis of data to clarify or validate the collected data through focus group technique.

The most important role of faculty in program evaluation involves what is called "the feedback loop of evaluation" or the implementation of evaluation findings. Unfortunately, even though a systematic evaluation design is developed and implemented and although accurate recommendations are made, it is not uncommon for evaluation reports to be shelved, with no implementation of recommendations. Barrett-Barrick (1993) states that promoting the use of evaluation findings among faculty is difficult because the importance of the report is often overlooked. It is important to remember that the purpose of program evaluation is to improve the program outcomes. Improvement of the program can occur only if faculty members take personal accountability to implement the recommendations and continue the evaluation process to determine if recommendations did improve the program.

EVALUATION OF LEARNING

A major component of the faculty role associated with program evaluation is the evaluation of student learning. In this context, the purpose of evaluation is to ascertain the learner's current level of knowledge and learning needs, to give feedback to improve learner achievement, to improve teaching effectiveness, to judge learning and teaching outcomes, and to provide data concerning program effectiveness. Much faculty time is devoted to designing measurements to collect data for measuring learning and then assigning a grade to reflect the degree of learning. Yet this process is a very small component of total program evaluation.

Evaluation of learning is defined as the systematic process of collecting and interpreting information as a basis for decisions about learners. It is more specific than program evaluation and obviously focuses on the learner. Evaluation of learning incorporates not only the objectives of the learning experience but also the characteristics of the learner. Evaluation of learning enables faculty members to determine the progression of students toward meeting the educational objectives. Specifically, the goal is to discover to what degree learners have attained the knowledge, attitudes, or skills emphasized in a learning experience. As a result of the dearth of available instruments to measure the student's brain to determine if learning has occurred, simulated or designed situations are developed to measure learning. Therefore, evaluation of learning is a value judgment based on the data obtained from the various designed measurements taken in the classroom and clinical settings. In addition, the evaluation methods should match the nature of the course and the outcomes. For example, if students are enrolled in a course that contains 45 clock hours of didactic learning and 150 clock hours of clinical experience, it would be important that most of the measurements used to evaluate this course would measure learning in the clinical area.

The process for evaluating learning is similar to the process for program evaluation, in that it is based on a planned design. Deliberate planning and thought are needed to decide what evaluation methods should be used in a course of study. First, faculty members need to identify what is to be evaluated. What are the outcomes of learning? Inherent in this process is the specification of the domain of learning. In the health professions, learning occurs not only in the cognitive or knowledge domain, but also in the affective or value domain, and in the psychomotor or competency domain. Each domain of learning requires different evaluation measures. For example, a multiple-choice exam measures a student's cognitive understanding of a concept but does not measure the student's ability to perform a clinical skill.

In addition, in measuring the domain of a learner, the faculty must determine the complexity of the learning. Complexity of learning is determined when one considers the characteristics of the learner (e.g., level of learning, prerequisite courses, past clinical experiences). Integrated into this determination is the identification of the content or concepts associated with the learning experience. All of these factors clearly describe the behavior to be measured that indicates that learning has occurred. One should construct a matrix that identifies all of the factors to ensure that all concepts are integrated and the best measurement is chosen.

Context-Dependent Measurement

Educators in the health professions are challenged to prepare graduates to practice in a managed care health environment and to care for patients with complex health needs. This challenge involves shifting the focus of teaching from content to process. Students need more than mastery of knowledge to be successful in practice. They must be able to solve problems, make decisions, and think critically. Therefore, it becomes as important to evaluate not only a student's learning of content but also a student's ability to think critically. This requires different evaluation methods than traditionally used. Oermann and Gaberson (1998) state that in assessing students' cognitive skills, the test items and evaluation methods need to meet two criteria: (1) introduce new information not encountered by students at an earlier point in the instruction and (2) provide data on the thought process used by students to arrive at an answer. This type of evaluation, called context-dependent evaluation, includes context-dependent test items, case method and study, discussion, debate, and other reality-based scenarios.

As stated earlier, evaluating higher-level thinking skills, although it involves more planning and time than most multiple-choice tests, is extremely important in health profession education. Ability to solve patient problems is an essential skill needed for successful practice—the expected program outcome. In evaluating these skills, the faculty member introduces new material in a format similar to a patient scenario. The student is asked to analyze the data, thus providing data on the thought process used to arrive at the answer. Therefore, the material must provide sufficient data for decision making. The intent is to evaluate the underlying thought process. Guidelines for writing context-dependent item sets include:

- Provide sufficient introductory information for the student to accurately analyze the situation.
- Have questions address the underlying thought process used to arrive at the answer, not the answer itself.
- Gear the information provided to the student's level of understanding and experience.
- Specify how the responses will be scored.

For example, to test decision making, the introductory material may present a situation up to the point of the decision, then ask students to make the decision, or it may describe a situation and decision and ask whether the students agree or disagree with the decision. The question is not measuring content but the students' decision-making skills.

Grading measurements that evaluate higher-order thinking differ from grading traditional tests because they require more time and analysis. The potential for subjectivity or grading biases exists in this type of evaluation. Providing a template that has been designed based on content validity reduces some of the subjectivity.

Classroom Assessment

Formative evaluation can provide valuable data when evaluating student learning and the teaching strategies being used. Classroom assessment is a type of formative evaluation that involves ongoing assessment of student learning and assists faculty in selecting teaching strategies (Melland & Volden, 1998). This technique involves both students and instructors in the continuous monitoring of student learning. The purpose of classroom assessment parallels the purpose of formative evaluation. The purpose is to collect data during the learning experience to make adjustments so that students can benefit from the modifications before the final measurement of learning occurs. This approach is learner centered, teacher directed, mutually beneficial, formative, context-specific, ongoing, and firmly rooted in good practice (Angelo & Cross, 1993).

Classroom assessment differs from other measurements of learning in that it is usually anonymous and is never graded. It is context specific, meaning that the technique used to evaluate one class or a content-related learning experience will not necessarily work in another experience.

The use of classroom assessment provides feedback about learning not only to the faculty but to the student as well. Assessment techniques (e.g., the muddiest point, one-sentence summary, chain notes) are simple to use, take little time, and yet are fun for the student. An example of a popular assessment technique is the muddiest point. Close to the end of the learning session, the student is asked to answer, "What was the muddiest point in this lecture?" (or whatever teaching strategy was used). The faculty then reviews the responses to determine if a concept is mentioned frequently or if a pattern emerges, indicating that a concept or content was misunderstood. Based on the results, the faculty may choose to address the muddiest point in the next class. Answering the question also causes students to reflect on the session and identify concepts needing further study.

Clinical Evaluation

Nursing and other health professions are practice disciplines, and therefore student learning involves more than acquiring cognitive knowledge. Learning includes the practice dimension where the student demonstrates the ability to apply theory in caring for patients. Clinical evaluation addresses three dimensions of student learning—cognitive, affective, and psychomotor—and is the most challenging of the evaluative processes. Inherent in this process is the need to demonstrate progressive acquisition of increasingly complex competencies. Evaluating student learning and student competency in clinical settings is challenging. The faculty must make professional judgments concerning the student's competencies in practice, as well as the higher-level cognitive learning associated with application. Yet, the clinical environment changes from one learning experience to another, making absolute comparisons among students even in the same clinical setting impossible. In addition, role expectations of the learners and evaluators are perceived differently. The evaluations of a student's performance frequently are influenced by one's own professional orientation and expectations. Evaluation in the clinical setting is the process of collecting data in order to make a judgment concerning the students' competencies in practice based on standards or criteria. Judgments influence the data collected; therefore, it is not an objective process. Deciding on the quality of performance and drawing inferences and conclusions from the data also involves judgment by the faculty. It is a subjective process that is influenced by the bias of the faculty and student and by the variables present in the clinical environment. These factors and others make evaluating the clinical experience a complex process.

In clinical evaluation, the faculty members observe performance and collect data associated with higher-order cognitive thinking, the influence of values (affective learning) and psychomotor skill acquisition. The judgment of a student's performance in the clinical area can either be based on norm-referenced or criterion-referenced evaluation. With norm-referenced evaluation, the student's clinical performance is compared with the performance of other students in the course, whereas criterion-referenced evaluation is the comparison of the student's performance with a set of criteria. Regardless of the type of evaluation used, providing a fair and valid evaluation is challenging. Although the use of criterion-referenced tools reduces the subjectivity inherent to this process, also using multiple and varied sources of data increases the possibility that a valid evaluation occurs (e.g., observation, evaluation of written work, student comments, staff comments). Also, making observations throughout the designated experience in an effort to obtain a sampling of behaviors that will reflect quality of care provided and the extent of student learning helps to validate the evaluation.

It has been established that even with the best-developed evaluation criteria, clinical evaluation is subjective, and therefore efforts must be made to ensure that the process is fair. Oermann and Gaberson (1998) addressed the following dimensions associated with fairness in clinical evaluation:

- identifying the faculty's own values, attitudes, beliefs, and biases that may influence the evaluation process
- basing clinical evaluation on predetermined objectives or competencies
- developing a supportive clinical environment
- basing judgments on the expected competency according to curriculum and standards of practice
- comparing the student's present behavior performance with past performance, other students' performances, or to the level of a norm reference group

The process of evaluating a student's performance in a clinical setting poses several challenges to evaluation theory. Extensive documentation exists in the nursing literature addressing clinical evaluation and providing examples of evaluation tools. Students are demonstrating their ability to apply knowledge in caring for patients in an uncontrolled environment, and therefore it is difficult for them to hide their lack of understanding or inability to put it all together. However, although this setting is ideal for learning, the variables that exist in the setting make each learning experience different. Faculty members also struggle with the concept of when the time for learning ends and the time for evaluation begins. Again, the literature provides guidelines addressing this issue.

A solution to the challenges of clinical evaluation may exist within the context of clearly defining the parameters of formative and summative evaluation. Although not without its flaws, this solution worked as long as the clinical experiences existed in the hospital setting and were defined by discrete units of time; however, educating students in a managed care environment has changed the settings and the focus of the clinical experience. Faculty members no longer have the security of the familiar hospital setting and the discrete time units. Patients receive health care in a variety of settings, such as day surgery, outpatient clinics, community settings, and in the home. Patients admitted to the hospital stay shorter periods, require more extensive care, and present with more complex situations. Thus, many past strategies that were successful in clinical evaluation are no longer applicable.

Clinical Concept Mapping

Clinical concept mapping was developed by an educational researcher as an instructional and assessment tool for use in science education (Novak, 1990). In general, the technique is a hierarchical graphic organizer developed individually by students. It demonstrates their understanding of relationships among concepts. Key concepts are placed centrally, and subconcepts and clusters of data are placed peripherally. All concepts are linked by arrows, lines, or broken lines to demonstrate the association between and among the concepts and the data (Baugh & Mellott, 1998).

Clinical concept mapping is applicable in evaluating students in the clinical setting because it facilitates the linking of previously learned concepts to actual patient scenarios. The diagramming of the concepts allows faculty members to evaluate the student's interpretation of collected data and how it applies to the student's patient and to management of patient care. It also provides data for faculty members to evaluate the student's ability to apply class content and concepts to implementing nursing care. Faculty members are also able to evaluate the student's ability to solve problems and to think critically. Clinical concept mapping can be applied to a variety of clinical settings (Bentley & Nugent, 1998) and to a variety of learning experiences. An in-depth discussion of concept mapping is in Chapter 6.

Portfolio Assessment

Portfolio analysis can serve an important component of the process of assessing student learning outcomes and the achievement of overall program outcomes. When used appropriately, portfolio assessment provides valid data for clinical evaluation of students and may be used to clearly demonstrate a correlation between competencies gained and curricular or program outcomes. A portfolio is a compilation of documents demonstrating learning, competencies, and achievements, usually over a period of time. Used extensively in business to demonstrate one's accomplishments, the portfolio is often used in education to track academic achievement of outcomes (Ryan & Carlton, 1990). Although portfolios are discussed here in relation to clinical evaluation, they can also be used in different aspects of program evaluation. Portfolios are valid measures in clinical evaluation in that students provide evidence in their portfolios to confirm their clinical competence and to document their learning. They may be used in either formative or summative evaluation. Portfolio assessments are a positive asset in clinical settings in which students are not directly supervised by faculty.

Nitko (1996) describes the use of portfolios in terms of best work and growth and learning portfolios. Best work portfolios provide evidence that students have mastered outcomes and have attained the desired level of competence (summative evaluation), thus contributing to the accreditation process. Growth and learning portfolios are designed to monitor students' progress (formative evaluation). Both types of portfolios reflect the philosophy of clinical evaluation.

Portfolios are constructed to match the purpose and objectives of the clinical experience. Faculty members need to clearly delineate the purpose and outcomes and to identify examples of work to be included. Likewise, the criteria by which the contents of the portfolio will be evaluated must be provided for the students. Students need to understand that portfolios are a reflection of their learning and an evaluation of their performance.

Although still in the exploratory stage, portfolios are evolving as effective measurements in outcome evaluation. If portfolios are used in clinical evaluation, then faculty members benefit from data that demonstrate the clinical progression of students through the curriculum toward the program outcomes. Although portfolio development has been shown to increase student responsibility for learning, increase faculty/student interaction, and facilitate the identification of need for curricular revision, they are time consuming to compile and present challenges related to document storage. In addition, faculty struggle with the lack of research-based evidence to establish validity and reliability of grading measures related to program outcome evaluation.

Clinical Journals

Teaching/learning in the clinical setting is broad and diverse, including much more than can be identified superficially. Journaling is a technique that has been successfully used to bring together those elusive bits of information and experience associated with the clinical experience (Kobert, 1995). Clinical journals provide an opportunity for students to not only document their clinical experience but also to reflect on their performance and knowledge and demonstrate a level of critical thinking. Journals provide an avenue for students to express their feelings of uncertainty and to engage in dialogue with the faculty concerning the experience. Journaling also can be structured to include nursing care, problem solving, and identification of learning needs. Whereas journals provide valuable evaluation data, the challenge is to obtain from the students the quality of journal entries needed.

Hodges (1996) addressed this issue in a proposed model in which four levels of journal writing were identified. These levels of journal writing progressed from summarizing, describing, and reacting to clinical experience, then to analyzing and critiquing the positions, issues, and views of others. Examples of journal entries that parallel this progression are moving from writing objectives or a summary to writing a critique or a focused argument. The key to this progression lies in providing a clear purpose for the journal entry. To think critically, students need to know what they are thinking about (Brown & Sorrell, 1993). Once faculty members have identified the desired outcome of the clinical journal, they can assist the students in attaining these outcomes by providing clear guidelines.

Although keeping a journal requires a substantial commitment of time by both faculty and students, it is a valuable evaluation tool for both groups. Controversy exists concerning whether journals should be used for evaluation of students' learning or to be graded (Holmes, 1997). Some educators maintain that grading journals negates the students' ability to be reflective and truthful concerning clinical experiences; however, as students document their evolution of clinical experiences, their journal entries are laden with expressions of self-evaluation (Kobert, 1995). If journals are to be graded, then clear and concise criteria that not only identify how they are graded but also what is to be included in the journal must exist. Regardless of the decision to grade or not to grade them, clinical journals provide important evaluation data concerning the student's performance in the clinical setting and can be used effectively to monitor the student's development in terms of program outcomes.

In summary, evaluation of learning is an important component of the faculty teaching role. Because the purpose of evaluation is to provide valid data concerning learning in all domains, a variety of measurements is needed. The key to successful evaluation is to match the evaluation tool with the learning in order to provide reliable and valid data on which to make judgments.

In addition to making a judgment concerning a student's performance in clinical practice, it is important to remember that the other purpose of clinical evaluation is to provide feedback to the student regarding his or her performance and to provide the student with an opportunity to improve in the needed areas. Clinical evaluation should be a consistent and frequent means of communicating the student's progress. Using an adopted clinical evaluation tool ensures that all students are counseled using the same criteria. The evaluation process needs to be constructed so that active student participation is included. Feedback should be stated in the specific terms of the measurement tool and the outcomes of the course. Comments should be based on data and should not contain general global clichés such as "will make a good nurse." Strengths, as well as areas needing improvement, should be documented. If a student needs to improve to pass the clinical experience, then the student should be given, in writing, those areas needing improvement with specific guidelines on what behavior is required to pass. Again, all comments should be stated in terms of the criteria on the evaluation tool.

EVALUATION OF TEACHING

Another area of evaluation in which faculty members are actively involved is in the evaluation of teaching. Inherent in this definition is the understanding that results of the evaluation will be used to provide feedback concerning teaching for the development of faculty and refinement of teaching skills. Students are given the opportunity to provide evaluative feedback related to faculty performance, and the purpose of this form of evaluation is to assess the quality of teaching in the classroom and in the clinical setting. This process is discussed in-depth in Chapter 30.

Other sources of teacher evaluation are peer evaluation and administrator evaluation. When conducting peer evaluation, it is important to remember that the definition of a peer or colleague should be determined before the evaluation. This definition is usually determined by some guidelines within the nursing education unit that may be based on academic experience, rank, and familiarity with the teaching material. It is also important to remember that peer or administrator evaluations are, at the most, an evaluation of a teaching episode. Additionally, although feedback can be given, it should be interpreted within the context of the teaching episode. A follow-up session between the evaluator and the faculty member should be planned to discuss the results of the observation. A copy of the written evaluation should be given to the faculty member for his or her portfolio for use in support of promotion and tenure applications, and not be shelved without attention to recommendations.

CONCLUSION

Clearly, evaluation is an important part of the faculty role as evaluations in the educational setting are undertaken to influence the actions and activities of individuals and groups, who have, or are presumed to have, an opportunity to tailor their actions on the basis of the results. Therefore, an understanding of evaluation and how it impacts the teaching-learning environment is critical. Proper use of evaluation techniques requires an awareness of both their limitations and their strengths and requires matching the appropriate measurement with the purpose or role of evaluation. This chapter has addressed some aspects of the role of evaluation in program development and student success. As faculty and program administrators are increasingly held accountable to external stakeholders, program evaluation becomes increasingly significant to a program's success and continued existence.

Nursing is entering a new era of teaching that will alter traditional roles between faculty and students. Inherent in this new era of teaching is the mandate to evaluate teaching and learning using less traditional methods to demonstrate success in meeting program outcomes and meeting the needs of the healthcare community.

REFERENCES

Angelo, T., & Cross, K. (1993). *Classroom assessment techniques: A handbook for college teachers* (2nd ed.). San Francisco: Jossey-Bass.

Barrett-Barrick, C. (1993). Promoting the use of program evaluation findings. *Nurse Educator, 18*(1), 10–12.

Baugh, N., & Mellott, K. (1998). Clinical concept mapping as preparation for student nurses' clinical experiences. *Journal of Nursing Education, 37*(6), 253–256.

Bentley, G., & Nugent, K. (1998). A creative student presentation on the nursing management of a complex family. *Nurse Educator, 23*(3), 8–9.

Bevil, C. (1991). Program evaluation in nursing education: Creating a meaningful plan. In M. Garbin (Ed.), *Assessing education outcome* (pp. 363–367). New York: National League for Nursing.

Bourke, M. P., & Ihrke, B. A. (2005). The evaluation process: An overview. In D. Billings & J. Halstead (Eds.). *Teaching in nursing* (pp. 443–464). Philadelphia: Saunders.

Brown, H., & Sorrell, J. (1993). Use of clinical journals to enhance critical thinking. *Nurse Educator, 18*(5), 16–18.

Chen, H. (1990). *Theory-driven evaluations.* Newbury Park, CA: Sage.

Gard, C. L., Flannigan, P. N. & Cluskey, M. (2004). Program evaluation: An ongoing systematic process. *Nursing Education Perspectives, 25*(4), 176–179.

Herbener, D. J., & Watson, J. E. (1992). Models for evaluating nursing education programs. *Nursing Outlook, 40*(1), 27–32.

Hodges, H. (1996). Journal writing as a mode of thinking for RN-BSN students: A leveled approach to learning to listen to self and others. *Journal of Nursing Education, 35,* 137–141.

Holmes, V. (1997). Grading journals in clinical practice. *Journal of Nursing Education, 36*(10), 89–92.

Kobert, L. (1995). In our own voice: Journaling as a teaching/learning technique for nurses. *Journal of Nursing Education, 34*(3), 140–142.

Melland, H., & Volden, C. (1998). Classroom assessment: Linking teaching and learning. *Journal of Nursing Education, 37*(6), 275–277.

Nitko, A. (1996). *Educational assessment of students* (2nd ed.). Englewood Cliffs, NJ: Prentice Hall.

Novak, J. (1990). Concept mapping: A useful tool for science education. *Journal of Research in Science Teaching, 27*(10), 937–949.

Oermann, K., & Gaberson, M. (1998). Evaluation of problem-solving, decision-making, and critical thinking: Context-dependent item sets and other evaluation strategies. In M. Oermann & K. Gaberson (Eds.). *Evaluation and testing in nursing education* (pp. 111–136). New York: Springer Publishing.

Ryan, M., & Carlton, K. (1990). Portfolio applications in a school of nursing. *Nurse Educator, 22*(1), 35–39.

Stufflebeam, D. L. (1980). The relevance of the CIPP evaluation model for educational accountability. *Journal of Research and Developmental Education, 5*(1),19–25.

Van Hoozer, N. L., Ostmoe, B. D., Weinholtz, D., Craft, M. J., Gjerde, C. L., & Albanese, M. A. (1987). *The teaching process: Theory and practice in nursing.* Norwalk, CT: Appleton-Century-Crofts.

CHAPTER 29

The Clinical Pathway: A Tool to Evaluate Clinical Learning

Martha J. Bradshaw

INTRODUCTION

The clinical pathway is a strategy that uses specific, essential evaluation criteria in unique clinical learning settings.

DEFINITION AND PURPOSE

The clinical pathway is an abbreviated form of clinical evaluation that provides a means for the instructor to evaluate student progress using specified criteria. Clinical pathways can be used to evaluate nursing practice and clinical learning that occur in time-limited, less traditional care settings. Learning activities are directed toward the same clinical outcomes as would be expected in traditionally structured patient care settings. The emphasis is on application of nursing principles in a new setting, versus gaining experience via repeated opportunities in a familiar setting. As students apply principles, they recognize the development of individual nursing judgment and decision making, and they begin to visualize themselves as professional nurses. Faculty can determine how well the student uses guided thinking in unfamiliar settings, yet at the same time provides familiar nursing interventions.

THEORETICAL FOUNDATIONS

Clinical pathways, also called critical pathways, are being used by nurses and other members of the healthcare team as a directed approach to goal-based outcomes; they are especially beneficial in case management and quality improvement (Dickerson, Sackett, Jones, & Brewer, 2001). Most nursing literature describes pathways for use in complex patient care situations, but pathways are also used for orientation of new nursing staff, quality improvement, and for student-precepted experiences (Kersbergen & Hrbosky, 1996; Kinsman & James, 2001). One of the advantages of a pathway is that it is a cost-effective means, in both time and money, by which the individual is directed to the goal(s) and progress is measured (Renholm, Leino-Kilpi, & Suominen, 2002). Pathways also enable all individuals involved to know exactly what the goals are, thus clarifying expectations and making energy expenditure more efficient (Kersbergen). Nursing faculty are able to collaborate on student evaluations by examining how well the student meets outcome criteria from more than one perspective. This principle is similar to how integrated-care pathways are used in interdisciplinary clinical situations, in that student progress and achievement of outcomes is the focus (Atwal & Caldwell, 2002).

CONDITIONS

In selected situations, student clinical learning activities are one-time experiences and may deviate from the more structured patient care experiences. In addition, many clinical experiences are short term because of decreases in hospitalization length and emphasis on wellness programs. Examples of these clinical experiences are community health fairs, outpatient surgery, and pediatric health screenings in day care settings. Whereas these unique clinical opportunities provide expanded observations and open up new areas of practice, one-time experiences do not always lend themselves to achievement of established clinical learning outcomes. If the learning outcomes are not readily identified, then the clinical instructor cannot easily evaluate clinical progress based on the experience. Therefore, instructors traditionally create one-time experiences as observation-only activities, or as task-focused activities that may not represent a professional nursing approach. In doing so, many valuable learning opportunities may be lost to the students. Instructors also lose the opportunity to determine the extent to which students are able to adapt to unique settings, apply principles, and enact new roles.

Use of a clinical pathway for student experiences enables continued learning by students and maximizes the benefits of the one-time clinical opportunities. Just as the critical pathway is an abbreviated version of a patient's plan of care, the student clinical pathway is an abbreviated version of the clinical evaluation tool. At the time of the clinical experience, the student uses the pathway as a guide for fulfilling selected roles and completing specific responsibilities. Simultaneously, the student is aware of the criteria by which evaluation will take place. Therefore, use of clinical time and experience is maximized. The clinical pathway makes unique clinical experiences more purposeful, thus improving student clinical learning outcomes (Kinsman, 2004). Student clinical pathways are based on the same purposes as are patient- or staff-oriented pathways: they are goal directed, designed to be efficient, and effective in terms of time and energy. The components of the clinical pathway are derived directly from the clinical evaluation tool used by faculty in student evaluation.

TYPES OF LEARNERS

Whereas the clinical pathway could be used with learners of all levels, it is best used with undergraduate students. The clinical pathway offers specific learning outcomes and can include recommended or structured activities that enable the student to meet these outcomes. Students in undergraduate clinical settings generally have more faculty supervision, which creates opportunity for direct observation and evaluation. The clinical pathway is designed for intended learning, even though students often acquire additional personal growth during the clinical experience.

The pathway also is quite suitable for students of all levels in brief clinical learning settings with a preceptor, such as a one-day event. The preceptor should not be expected to conduct an in-depth evaluation of the student, but preceptor feedback is exceedingly helpful in compiling comprehensive information on a student. Therefore, a succinct and purposeful tool can be easily completed and provide needed information. Preceptors also feel more empowered in their ability to make decisions about students and promote accountability for care (Kersbergen & Hrbosky, 1996).

RESOURCES

The basis for a clinical pathway is the learning outcomes for the course. Evaluation tools used by all clinical instructors are directed toward course outcomes. Instructors supervising students in selected experiences identify outcomes and expected behaviors from the evaluation tool. Based on anticipated clinical learning opportunities, the instructor develops a clinical pathway that guides the student in what will be accomplished during the experience and the activities or behaviors the instructor expects to observe in each learner.

USING THE METHOD

Implementation of an education-focused clinical pathway enables the faculty to develop student learning experiences that are directly related to the outcomes for the total clinical course. Two examples demonstrate how pathways are derived from the clinical evaluation tool and how components of the tool can be applied to more than one setting. Hearing and vision screening with school-age children can be conducted with nursing students at any level in the educational program. Such screenings have a place in a fundamentals course, a course on nursing care of children, or in a community nursing course. A more sophisticated version of the screening (to include patient referral) can be developed for nurse practitioner students.

When students are assigned to a unique, one-time clinical experience, they may have some apprehension about being responsible for patient care in a new setting. Knowing that they have only one opportunity to demonstrate competence, students benefit from the direction that a pathway provides. In fact, many students like the opportunity to test themselves in the new setting. Time and opportunity do not permit the students to meet all criteria on the standard, comprehensive course evaluation tool. To maximize the learning experience, a sample pathway (see **Table 29-1**) was developed based on the following items from the course clinical evaluation tool:

- Demonstrates preparation for assignment.
- Performs nursing skills correctly.
- Maintains professionalism.
- Demonstrates professional inquiry activities.

As can be seen by the example in Table 29-1, other expectations are specified under the broad clinical outcomes. The pathway expectations are derived from the clinical evaluation tool and applied to the situation, such as communications with children or use of critical thinking. The expectations also indicate specific behaviors related to the clinical activity that must be demonstrated by the student, such as ability to complete vision screening.

Additional information that leaves no room for guesswork regarding preparation and professional behaviors is provided in the pathway for the student. Also, the standard for acceptable behavior (pass) is indicated as part of the directions, so that in the event a student demonstrates unacceptable behaviors, he or she has a clear understanding of how the final evaluation was determined (see **Exhibit 29-1**).

In developing the pathway, the focus is on outcomes (student learning), not process (tasks or activities). Therefore, the instructor may designate specified activities or behaviors that direct the student to the outcomes; not all behaviors must be seen in order to attain the goal. Furthermore, other, unanticipated activities related to the patient situation that enable the student to meet the outcomes may present themselves.

Table 29-1   Course Outcomes Applied to Clinical Pathways

Learning outcomes of clinical pathways	Clinical learning outcomes of course
Demonstrates professional behaviors and inquiry activities.	1. Demonstrates professional behavior and accountability.
	2. Demonstrates preparedness for assignment.
Demonstrates preparation and use of principles in screening techniques.	3. Provides a safe environment.
	4. Complies with the regulations of the school of nursing and clinical agency.
	5. Performs nursing skills or interventions appropriate to the patient's health.
Assesses behaviors of patient and family/support in ambulatory surgery and provides appropriate nursing interventions.	6. Demonstrates safe administration of medications.
	7. Establishes rapport and demonstrates good communication skills.
Provides nursing interventions for a patient in the ambulatory surgery/operative unit.	8. Demonstrates collaboration with other care disciplines.
	9. Demonstrates patient and family teaching.
	10. Demonstrates appropriate documentation.
	11. Maintains confidentiality and respect for others.
	12. Completes assignments on time.
	13. Seeks assistance/guidance appropriately.
	14. Adapts to changing or stressful situations.
	15. Uses critical-thinking skills.
	16. Demonstrates professional inquiry activities.

An evaluation sheet provides feedback to the student regarding the experience and serves as the evaluation measure and anecdotal record for the instructor. Information regarding clinical activities and evaluation is found in the clinical section of the course syllabus. In that section is the detailed information indicating that the one-time activity is a clinical day of equal importance to a day caring for a hospitalized patient. Clinical instructors use the information from the pathway when formulating a final clinical evaluation report on each student.

Exhibit 29-2 is a clinical pathway developed for use with nursing students in an ambulatory surgery unit. In addition to typical nursing activities related to an operative experience, an emphasis of this experience includes patient and caregiver interaction, alleviation of anxiety, provision of information about the procedure, and presentation of postoperative teaching prior to discharge. The ambulatory surgery pathway also is constructed to indicate to the students what the expectations are for patient care. Prior to use of the pathway, students may

EXHIBIT 29-1

Clinical Pathway: Hearing and Vision Screening

The clinical pathway identifies the specific nursing activities that will enable the student to meet the objectives for this one-time clinical experience. The student will be evaluated based on completion of items on this pathway. *A student who fails this clinical pathway* (i.e., fails to pass at least 7 of the 12 items on the clinical pathway) *has failed the clinical day.*

Objectives and Student Nursing Activities:
1. *Demonstrates preparation and use of principles in screening techniques:*
   - Attends clinical experience promptly, appropriately attired, and with own supplies.
   - Establishes a positive working relationship with patient(s).
   - Initiates and completes screening in timely manner.
   - Correctly follows sequence of steps in screening assessment(s).
   - Shows familiarity with equipment, screening criteria, and documentation.
   - Individualizes assessments as needed based on unique attributes of each patient.
2. *Demonstrates professional behaviors and inquiry activities:*
   - Uses principles of therapeutic and professional communications when interacting with patient(s).
   - Shows appropriate level of independence and self-direction.
   - Demonstrates critical-thinking and problem-solving skills regarding screenings or patient interactions.
   - Documents or reports results of screening exam.
   - Seeks guidance or advice from instructor as needed.
   - Discusses screening results and/or patient responses with instructor and fellow students.

Student Preparation
   - Complete check-off on hearing and vision screening equipment in the skills lab. If needed, practice again before clinical experience.
   - You are permitted to bring your H&V booklet or some guidelines written on a card. This does not take the place of preparation and familiarity with the procedure. If you make too many references to the guidelines, your instructor will consider you unprepared. Bring these pathway sheets to give to your instructor.

be unsure of what they are permitted to do, and thus miss many learning opportunities.

Because the ambulatory surgery pathway is broader in scope, it uses both basic care items (same as in Table 29-1) and specific items:

EXHIBIT 29-2

Clinical Pathway: Ambulatory Surgery Experience

For this one-time clinical experience, the clinical pathway identifies the specific nursing care activities on which the student will be evaluated. Items on this pathway will enable the student to meet the objectives for the ambulatory surgery experience for NUR (listed below). *A student who fails the Ambulatory Surgery experience* (i.e., receives a failing evaluation on two of the three sections of the clinical pathway) *has failed a clinical day.*

Objectives and Student Nursing Activities:
1. **Assesses behaviors of patient and family/support in ambulatory surgery and provides appropriate nursing interventions:**
   • Introduces self to patient and family/support person; establishes a working relationship.
   • Identifies behaviors related to hospitalization and surgery; discusses conclusions regarding behaviors with instructor, giving specific examples.
   • Indicates how patient behaviors influence preoperative, surgical, and postoperative periods.
   • Gives specific examples of family/support coping abilities.
   • Makes conclusions and interventions that are correctly based on patient's developmental level.
2. **Provides nursing interventions for a patient in the ambulatory surgery/operative unit:**
   • Demonstrates preparedness regarding knowledge of surgical procedure; discusses procedure and pertinent information with instructor.
   • Reviews patient's health history, lab, and other data as available on unit.
   • Teams with staff RN to provide care for patient.
   • Conducts assessments, including vital signs, in a timely manner, using correct technique.
   • Recognizes comfort and safety needs, specific for operative patients.
   • Provides interventions promptly.
   • Administers medications, based on the "five-rights" and according to school of nursing guidelines.
   • Practices professional therapeutic communication skills in the areas of teaching, reassurance, and collaboration.
3. **Demonstrates professional behaviors and inquiry activities:**
   • Selects appropriate priorities for patient and family/support.
   • Conducts self in dignified, professional manner, including conversation and general appearance.
   • Shows organization and good use of time.
   • Demonstrates initiative to be involved in patient care and to further own learning.

continues

EXHIBIT 29-2 *(continued)*

• Evaluates outcomes of patient's surgical experience; discusses patient responses and readiness for discharge/transfer with instructor.

Ambulatory Surgery Experience Clinical Pathway: Evaluation

Note: The student must receive a passing evaluation for at least two of the objectives in order to receive a passing grade for this clinical day.

1. Assess behaviors of patient and family/support in ambulatory surgery and provide appropriate nursing interventions.

Pass/Fail   Comments:

_____

_____

_____

_____

2. Provide nursing interventions for a patient in the ambulatory surgery/ operative unit.

Pass/Fail   Comments:

_____

_____

_____

_____

3. Demonstrate professional behaviors and inquiry activities.

Pass/Fail   Comments:

_____

_____

_____

_____

Instructor _____ Date_____

• Provides a safe environment.
• Establishes good rapport and maintains good communication.
• Recognizes skill and knowledge limitations and seeks assistance appropriately.
• Demonstrates safe administration of medications.
• Uses critical thinking in decision making and applying various problem-solving methods.

For this clinical experience, the student may be evaluated either by a different instructor or by a staff preceptor. Evaluation information is shared with the clinical instructor, added to other evaluation data, and used as part of the final course evaluation. One benefit of using the pathway in total course evaluation is that it provides the instructor with a glimpse at behavior patterns in a student, regardless of setting. In the event that the pathway does not provide beneficial evaluative feedback, the faculty must determine if the clinical experience and learning opportunities cannot be measured the way the pathway was constructed, or if the course evaluation tool needs to be revised to better reflect student learning outcomes (Kinsman, 2004).

POTENTIAL PROBLEMS

Any difficulties encountered in using the clinical pathway are related to the nature of this evaluation measure. It is intended to evaluate the student in a one-time experience, based on selected criteria.

Potential problems with this method include:

- Inability of the instructor to observe and evaluate all behaviors. The type of clinical activity and spontaneous events govern the student's participation in care and types of care provided.
- The new environment may have a negative effect on the students' behavior. Some students adapt more quickly than others to working in new settings. This is especially true of more experienced students and field-independent students who are able to sort out and select relevant information about the clinical setting. Students who are less able to adapt are therefore hampered in their performance and may appear to be weak in clinical judgment or nursing skills.
- It is easy to rubber stamp evaluation remarks. For the instructor who has 40 or 50 students progressing through the one-time experience, the evaluation remarks become repetitive and tiresome. Instructors must endeavor to make individual comments that are an accurate description of the student. Remarks that reflect abilities in other clinical settings will validate the student's total clinical evaluation.
- To some instructors, the clinical pathway may be seen as too behavioral. In some cases, this is the intent of the pathway: to evaluate psychomotor skills. An immunization pathway is an example of psychomotor evaluation. The clinical pathway can be constructed in such a way to provide opportunities for the student to use critical-thinking and problem-solving abilities in ways that the instructor can readily observe and evaluate. An example is priority setting and decision making related to immediate patient care needs. This is an advantage of the pathway in that it facilitates evaluation in spontaneous situations.

CONCLUSION

Clinical pathways are a means by which an instructor can objectively and effectively evaluate student learning and progress toward clinical outcomes. An advantage to use of pathways in one-time experiences is that the pathway serves as a criterion-based frame of reference for both the student and the instructor because the criteria are the same as for other clinical experiences in that course. The faculty member thus has an objective measure of student learning and performance, and the student always knows the measure on which he or she will be evaluated.

Clinical pathways are limited to brief experiences and are not designed to show professional growth and progress in learning over time. However, a pathway could be designed to appraise critical thinking and professional behaviors associated with spontaneous incidents, such as a problem patient. Nurse educators can use pathways as a creative means to address student performance in a variety of situations.

REFERENCES

Atwal, A., & Caldwell, K. (2002). Do multidisciplinary integrated care pathways improve interprofessional collaboration? *Scandinavian Journal of Caring Sciences, 16,* 360–367.

Dickerson, S. S., Sackett, K., Jones, J. M., & Brewer, C. (2001). Guidelines for evaluating tools for clinical decision making. *Nurse Educator, 26,* 215–220.

Kersbergen, A. L., & Hrbosky, P. E. (1996). Use of clinical map guides in precepted clinical experiences. *Nurse Educator, 21*(6), 19–22.

Kinsman, L. (2004). Clinical pathway compliance and quality improvement. *Nursing Standard, 18,* 33–35.

Kinsman, L., & James, E. L. (2001). Evidence-based practice needs evidence-based implementation. *Lippincott's Case Management, 5,* 208–219.

Renholm, M., Leino-Kilpi, H., & Suominen, T. (2002). Critical pathways: A systematic review. *The Journal of Nursing Administration, 32,* 196–202.

CHAPTER 30

Student Evaluation of Teaching

Jill M. Hayes

INTRODUCTION

As the arena of health care continues to experience a critical nursing short-age, educational programs of nursing increasingly face pressure to increase enrollment and the retention of existing students and improve the numbers of students successfully completing their program of study and licensure examinations. Innovative efforts are under way to recruit the most eligible students into nursing educational programs and to design programs that meet the unique needs of the current student population. Curricula are planned to include flexible scheduling to accommodate the nontraditional students, and students may enroll in part- or full-time study. Nursing educational programs are accountable to external agencies for funding and/or for approval of the program through formalized accreditation standards. Although accreditation is voluntary (Gard, Flannigan, & Cluskey, 2004) most nursing educational programs seek accreditation as a response to the public sector's demands for demonstrated accountability, requirement of federal funding agencies, and to provide their graduates with opportunities for educational mobility into higher degree programs.

Program evaluation, discussed in depth in Chapter 28, requires comprehensive assessment of every aspect of the program. A significant component of that assessment is the evaluation of teaching effectiveness. A subcomponent of this assessment is the mechanism to obtain evaluative feedback of teaching effectiveness from the direct consumer of teaching and instruction—the student.

Student evaluation of teaching effectiveness has long been recognized as valid and reliable (Miller, 1988; Raingruber & Bowles, 2000) and considered a significant input into the quality of faculty performance and overall program quality. Because nursing education is multidimensional, feedback on the effectiveness of teaching/learning strategies must be sought from all arenas in which nursing educational experience occur—the classroom, the simulation laboratory, clinical settings, and precepted experiences (Raingruber & Bowles).

BACKGROUND

Historically, research in education has focused on teaching strategies to enhance student and faculty success in their respective roles. In addition, numerous attempts have been made to evaluate teaching effectiveness to promote the development of expert faculty, meet the accountability requirements for funding sources, and to satisfy consumer demand for a quality educational experience.

Prior to further discussion of evaluation, definitions of the terms commonly employed in such a discussion will be helpful. Evaluation is viewed as "a means of appraising data or placing a value on data gathered through one or more measurements" (Bourke & Ihrke, 2005, p. 443). Evaluation also is utilized to render a judgment relative to a process or product, identifying the strengths and weaknesses of the features or dimensions of the product. Formative evaluation takes place during the activity, focusing on the progress being made toward achieving the stated objectives or outcomes of the activity. Summative evaluation refers to data collected following completion of the activity and focuses on the extent to which the objectives or outcomes have been met.

According to Miller (1988) efforts to evaluate faculty effectiveness have been primarily summative in nature, directed toward satisfying funding agency requirements, and facilitating faculty attainment of tenure and promotion. Formative evaluation, when it occurs, is intended to assist the faculty to grow and develop in their roles. Outcomes measured through student evaluation to meet these goals strive to identify the amount of learning that occurs, the resultant ability of students to integrate and apply knowledge gained, and a cost-benefit analysis of the program. Student ratings are considered highly reliable, highly correlated with other types of observational evaluation, and positively correlated with student achievement.

Hoyt and Pallett (1999) consider faculty evaluation as providing data on two aspects of faculty performance to be direct and indirect contributions. Indirect contribution is described as activities that contribute to the learning environment such as collegiality, curriculum development, and sharing of effective teaching strategies with colleagues. Direct contribution activities are described as those contributing to the achievement of program goals. The area of direct contributions is where student evaluation and/or feedback is considered an important element.

THEORETICAL FRAMEWORK

As stated earlier, research in evaluation began with a focus on the identification of behavioral learning objectives, the development of tools to measure those behaviors, and then the evaluation of students to determine if the objectives had been met—summative evaluation. As the process of evaluation evolved, more emphasis was placed on formative evaluation and the compilation of both formative and summative data to enhance educational program effectiveness. Perhaps because nursing has historically sought to identify sound theoretical frameworks by which to collect and interpret data to build on the body of professional knowledge, theoretical frameworks or models have been integrated into evaluative research in recent research. Although several models are useful guides to the evaluative process, the concepts of the CIPP (context, input, process, product) model (Stufflebeam & Associates, 1971; Stufflebeam & Webster, 1994) are easily applicable when attempting to collect data useful in decision making relative to the evaluation of nursing educational programs.

Within this model, context refers to the target population of any teaching/learning activities—in the case of nursing education and student evaluation, this would refer to the student population currently enrolling in these programs and the need to assess their unique needs. Input evaluates the target system's capabilities, including program strategies and mechanisms to implement those strategies—in the case of student evaluation of teaching effectiveness, this would consider the overall educational program design, curricular arrangement of courses, and teaching and learning strategies. Process evaluation would involve the assessment of the curricular implementation—how courses are designed and implemented, course sequencing, clinical site selection, etc. Product evaluation would assess the end product—the graduates' success relative to program outcomes and pass rate on licensure examinations. Using this model, a discussion of student evaluation demonstrates the ease of use of this model and how it would facilitate decision making relative to student feedback on programmatic quality and teaching effectiveness. Evaluation of teaching in nursing education must consider the current target population (context) and assess their unique needs within the arena where the teaching/learning will occur. This will include consideration given to the type of setting and the level of the student within the program structure—such aspects as acute care settings versus outpatient settings; high acuity patients versus ambulatory; novice student versus advanced beginner. Decisions then must be made related to what teaching/learning strategies would be appropriate to the particular setting, content being presented, and the expected student learning activities (input). Process evaluation examines the teaching/learning strategies selected and the effectiveness in transmitting required knowledge. Product evaluation would examine expected educational outcomes of the learning experience and correlate these with student success in meeting expected outcomes, course design (input), and teaching/learning strategies employed (process). Student evaluation is pertinent to all aspects of this decision-making model, and elements of the model are identifiable in the two instruments to be discussed later in this chapter.

IMPLEMENTATION

Nursing education is viewed as multidimensional and is strongly influenced by the particular setting in which it occurs. Raingruber and Bowles (2000) proposed that student evaluative feedback must be sought in all four major areas in which the educational experiences occur: clinical settings, simulation laboratory settings, preceptor-led experiences, and didactic/classroom settings. The evaluation of faculty should be guided by a need to provide feedback on faculty performance, opportunities for student input into the curriculum, information for personnel decisions, and a focus for educational research. In addition, evaluation is considered to be significant for its impact on faculty and student satisfaction, faculty promotion and tenure decisions, and the overall quality of instruction provided. These authors also acknowledge the significant reliability and validity of student evaluative data.

In an effort to enhance the evaluative process and its meaningfulness in terms of program quality and faculty and student success, recent educational research has focused on identifying the characteristics of effective teachers and the perceptions of nursing students related to what constitutes effective teaching. According to Raingruber and Bowles (2000), adequate measures of faculty performance must address the following: clinical competency, continuing education activities, national certifications, participation in curriculum development, research/scholarship activities, community service, and self- and peer evaluation. Most research supports the need for student evaluation as a valuable supplement to evaluation of overall faculty performance and as essential to program success. To this end, the authors advocate for the development of evaluative instruments that address the diverse settings in which teaching occurs and attempt to capture or match the essential skills required for effective instruction in the four major settings in which nursing education occurs. Individual factors identified as important to assess are: method of instruction, course design, course objectives, mode of delivery, feedback mechanism, and clinical competencies. Through their research, characteristics of effective teaching were identified. Overwhelmingly, in all settings, the significance of faculty attitude toward students stood out as essential to student learning. Within the context of attitude, faculty enthusiasm, ability to establish strong, positive interpersonal relationships with students, staff, and patients, and to create an atmosphere of mutual respect were viewed as characteristic of effective teaching. These characteristics mirror those discussed by Miller (1988), which included concern for students, enthusiasm, fairness, and encouragement of student participation. In addition, study findings also identified the following as essential to student satisfaction and success: subject mastery, stimulation of interest, clarity of explanation, availability to students, preparation and organization, and speaking ability. Theis (1988) surveyed nursing students in an attempt to determine whether students could identify unethical behaviors among nurse educators. The presence or absence of an atmosphere of mutual respect was indicated to be the determinant as to whether students perceived unethical behavior in nursing faculty—the absence of this element in the educational environment resulted in students reporting more unethical behavior on the part of nurse educators.

Tang, Chou, and Chiang (2005) recognized the contribution of faculty attitude toward students to student success. Teachers receiving low scores on interpersonal relationships and personal characteristics received significantly lower scores on teaching effectiveness, in spite of relatively positive scores on professional competency. A need for a feeling of mutual respect and concern for students' unique needs contributes significantly to student success. Bietz and Wieland (2005) support this premise, advocating for behavior supportive of student learning needs as essential to student perceptions of teaching effectiveness.

Within the process of programmatic assessment, an important element is the teaching/learning environment created by the faculty and administration. This will include physical facilities, instructional resources (to be discussed in Chapter 31), faculty, and the teaching/learning environment. Schaefer and Zygmont (2003) analyzed the type of learning environment created in nursing education and categorized them as either student-centered or teacher-centered. Results of quantitative analysis of the findings demonstrated a predominance of teacher-centered environments, which, in turn, will impact students' perceptions of teacher effectiveness. However, qualitative data analysis indicated a desire on the part of faculty to create student-centered learning environments, but it indicated an inability to achieve this, arising most often from a tendency on the part of faculty to teach the way they were taught. Student-centered environments are viewed as promoting critical and reflective thinking, creativity, and a foundation of trust, as well as higher student and faculty satisfaction and more active engagement of the student. The authors advocate a move to student-centered environments by supporting faculty in this endeavor to better meet the needs of the current nursing student population. Student-centered environments have been shown to be better suited to the student of today and the demands of the current healthcare environment for graduates with the ability to think critically and creatively within their work environment. According to Tanner (2005), nursing education and practice would greatly benefit from students who anticipate positive clinical learning experiences, practice for the love of it for knowledge's sake, and not out of fear of the consequences for not preparing, and for learning experiences that are positive and beneficial. Characteristics of effective teaching are described as the ability to strengthen links between theory and practice, provide information on a continuum of simple to complex, present information as an inductive process, and create trusting relationships inclusive of appropriate constructive feedback in a timely and caring approach.

Although student evaluation of teaching effectiveness is viewed as highly reliable and the most common mechanism used, there remains a recognized need to enhance the process of faculty evaluation with meaningful measures (Raingruber & Bowles, 2000). In the academic environment, faculty performance is increasingly being evaluated for reasons other than the measure of student satisfaction. These measures are being utilized to respond to funding agencies' requirements, consumer demand, and faculty reward systems. As the use of these data increases, additional measures that are objective and provide accurate information must be employed. Such supplemental measures as self-evaluation, peer evaluation, and administrative evaluation are being explored.

Bietz and Wieland (2005) present two clinical evaluation instruments with established validity and reliability and advocate their use in obtaining feedback on students' perceptions of teaching effectiveness in clinical settings. The Nursing Clinical Teaching Effectiveness Inventory (NCTEI) is a 48-item Likert-scale instrument that is utilized to determine students' perceptions of effective clinical teaching behaviors (Knox & Mogan, 1985; Mogan & Warbinek, 1994) (as cited in Bietz & Wieland, 2005). The five specific areas of clinical teaching addressed in the instrument are teaching ability, interpersonal relationships, personality traits, nursing competency, and evaluation. Higher scores on the instrument are indicative of a higher level of teaching ability. Applying the CIPP model to this instrument, it is easy to see that teaching ability corresponds to process as do interpersonal relationships and personality traits; nursing competency corresponds to input; and evaluation corresponds to product. A second tool discussed by Bietz and Wieland (2005) as being useful in assessing teaching effectiveness in nursing education is the Effective Clinical Teaching Behaviors (ECTB) tool (Zimmerman & Westfall, 1988 [as cited in Bietz & Wieland, 2005]). This instrument is a 43-item Likert-scale tool with established reliability and validity. Similar behaviors are identified in this instrument as in the NCTEI and higher scores are indicative of more frequently observed effective teaching behaviors.

Other tools exist for use in the evaluation of faculty performance in all settings, many of which are developed by nursing educational programs in response to the demand of accrediting agencies for outcome data and/or the need to meet individual institutional requirements for faculty evaluation. These tools often are developed as required, and efforts to establish validity and reliability are time consuming and the results tenuous at best. Research in nursing should emphasize the development of accurate, valid, and reliable tools to collect data on teacher effectiveness to meet accrediting requirements, consumer demand for a quality product, and the demand of healthcare agencies for competent nurses.

CHALLENGES

Challenges to valid and reliable evaluation of teaching effectiveness exist within the instrument in use, the student population enrolling in nursing educational programs, and the analysis of data collected. Overall challenges to effective evaluation are identified as lack of training for effective self-, peer, and administrative evaluation; demand for a time commitment for both peer and administrative evaluation; a need for multiple observational experiences for adequate evaluative feedback; and validity and reliability of tools specific to teaching activities in all major arenas where nursing educational experiences occur (Raingruber & Bowles, 2000).

As stated, valid and reliable instruments are time consuming to develop and often characterized as setting specific—clinical teaching, classroom teaching, and seminar teaching. Poorly constructed and nonstandardized evaluative tools, associated with an inability to account for extraneous factors such as class size, all lead to inadequate reliability and validity of the instruments currently in use. Research focused on instrument development, although incorporated into advanced degree programs for nursing faculty, is lacking but clearly needed to provide for accurate, meaningful faculty evaluation.

Current nursing education literature is rife with discussions related to the characteristics of the nursing students of today and their impact on nursing education. The nursing students encountered today differ significantly from the nursing students of the late 20th century. According to The American Association of Colleges of Nursing (AACN) (2003), the average student enrolling in nursing education today possesses prior degrees, is more mature and older chronologically, has more pressure from personal responsibilities and accountabilities, is embarking on a second career, and is more assertive. Anderson (2002) further characterizes this student as more actively engaged in learning, more self-directed, possessing more life experience, more goal focused, and possessing a higher level of potential talent for future career choices. Bietz and Wieland (2005) posit the idea that, considering the characteristics of the current nursing student, educators are compelled to develop new strategies and approaches to the presentation of content to meet these students' unique learning needs. These characteristics also have significant implications for the context of nursing education (curriculum design, settings selected for educational experiences); input (course sequencing, instructional strategies, content presented); process (teaching/learning activities employed in the particular settings, competencies of the faculty, interpersonal relationships); and product (student-expected outcomes, learning behavioral outcomes).

It is clear how the aforementioned characteristics of students lead to the elements of teaching effectiveness identified in recent research literature.

Raingruber and Bowles (2000) identified the importance of faculty attitude, interpersonal relationship building with students, staff, and patients, and an atmosphere of mutual trust to students' perceptions of effective teaching. Multiple theories of learning abound in an attempt to develop an understanding of how learning occurs and what activities are best suited to facilitating learning in a group of individuals, and adult education models provide assistance to faculty in the planning of curricula and associated teaching/learning processes to present content. Within the context of adult education, Knowles (1980) too characterizes adult learners as individuals who perform best when required to use their life experiences when learning new material, desire to apply new knowledge to solve real life problems, and are motivated to learn by pragmatism and a need to solve problems. Further assumptions relative to adult learners include: they are self-directed, their life experiences serve as a resource for other learning, and their readiness to learn arises from the need to perform life tasks and solve problems. Additionally, Jackson and Caffarella (1994) characterize adult learners as those who have preferred styles of personal learning, prefer being actively involved in their learning, desire to be connected to and supportive of each other in the learning process, and have responsibilities and life circumstances that provide a social context within which learning occurs. When students of today are characterized as adult learners— self-directed and possessing life experience, more personal responsibilities, and possessing a higher level of potential talent for future career choices—it is easy to see the applicability of the premise that faculty attitude and an environment of mutual trust are important.

Student characteristics impact the teaching/learning environment, and faculty must be equipped and willing to adjust their approach to education to meet the unique needs of these students—most often best met through student-centered learning environments. Failure to do so will result in poor student evaluations, reduced student and faculty satisfaction, and a lower level of student and faculty success. In addition, students are viewed as poorly qualified to evaluate subject matter presented, course and curriculum design, individual commitment of faculty to teaching, institutional support of faculty, evaluative methods for student work, and methods and materials used for content delivery (Hoyt & Pallett, 1999).

The connection between the perceptions of students in programs of higher education, such as nursing, as to what constitutes effective teaching and the characteristics of adult learners is clear. If curricula are developed without considering the need for these students to be actively engaged in their learning and their need to be connected and supported, then students will not perceive that their needs are being addressed, and evaluative feedback will be less than positive. When content is developed, the teaching/learning strategies employed to present the content should reflect consideration of the need for students to apply this new knowledge immediately to solve problems, to be supported in the learning process, and to learn in an environment that is individualized and personalized for self-directed, mature students who desire to be actively engaged in the learning process. Attention to these unique student needs will potentially be reflected in more positive evaluative feedback and enhanced student and faculty satisfaction.

Challenges also exist within the processes of data analysis and interpretation and the use of evaluative findings. The instruments currently in use have questionable reliability due to the difficulty in accounting for the impact of class size, course level, and whether the course is a requirement of the curriculum or an elective when data is interpreted. In addition, analysis must take into consideration the setting in which the teaching occurs, the mode of delivery of content, and the teaching strategies employed. Since teaching/learning in nursing often occurs within a social context, additional factors of space, access to educational experiences, privacy issues, agency policies governing and constraining student activities, and staffing plans must all be considered. Few if any instruments that account for these factors exist, and all have the potential to significantly impact the quality of any educational experience.

CONCLUSION

Clearly, student evaluation of teaching is an essential element of successful faculty performance and professional development, student success, and programmatic success. Much effort has been expended to develop tools to capture the essence of teaching, but much still remains to be done. Although student evaluation of teaching effectiveness is viewed as highly reliable and the most common mechanism, there remains a recognized need to enhance the process of faculty evaluation with additional measures (Raingruber & Bowles, 2000). In the academic environment, faculty performance is increasingly being evaluated for reasons other than the measure of students' satisfaction. In addition, these measures are being utilized, as discussed earlier, to respond to funding agency requirements, consumer demand, and faculty reward systems. As the use of these data increases, additional measures of faculty performance must be employed. Supplemental measures such as self-evaluation, peer evaluation, and administrative evaluation are being explored.

Considering the characteristics of the nursing students of the 21st century and their stated need for concerned and caring faculty (Norman, Buerhaus, Donelan, McCloskey, & Dittus, 2005), further investigation is needed to identify characteristics of effective teaching from the students' perspective, and then to match those needs to the other demands placed on faculty in higher education.

REFERENCES

American Association of Colleges of Nursing. (2003). Accelerated programs: The fast track to careers in nursing. *AACN Issue Bulletin*, 1–6.

Anderson, C. A. (2002). A reservoir of talent waiting to be tapped. *Nursing Outlook, 50*(1), 1–2.

Bietz, J. M., & Wieland, D. (2005). Analyzing the teaching effectiveness of clinical nursing faculty of full- and part-time generic BSN, LPN-BSN, and RN-BSN nursing students. *Journal of Professional Nursing, 21*(1), 32–45.

Bourke, M. P., & Ihrke, B. A. (2005). The evaluation process: An overview. In D. M. Billings & J. A. Halstead (Eds.), *Teaching in nursing: A guide for faculty* (2nd ed., pp. 443–464). St. Louis, MI: Elsevier Saunders.

Gard, C. L., Flannigan, P. N., & Cluskey, M. (2004). Program evaluation: An ongoing systematic process. *Nursing Education Perspectives, 25*(4), 176–179.

Hoyt, D. P., & Pallett, W. H. (1999). Appraising teaching effectiveness: Beyond student ratings. *Idea Paper No. 36*. Manhattan, KS: Idea Center, Kansas State University.

Jackson, L., & Caffarella, R. S. (1994). *Experiential learning: A new approach*. San Francisco: Jossey-Bass.

Knowles, M. S. (1980). *The modern practice of adult education*. Chicago: Follett.

Miller, A. (1988). Student assessment of teaching in higher education. *Journal of Higher Education, 17*, 3–15.

Norman, L., Buerhaus, P. I., Donelan, K., McCloskey, B. & Dittus, R. (2005). Nursing students assess nursing education. *Journal of Professional Nursing, 21*(3), 150–158.

Raingruber, B., & Bowles, K. (2000). Developing student evaluation instruments to measure instructor effectiveness. *Nurse Educator, 25*(2), 65–69.

Schaefer, K. M., & Zygmont, D. (2003). Analyzing the teaching style of nursing faculty: Does it promote a student-centered or teacher-centered learning environment? *Nursing Educational Perspectives, 24*(5), 238–245.

Stufflebeam, D. L., & Associates. (1971). In D. M. Billings & J. A. Halstead (Eds.), *Teaching in nursing: A guide for faculty* (2nd ed., pp. 449–450). St. Louis, MI: Elsevier Saunders.

Stufflebeam, D. L., & Webster, W. J. (1994). In D. M. Billings & J. A. Halstead (Eds.), *Teaching in nursing: A guide for faculty* (2nd ed., pp. 449–450). St. Louis, MI: Elsevier Saunders.

Tang, F., Chou, S., & Chiang, H. (2005). Students' perceptions of effective and ineffective clinical instructors. *Journal of Nursing Education, 44*(4), 187–192.

Tanner, C. A. (2005). The art and science of clinical teaching. *Journal of Nursing Education, 44*(4), 151–152.

Theis, E. C. (1988). Nursing students' perspectives of unethical teaching behaviors. *Journal of Nursing Education, 27*(3), 102–106.

CHAPTER 31

Evaluation of Teaching Resources

Jill M. Hayes

INTRODUCTION

The critical nursing shortage that the healthcare industry is currently experiencing and that is predicted to worsen is occurring simultaneously with budgetary constraints in health care and the academic environment. The shortage of registered nurses is attributable to myriad issues such as the increasing demand for healthcare services by the aging "baby boomers," aging of the nursing workforce, and a decline of interest in a career of professional nursing, to name but a few.

Budgetary constraints in academe contributed to more than 5,000 qualified students being denied admission to nursing programs across the country in 2002 (American Association of Colleges of Nursing [AACN], 2003). Yet vacancy rates in hospitals and in healthcare organizations are reported to average 14% nationwide and are predicted to reach 20% by the year 2010 (Baggot, Hensinger, Parry, Valdes, & Zaim, 2005). Some reasons for this shortage include shortage of nursing faculty, decreasing opportunities for clinical sites for student educational experiences, and inadequate classroom space. The shortage of nursing staff in health organizations in turn frequently leads to an inability of these organizations to accommodate nursing students for clinical educational experiences, thus reducing enrollment capacity in nursing educational programs. Other healthcare professions are facing similar issues. According to Bogdanowicz (2006), the educator shortage in dentistry educational programs is approaching crisis proportions and is resulting in concern for the quality of care provided. The process is cyclical, and clearly, multiple factors contribute to the shortage of nurses, and both the academic and healthcare arenas are being pressured to address this critical issue. Within the context of this crisis is a growing acknowledgment of the need for all parties involved to carefully evaluate resources utilized by programs of nursing education, professional programs, and all postsecondary educational programming.

BACKGROUND

The evolution of nursing education, more than that of all health professions with the exceptions of dentistry and medicine, has a clear and often articulated history. Nursing education first occurred within the hospital setting and was directed by faculty with a dual role, that of providing service to the healthcare institution while educating new nurses (Finke, 2005). Nursing students were expected to learn while at the same time staffing the hospital. The commitment of educational resources included some classroom and simulation laboratory space, usually housed in the school of nursing located within the hospital campus, and the patient care environment of the hospital.

As other health professions made the transition into the academic environment, nursing education also began moving into the university setting in the middle of the 19th century, with clinical practice remaining an integral part of the overall educational experience. Faculty were compelled to learn and use instructional resources in the classroom and simulation laboratory, as a supplement to clinical practice, in the presentation of content. In addition, faculty were actively engaged in the clinical practice component of the students' educational experiences and had a lesser role in the service aspect of the healthcare environment. Healthcare organizations were asked to provide sites for clinical experiences as an adjunct to the educational program.

More recent changes in higher education have contributed to a demand for new teaching/learning strategies to be incorporated into the program. The student population continues to evolve, and this is associated with a need for faculty to constantly revise, adjust, and update the strategies used to present content in all four areas where nursing education occurs: simulation laboratory settings, clinical settings, classroom settings, and preceptor-led educational experiences (Raingruber & Bowles, 2000). Lecture is no longer the only acceptable format for presentation of content. Faculty are increasingly required to incorporate technology into their course presentations, which includes modes of distance learning delivery and computer mediated presentations, and this technology is viewed as contributing to active engagement of the student in the learning process. Increasingly, faculty and administration are exploring innovative simulation activities that provide students with valuable learning experiences for students prior to their engagement in clinical practice with actual patients.

As the needs of students change, the numbers of students entering into nursing education increase, and faculty strive to ensure valuable educational experiences and positive learning outcomes in programs of higher education, new and varied teaching/learning strategies will be developed and introduced into the educational settings. However, a balance must be sought between the need for a variety of educational resources to support these new innovative instructional strategies and the budgetary constraints currently being imposed on institutions of higher education, and in the case of nursing education, the clinical practice settings. This, in turn, requires consistent and meaningful evaluation of needed resources and their contribution to the students' educational experiences.

THEORETICAL FRAMEWORK

Jeffries (2005) proposes a framework to utilize when designing, implementing, and evaluating simulation activities in the education of nursing students, and this model is well suited to the evaluation of any instructional resource. Within the context of this model, antecedent factors that are to be considered when evaluating teaching/learning resources include instructor/teacher's use of the strategy relative the various areas of expertise, faculty members' historical or traditional teaching styles, and familiarity with the teaching strategy. Additionally, students participating in the educational activity should also be considered relative to their program of study, level in the program, and their ages. The educational philosophy commonly held by the institution impacts the use of educational strategies in the classroom, learning laboratory, and clinical setting by the nursing faculty, and it requires evaluation in terms of factors such as what active learning strategies are used, the type of student/faculty interactive activities that occur, and the type and format of collaborative teaching activities employed. Prior to selecting and implementing an instructional intervention, teacher and student and institutional factors must be considered. Antecedent factors play a significant role in the planning of instructional interventions to present required content. In any academic setting, following the intervention, evaluation of the value of the resources/strategies utilized should focus on the outcomes of that intervention—the knowledge gained, skill performance demonstrated, learner satisfaction with the intervention, level of critical thinking demonstrated, and the overall confidence of the student in the performance of the acquired skills. According to Jeffries, simulations are increasingly being used in nursing education. This feedback is then used to enhance future instructional interventions. In addition, evaluation of the resource(s) relevant to their value to the educational experiences of the students, feasibility of the cost involved in their purchase, and the readiness of faculty to utilize them all contribute to the activity's impact on program outcomes—summative evaluation. Resource evaluation, in professional educational programs such as nursing, of necessity should focus on the skill performance and learner satisfaction following participation.

IMPLEMENTATION

Resource evaluation in the current environments of institutions of higher education must address how best to implement and use teaching/learning resources in the presentation of required content. This evaluation must focus on which outcomes best fit with the use of which resources, and what is the best method to promote faculty and student development within the context of current budgetary restraints. Resource evaluation in nursing education must involve all resources utilized to enhance the students' learning experience. This includes faculty resources, material resources, physical plant resources, and instructional resources.

Faculty evaluation as typically formalized by the program administrator may include processes of peer evaluation, self-evaluation, classroom and clinical observations, and student evaluation. According to Miller (1988) faculty evaluation commonly is summative in format; it is usually an annual performance evaluation completed by the program administrator and focusing on the faculty member's performance within the tripartite mission of the university—teaching, service, and scholarship. Formalized student evaluations are incorporated into this evaluation along with peer and self-evaluation. Dependent upon the primary mission of the university—research or teaching—the three elements are weighted and the faculty counseled on identified areas of strengths and weaknesses. Raingruber and Bowles (2000) propose that student evaluations be solicited in all four areas in which nursing education occurs—classroom, clinical areas, laboratory, and precepted educational experiences—and address clinical competency, scholarship, service, and knowledge base in area of expertise. Multiple observational opportunities should be offered to ensure the accuracy of the data obtained.

Although student evaluations are recognized as highly reliable and valid (Raingruber & Bowles, 2000), when utilizing the aforementioned model, the evaluation of faculty should primarily focus on teacher factors such as knowledge base in the area of expertise, readiness to explore and use new instructional strategies, and the support available to facilitate this innovative practice. According to Jeffries (2005), faculty are critical to the successful implementation of any instructional resource. Dependent upon the philosophical perspective on teaching held by the institution, the department, and/or the faculty member, the faculty member will employ student-centered or teacher-centered activities in the educational setting. Faculty steeped in the traditional pedagogical method of structured lectures—a teacher-centered strategy—will utilize teaching/learning strategies that support that form of instruction such as overhead technology, handouts, and PowerPoint presentations. In addition, resistance to the adoption of new technology/simulation resources into instructional activities may well occur.

This will, in turn, impact outcomes of student learning and learner satisfaction. Faculty whose teaching/learning philosophies are characterized by a readiness to engage in student/faculty interaction in the classroom, collaborative learning, and active participation in the learning process may utilize technology and simulation activities to facilitate their students' educational experiences and thus impact educational outcomes. In addition, Jeffries (2005) proposes that increasing use of simulation activities in the classroom and the learning laboratory will somewhat alleviate the impact of the current faculty shortage. Creative use of technology to simulate real clinical experiences will reduce the dependency of nursing educational programs on actual clinical experiences while continuing to provide valuable educational experiences for their students.

According to the AACN (2003) the current nursing faculty shortage is contributed to by the aging of the current faculty workforce, diminishing enrollment in masters of nursing education programs, longer time requirements to achieve a doctoral preparation in nursing, and increasing competition for doctorally prepared faculty. Once an individual has successfully completed doctoral studies, educational institutions must then be willing to invest additional resources to train the new educators. The multifaceted role of a nurse educator necessitates training in the design of curriculum, programmatic evaluation, and skills in developing and implementing strategies to meet program outcomes and thus accreditation requirements. Collaborative innovations between the service and academic environments will assist with the alleviation of the impact of this shortage. However, educational programs in nursing must also pursue creative and innovative methods of developing competent practitioners and use simulation activities to contribute meaningful educational experiences to the curriculum. Feedback from the outcome evaluation must be recognized as valuable data to influence teacher/student factors and educational practices. Teacher evaluation should include this feedback data to assist in the development of faculty expertise and the structure of educational practices.

When evaluating faculty performance relative to resources utilized, it is imperative to remember that a faculty member's utilization of innovative teaching resources must be supported and facilitated by the institution (Jeffries, 2005). This support may range from the provision of financial resources to purchase needed equipment, to the provision of adequate facilities to house and utilize the resources, to training and support in the use of such resources. Faculty development workshops provide faculty with the opportunity to develop new skills and also provide tangible evidence of administrative support for the use of such resources.

Physical plant resources must be considered as critical elements of successful nursing education—classroom space, simulation laboratory space, and clinical sites. In this time of budgetary constraints, classroom space often is inadequate. Large classrooms necessitate the use of varying teaching/learning strategies. For example, active engagement of students with group work is difficult when 50 nursing students are crowded into a classroom designed to accommodate 30–40 students. In addition, the incorporation of technology as an instructional strategy requires that the equipment be available and be user friendly for faculty and students alike. This requires substantial financial commitment on the part of the institution to provide the needed and updated equipment, as well as support of the faculty in the design, setup, and use of the equipment. These factors, all considered as a part of educational practices, must be considered when evaluating the use and value of instructional resources.

CHALLENGES

The procurement of adequate and valuable sites for clinical learning in nursing education continues to be a critical factor in nursing education (Mathews, 2003). Questions center on what competencies are needed for effective teaching in the clinical setting; how best to ensure nursing faculty who possess needed competencies; how to supplement faculty deficiencies in either numbers or clinical competency to maximize student educational experiences to meet the needs of the healthcare industry; how to ensure adequate numbers of qualified clinical faculty; and how to ensure adequate physical facilities for a diversity of clinical educational experiences. Once again, the theoretical model proposed by Jeffries (2005) may be utilized to evaluate clinical resources. Philosophy and mission of the nursing program impacts the educational practices utilized to promote successful program outcomes. According to Jeffries (2005), sound educational practices, based on pedagogical principles, are crucial to good teaching, student learning, and learner satisfaction. Active learning, timely feedback, and collaborative learning are viewed as critical to successful student learning outcomes. Simulation activities with appropriate teaching/learning resources have been shown to be effective tools in nursing education, resulting in positive program outcomes, knowledge and skill acquired, and learner satisfaction. However, participation in clinical experiences in diverse settings is mandated by accrediting agencies, such as AACN, the National League for Nursing Accrediting Commission (NLNAC), and the state boards of nursing. With ever-increasing enrollments in nursing education, an ongoing shortage of nursing staff in health care and nursing faculty in academia, coupled with ongoing budgetary constraints, nursing education programs struggle with finding adequate clinical sites to provide meaningful nursing education.

Mathews (2003) proposes the establishment of creative collaborative relationships between academia and the service industry to enhance student educational experiences. The establishment of partnerships that provide adjunct/joint faculty appointments enhance the availability of faculty and opportunities for the development of nurse educators in the service sector. The faculty shortage is attributed in part to salary disparity between academia and the service industry, limited access to scholarships to fund advanced education for staff nurses, inadequate access to information related to advanced degree programs, and the aging of the current faculty workforce. Joint appointments provide opportunities for creative job designs for staff nurses and an increase in the numbers of qualified educators to participate in student clinical educational experiences. In addition, partnerships between academia and service promote careers in nursing education and recognition of clinical expertise and aid in the retention of nurse educators in the service industry. Student evaluation of clinical sites contribute valuable data for program and faculty evaluation. As clinicians are encouraged to contribute their expertise to the students' educational experience through these collaborative partnerships, evaluation data on learner satisfaction, critical thinking, knowledge and skill acquisition, and the learners' self-confidence in their roles will contribute significantly to the selection and utilization of innovative learning resources and academic institutions' willingness to provide and support these resources.

As technology becomes more evident in today's society, students in nursing and other disciplines enter educational programs as computer savvy consumers. Feedback on the introduction of these instructional strategies bring mixed results. According to Ndiwane (2005), instructional technology tools such as individual devices to store and communicate data enhance student learning and reduce student dependence on faculty presence in the clinical settings. Jang, Hwang, Park, Kim, and Kim (2005) advocate for the use of web-based instruction to enhance the flexibility of nursing educational programming, reduce faculty travel time and cost, and enhance student educational experiences through opportunities for self-analysis, critical reflection, and sharing information with peers. Although research on web-based instruction and the use of other instructional technology has produced mixed results, many efforts have demonstrated significant improvements in learner motivation, course satisfaction, and stimulation of learning.

Medley and Horne (2005) advocate for increased use of technological simulation activities in undergraduate nursing education, citing improved skill acquisition, enhanced decision making and critical thinking, and team building. Challenges identified related to the implementation and utilization of technology arise from faculty underestimation of their potential to enhance nursing education and their underuse by faculty. Clinical practice in nursing education programs, although viewed as critical to professional development, is associated with increasing challenges arising from inadequate faculty resources, increasing numbers of students, decreased lengths of stay for patients in the hospital, high patient acuity in hospital settings, and the current nursing shortage in healthcare delivery settings. All these factors create a need for students who are highly competent in clinical practice and yet also contribute to increasing difficulties in the preparation of such a student. Complex high tech simulation learning resources are viewed as a highly valued supplement to the education of competent practitioners.

CONCLUSION

Students today are characterized as adult learners and virtual learners (Ostrow and DiMaria-Ghalili, 2005). Both types are described as adaptable, self-directed, and with a strong desire for immediate application of knowledge. Based on principles of adult learning theory, these students require a learning environment that enables them to incorporate their life experiences into their education and allows them to be actively engaged in the learning process and immediately apply new knowledge to problem solving, be it in the clinical environment or any other environment that enhances their education (Knowles, 1980). To meet the needs of these students, technology-based instruction that is reliable, ensures complete and organized information, includes a detailed orientation to the instructional tools, and provides prompt feedback to the student results in positive learning outcomes (Ostrow & DiMaria-Ghalili). The faculty role vis-à-vis the technology is characterized by an ability to promote and develop a sense of community, encourage student engagement in the learning process, empower students to develop and maintain a learning community, and enlist student cooperation and active learning. Educational practices conducive to positive learning outcomes are characterized as those that ensure a creative interactive learning environment, time devoted to the specific task, provide prompt feedback and active learning, and are viewed as contributing significantly to positive educational outcomes. Feedback data from formative and summative evaluation must be used to enhance or alter teacher effectiveness and educational practices.

REFERENCES

American Association of Colleges of Nursing. (2003). *Faculty shortages in baccalaureate and graduate nursing programs: Scope of the problem and strategies for expanding the supply.* Washington, DC: Author.

Baggot, D. M., Hensinger, B., Parry, J., Valdes, M. S., & Zaim, S. (2005). The new hire/preceptor experience. *Journal of Nursing Administration, 35*(3), 138–145.

Bogdanowicz, H. (2006). Dental community faces shortage of educators as numbers steadily decline. Retrieved February 15, 2006, from http://www.aae.org/pressroom/releases/newseducators.htm

Finke, L. M. (2005). Teaching in nursing: The faculty role. In D. M. Billings & J. A. Halstead (Eds.), *Teaching in nursing: A guide for faculty* (2nd ed., pp. 443–464). St. Louis, MI: Elsevier Saunders.

Jang, K. S., Hwang, S. Y., Park, S. J., Kim, Y. M., & Kim, M. J. (2005). Effects of a web-based teaching method on undergraduate nursing students' learning of electrocardiography. *Journal of Nursing Education, 44*(1), 35–39.

Jeffries, P. R. (2005). A framework for designing, implementing, and evaluating simulations used as teaching strategies in nursing. *Journal of Nursing Education Perspectives, 26*(2), 96–103.

Knowles, M. S. (1980). *The modern practice of adult education.* Chicago: Follett.

Mathews, M. B. (2003). Resourcing nursing education through collaboration. *Journal of Continuing Education in Nursing, 34*(6), 251–257.

Medley, C. F., & Horne, C. (2005). Using simulation technology for undergraduate nursing education. *Journal of Nursing Education, 44*(1), 31–34.

Miller, A. (1988). Student assessment of teaching in higher education. *Journal of Higher Education, 17*, 3–15.

Ndiwane, A. (2005). Teaching with the Nightingale tracker technology in community-based nursing education: A pilot study. *Journal of Nursing Education, 44*(1), 40–42.

Ostrow, L., & DiMaria-Ghalili, R. A. (2005). Distance education for graduate nursing: One state school's experience. *Journal of Nursing Education, 44*(1), 5–10.

Raingruber, B., & Bowles, K. (2000). Developing student evaluation instruments to measure instructor effectiveness. *Nurse Educator, 25*(2), 65–69.

Index

evaluation of teaching *(continued)*
  program evaluation, 411–412, 415–416
  by students, 424–425, 437–445, 450
  teaching resources, 447–454
  web-based instruction, 284, 301–302
evidence-based practice, 50, 314
exaggeration, as source of humor, 85
expectations for group discussion,
  establishing, 100–101
expectations with multimedia-based learning,
  239
experience-based learning. *See also* clinical
  setting; simulation
  in distance education, 274
  one-time clinical experiences, for
    evaluation, 428, 430
  preceptorships, 341–354
    case studies, 354–359, 402–403
    implementing, 346–351
    potential problems, 351–353
  preparing for, 188
  service-learning, 363–375
  through creative movement, 183–194
  uncovering painful material, 190
expert practitioners, defined, 141
expertise, problem-based learning and,
  133–134
expository lectures, 116
expository writing, 62
exposure to concepts, 60–61
eye contact, 121

F

faculty
  blocks to creativity, 71–72
  concept mapping, 381, 386
  consideration of student's values, 96–97
  constructionist theory, 379
  development of, 308
  disability regulations, awareness of, 29
  distance education, 271. *See also* distance
    education
  diversity of, 23
  electronic communication. *See* electronic
    communication
  evaluation of. *See* evaluation of teaching
  evaluation responsibilities, 414–416. *See
    also* evaluation of students

  feedback from. *See* feedback from faculty
  humor and, 80
  lecturer types, 116–117
  multimedia and, 240–241
  personal values of, 97–98
  philosophical approaches, 303–309
  preceptorships, 341, 344, 350
  preparing for teaching. *See* preparation
  problem-based learning, role in, 133–134
  role in debate, 153
  role in simulation, 202, 209
  role modeling, 66, 306
  skills laboratories, 316, 317, 320
  teacher-practitioner model, 325–338
    advanced-practice clinics, 333–336
    entry-level clinics, 327–332
  unpredictable problems with students,
    393–405
    student dishonesty, 402–403
    student incompetence, 399–400
  web-based instruction, 283–284, 286, 294
fairness, defined, 29
falling backward (trust exercise), 193
fear. *See* anxiety
feedback from faculty, 9, 12. *See also*
  evaluation of students
  handling student incompetence, 399–400
  multimedia, 239
  peer evaluation of teaching, 425, 442
  philosophies of clinical instructions,
    306–307
  preceptorships, 341, 350–351, 352. *See also*
    preceptored clinical experience
  skills laboratories, 316
  student rights and responsibilities, 403–404
  transition into professional roles, 343–345
  web-based instruction, 286
feedback to faculty. *See* evaluation of
  teaching; program evaluation; student
  evaluation of teaching
feelings, value-sensitive subjects and, 99–104
feminist movement, 21–22
field dependent–field independent style, 5–6
financial support. *See* support
financially challenged students, 30
first clinical encounters, 328, 336. *See also*
  preceptored clinical experience
follow-up to games, 167–168